Practical Exotic Animal Medicine

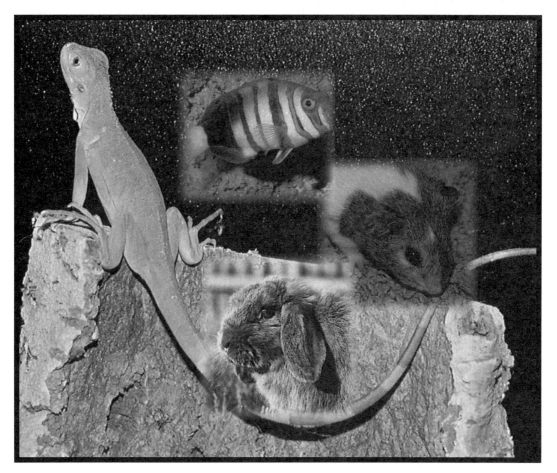

Karen L. Rosenthal, DVM, MS, Editor and Reviewer

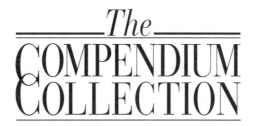

The
COMPENDIUM
COLLECTION

FOREWORD

The Compendium Collections gather together the best, most practical information from the pages of the *Compendium on Continuing Education for the Practicing Veterinarian*. As the knowledge base within veterinary medicine has expanded, so too have the sources from which to cull information. In order to provide our readers with the latest, most applicable answers, we have drawn from other pertinent veterinary material for this collection. Included are five articles from *Veterinary Technician* and two articles from the out-of-print VLS book, *Dermatology for the Small Animal Practitioner* (Nesbitt GH, Ackerman LJ (eds), 1991). In addition, the article "Husbandry of Rodents and Hedgehogs" by Beth A. Breitweiser was written specifically for this publication.

Although not from the pages of *Compendium*, these additional articles were found by our editors to be in keeping with the editorial and educational standards that have been established by previous Collections. The information provided herein, therefore, provides a well-rounded reference for the practitioner involved with or interested in exotic animal medicine.

Published by Veterinary Learning Systems
Trenton, New Jersey

ISBN 1-884254-33-0

PREFACE

I am privileged to present a series of papers on the biology, husbandry, surgery, and medicine of exotic animals. We have included information on the most common of the animal species that are seen in an exotic animal practice. (Birds are addressed separately in another, new Compendium Collection, *Practical Avian Medicine*.) A wide spectrum of opinions has been assembled by bringing together an array of well-respected authors who work in universities, other institutions, and private practice.

These days, staying current in veterinary medicine is an exercise in information gathering that can quickly slide into an exercise in futility. This is due to the information onslaught and the Herculean effort it takes to find and reign in all of the data available, especially in the wide-ranging field of exotic animal medicine. There are many reasons for this. Mainstream journals that we all get rarely have the exotic animal articles we need. Our patients include hundreds of different species and, since most of us did not leave school with even a rudimentary knowledge of exotic animals, it is difficult to know where to find information on them. Fifteen years ago, a handful of schools offered courses on exotics, and still there are many schools that totally ignore in their curriculum this fastest growing segment of the pet population. This Compendium Collection has assembled much of this information into one package. And if more information is desired, the extensive literature reviews act as a springboard for further exploration.

Most of the articles in this collection that have been published previously have been updated by the authors to reflect new information and references now available. Although most of the material comes from previous *Compendium* offerings, we also have included a few from *Veterinary Technician* and from the out-of-print book, *Dermatology for the Small Animal Practitioner* (Nesbitt G, Ackerman L (eds): Trenton, NJ, VLS Books, 1991). While the main purpose of each contribution is to inform, I think all the authors would agree that the articles are also meant to stimulate thought and discussion and to encourage new ways of viewing exotics problems. I would hope this will motivate others to develop new diagnostic approaches and treatments.

As we feel compelled, sometimes in a self-gratifying way, to know as much as we can about the animals we treat, we cannot forget that clients' expectations of medicine are for increased sophistication, even in the area of exotic animals. This also pushes us to excel. The day may not yet be here when a hamster-owning client goes elsewhere because you did not offer a CT scan to diagnose its abdominal mass; but, then again, who would have thought 20 years ago of reading a detailed article on the dermatologic conditions of rabbits, rodents, and ferrets, or caring about the medicine of a chinchilla. It is my hope that this Compendium Collection helps you obtain some of the goals you have set for yourself in the area of exotic animal medicine.

I am grateful to all the authors for their time and effort. Without them, there would be no Compendium Collection, but only a 500-word introduction!

Karen L. Rosenthal, DVM, MS
Diplomate, ABVP-Avian Practice
Staff Veterinarian
Avian and Exotic Animal Service
The Animal Medical Center
New York, New York

CONTENTS

REPTILES AND AMPHIBIANS

REPTILIAN PARASITES

SMALL MAMMALS

MANAGEMENT OF RODENTS

DERMATOLOGY

HEMATOLOGY

MARINE AND FRESHWATER FISH

MEDICAL MANAGEMENT OF PRIMATES

Medical Management of Reptile Patients

KEY FACTS

- A thorough, in-depth history is paramount in assessing reptile patients.
- The proper environment and nutrition are critical if a reptile is to survive in captivity; problems in these areas are common precursors to reptilian maladies.
- Samples for cytologic and microbiologic evaluation are of primary clinical importance.
- The reaction to therapy is profoundly affected by the state of debilitation, energy balance, hydration, and ambient temperature.

Avian & Exotic Animal Hospital
San Diego, California
Jeffrey R. Jenkins, DVM

REPTILES have found their way into the homes of the American public and thus into many veterinary practices. Some reptiles are considered as collected specimens and others as beloved pets. The most common reptiles kept as pets are iguanas, box turtles, and constrictor snakes. Reptile patients are a treatment dilemma for many veterinarians. This article presents a synopsis of the diagnostic approach and therapeutics commonly used in managing reptiles. Information concerning individual species and specific disease conditions is not provided.

HISTORY

A thorough, in-depth history is paramount in assessing a reptile patient. A comprehensive history should include the origin of the animal, both initially (wild caught or captive bred) and recently (e.g., private collector or pet shop), and the period the animal has spent in captivity. Wild specimens are commonly infested with parasites, but parasites are rarely a problem in captive-bred reptiles. Newly imported reptiles are more likely to evidence the compounding problems of stress, poor care, and maladaptation.

The proper environment and nutrition are critical if a reptile is to survive in captivity; problems in these areas are common precursors to reptilian maladies (Figure 1). A complete description of the environment in which an ani-

mal is housed should include the size and construction of the cage, substrate used, light cycle, heat source and temperature maintained in the cage, relative humidity, and any embellishments (e.g., hiding boxes, plants, limbs, or rocks).

Caging should be large enough to allow the animal to exercise but small enough to facilitate control of the environment. Substrate should be easy to clean; newspaper, artificial grass, or indoor-outdoor carpeting is recommended for most captive reptiles.

Reptiles have a primitive endocrine system that depends on the light cycle. A light-to-dark cycle of 14 hours to 10 hours is recommended for all growing reptiles and for adults during the summer months. The cycle may be reversed for winter months. Exposure to direct sunlight or light that provides a source of ultraviolet rays is recommended to promote vitamin D metabolism.

Reptiles strive to maintain an optimum temperature via behavior and limited physiologic mechanisms. Preferred temperatures are discussed in the literature.[1,2] The most commonly kept reptiles are diurnal in behavior and benefit from a radiant heat source. Such a source is best provided in the form of an incandescent light bulb, which allows basking in a thermal gradient and thus produces a more natural condition for temperature regulation. Bulbs should

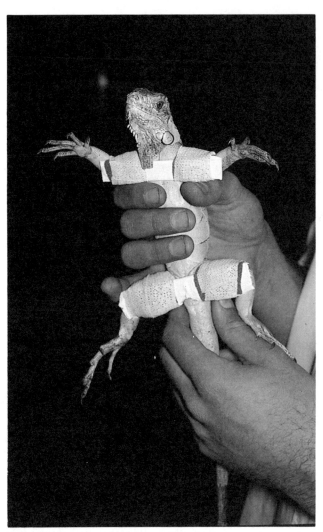

Figure 1—Fractured femurs and humeri in a young iguana. The underlying cause of the four fractured bones was environmental and nutritional. Such fractures typically heal with simple coaptive devices.

be located such that the reptile cannot burn itself.

Many reptiles prefer to lower body temperature at night and during cold seasons. With some species, lowering the temperature to room temperature (turning out the light) at night is appropriate; other species need reduced heat, which may be provided by a low-wattage colored light or a well-protected heating pad or tape. Hot rocks and stones sold in the pet trade are a poor heat source and are not recommended.

Barring extremes, relative humidity is usually not a cause of concern. Rarely, tropical species kept at a humidity lower than 50% have problems with ecdysis (shedding skin). Skin infection caused by high relative humidity is a more common problem.

Many species are shy and require cover or a place to hide. The ball, or royal, python (*Python regis*) may refuse food for months if placed in a stressful environment. Own-

ers should provide hiding boxes that are easy to clean and facilitate access to snakes. Small, opaque plastic boxes or cases with an entry hole slightly larger than the snake's largest diameter work well.

Assessment of proper diet requires knowledge of the biology of the species involved. Some generalizations can be made. Carnivorous species that eat whole prey seldom have problems related to inadequate diet and do not require supplementation if the prey species is well fed. For the welfare of the rodent and the safety of the reptile, rodents should be killed humanely before being fed.

Nutrition is more often a problem in omnivorous and insectivorous reptiles. A balanced variety of foods or insect prey should be supplemented with any quality of bird or reptile vitamin that contains vitamin D_3 and a calcium supplement. The diets of large insectivorous species should be augmented with pinkie mice. The origin of a problem also may be related to the water, its source, how often it is cleaned and changed, or the manner in which it is supplied.

Finally, the history should include information concerning recent activity. Alterations in behavior, eating, molting, and defecation should be noted. Exposure to other animals, especially those new to the collection, is important. Exposure to ectoparasites (mites or ticks) may be equivalent to exposure to a new animal.

In-depth history evaluates the reptile's level of stress, the limitations placed on the immune response to opportunistic pathogens, and the origin of a disease problem. Correction of underlying dietary and environmental defects is of foremost importance in the treatment of reptile patients. In many cases, such correction is the only therapy required.

PHYSICAL EXAMINATION

Bearing the history in mind, the practitioner should undertake a thorough inspection of the patient. Reptiles are not well suited to physical examination. Restraint alone is difficult in some species. Iguanas and varanid lizards, especially large specimens, are given a free nail trim before attempted examination. Like cats, most reptile species appreciate a light touch and may become irascible if tightly grasped.

EXPERIENCE helps in identifying animals that are likely to strike or bite. Many species of exotic tortoises are impossible to coax from the shell; there is little to examine beyond shell and body weight. Obtaining information may require chemical restraint.

A top-down, or systemic, approach should be taken to avoid overlooking any information. Concerning exotic patients, the adage is true: ''For every detail you miss by not knowing, you miss 10 by not looking.'' Special attention should be paid to the patient's attitude and level of awareness. Snakes and lizards should be observed for a normal

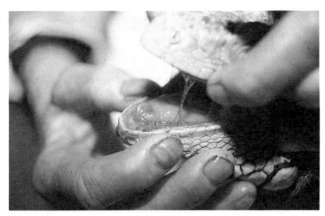

Figure 2—Stomatitis in an iguana. The oral cavity is carefully examined.

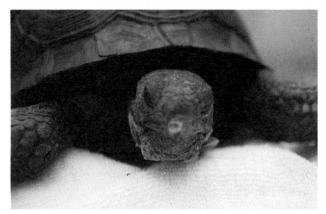

Figure 3—Cytologic evaluation and culture of this desert tortoise's nasal discharge will help differentiate bacterial infection from the syndrome believed to be caused by mycoplasma.

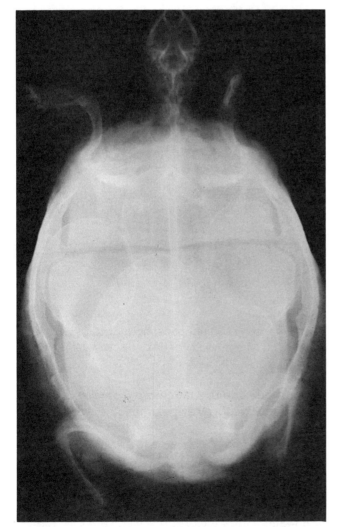

Figure 4A

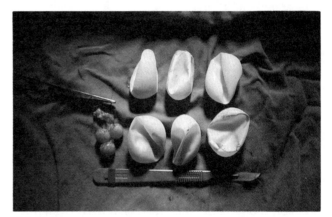

Figure 4B

Figure 4—(**A**) Radiographic view of an egg-bound box turtle. (**B**) Eggs surgically removed from the turtle.

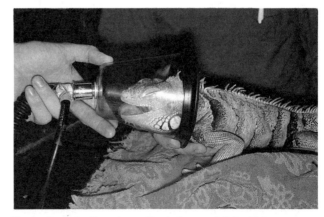

Figure 5—Induction of anesthesia in an adult iguana.

rate of tongue flicking. The oral cavity is carefully examined to determine the color of the mucous membranes, the presence of discharge, or hemorrhages along tooth lines (Figure 2).

Skin and scales should be checked for parasites. The areas in folds under the jaw and along the dewlaps, in heat pits, under large scales, and around the eyes and ears are examined. The practitioner should palpate for bladder

Drugs for Reptiles and Amphibians

Antibiotics

Amikacin sulfate Dosage: 2.5 mg/kg subcutaneously or intramuscularly every 72 hours for five to seven treatments. 1.0 mg/kg in the blood python *Python curtis*, and 2.0 mg/kg in the black-headed python *Aspidites melanocephalus* and rock python *Liasis macloti*. May be used with a β-lactam antibiotic, such as ampicillin, carbenicillin, piperacillin, or cefotaxime. Poor lipid solubility; may be less nephrotoxic than some other aminoglycosides. Neurotoxicity has been reported.

Ampicillin trihydrate Dosage: 10 mg/kg subcutaneously or intramuscularly every 12 hours for 14 treatments. Poor results if used alone. May potentiate aminoglycosides; is considered safe.

Carbenicillin Dosage: 200 to 400 mg/kg intramuscularly every 24 hours for 14 to 21 treatments. Used primarily with aminoglycoside antibiotics because of the rapid development of resistance. May have a deactivating effect on gentamicin. (Gentamicin is often not used because of the apparently greater nephrotoxic effect than that of amikacin.)

Chloramphenicol succinate 20 mg/kg intramuscularly or subcutaneously every 12 hours for 14 to 21 days. Bacteriostatic; may require long treatment period.

Doxycycline Dosage: 5 to 10 mg/kg orally daily for 10 to 45 treatments. May alleviate the clinical signs of the respiratory syndrome of desert tortoises; is bacteriostatic.

Enrofloxacin Dosage: 5 to 10 mg/kg every 24 to 48 hours for 10 to 14 treatments. May cause discoloration of skin or tissue necrosis in some animals if given subcutaneously. Alleviates the clinical signs of the respiratory syndrome of desert tortoises. May be used as a nasal flush (50 mg/250 ml sterile water or saline); each nostril is flushed with 1 to 3 ml every 24 to 48 hours until no discharge is visible.

Piperacillin Dosage: 50 to 100 mg/kg intramuscularly every 24 hours. Excellent as a broad-spectrum bactericidal antibiotic. Unsurpassed first-choice antibiotic (combined with amikacin or tobramycin) for septic patients. The low dose is usually used in combination with another drug.

Tobramycin Dosage: 2.5 mg/kg intramuscularly every 72 hours. May be more nephrotoxic than amikacin. Potentiated by β-lactam antibiotics.

Trimethoprim-sulfadiazine Dosage: 30 mg/kg intramuscularly or subcutaneously every 24 hours for 10 to 14 treatments. Apparently is very safe (I have maintained snakes with cryptosporidiosis on this dosage for more than 90 days). Also used to treat coccidiosis.

Tylocin Dosage: 5 mg/kg intramuscularly every 24 hours for 10 to 60 days. May alleviate clinical signs of the respiratory syndrome of desert tortoises.

Antifungal Agents

Amphotericin B Dosage: 1.0 mg/kg (diluted with water or saline) intratracheally every 24 hours for 14 to 28 treatments. Used to treat fungal lung infection.

Ketoconazole Dosage: 50.0 mg/kg orally every 12 hours for 14 to 28 days. Used to treat deep fungal or yeast infections.

Nystatin Dosage: 100,000 IU/kg orally every 24 hours. Used to treat gastrointestinal yeast infections.

Steroids

I discourage the use of steroids or other immunosuppressive drugs in lower invertebrates. Septic patients may be exceptions.

Dexamethasone sodium phosphate Dosage: 0.10 to 0.25 mg/kg intravenously or intramuscularly. May be used to treat sepsis.

Prednisolone sodium succinate Dosage: 5 to 10 mg/kg intravenously. May be used to treat sepsis.

Parasiticides

Fenbendazole Dosage: 50 to 100 mg/kg orally, repeated in 10 to 14 days. Used to treat nematode infestation.

Ivermectin Dosage: 0.20 mg/kg intramuscularly, subcutaneously, or orally; repeated in 10 to 14 days. Used to treat nematode and arthropod parasite infestation. May be lethal to and must be avoided in turtles and tortoises. In chameleons, may cause skin discoloration at the injection site.

stones, obstipation, retained eggs, and enlarged organs. The abdomens of turtles and tortoises can be palpated by placing a finger in the space cranial to each hindleg and gently rocking the animal from side to side. Common sites of problems include the sense organs, vent, and sexual organs.

CLINICAL PATHOLOGY

There is controversy concerning reptilian hematology and serum chemistry and how they are affected by suboptimum environment or the state of decompensation.[1] Significantly abnormal values may help in diagnosing systemic illness and thus assist in restoring the patient to health. Samples for cytologic and microbiologic evaluation are of greatest clinical importance (Figure 3). Discharges, aspirates and biopsies of masses, and samples of regurgitated material and diarrhea should be examined.

RADIOLOGY

Radiology enables the practitioner to see through thick hides and bony shells and makes information about the patient available immediately (Figure 4). Textbooks may aid in the evaluation of radiographs.[2,3] High-detail screens and film are necessary in examining small patients.

Diagnostic radiographs depend on proper positioning. Lizards and snakes should be positioned ventrodorsally or dorsoventrally with limbs extended. Lateral radiographs should be taken with forelimbs and hindlimbs extended cranially and caudally, respectively, and just ventral enough to avoid overlapping of the neck, head, or tail. Turtles and tortoises are treated similarly, and a craniocaudal view should be taken to visualize the lung field. Paper or plastic tubes aid in positioning snakes; pieces of foam are helpful in wedging and positioning turtles, tortoises, and lizards.

THERAPEUTICS

Limited research has been performed in reptilian pharmacokinetics. Even less has been done to examine the absorption, distribution, and excretion of drugs in maladapted or decompensated reptiles. The state of debilitation, energy balance, and hydration as well as the ambient temperature have a profound effect on the reaction obtained from therapy.[4,5] These factors must be considered in choosing a therapeutic agent. In some cases, it may be advantageous to postpone drug therapy until the patient returns to a more physiologically normal circumstance.[6,7]

The pathogenesis of bacterial disease in reptiles involves suppression of a rudimentary immune system and invasion by opportunistic bacteria. Evidence indicates that most of these conditions are caused by gram-negative bacteria, especially *Pseudomonas* species, which are ubiquitous among captive reptiles.[8,9] The chosen antibiotic thus should be aggressively bactericidal rather than bacteriostatic and

should perform well against *Pseudomonas*.

AMINOGLYCOSIDE antibiotics and aminoglycoside-β-lactam combinations fulfill this requirement. In vitro sensitivity to antibiotics of the penicillin family may be good, but their usefulness is limited because resistance apparently develops rapidly. Chloramphenicol and tetracycline perform poorly in reptiles. The semisynthetic tetracycline doxycycline apparently controls the signs of the upper respiratory tract syndrome of desert tortoises. This finding confirms recent evidence that the disease is caused by a mycoplasmal organism.

The new quinolone antibiotic enrofloxacin has demonstrated great promise. Several cases of infection that failed to respond to aminoglycosides and aminoglycoside-β-lactam combinations have responded to enrofloxacin. My best success in treating desert tortoise respiratory syndrome has involved giving enrofloxacin systemically and topically in the form of a nasal flush. This therapeutic regimen has continued to be very successful in the treatment of this syndrome. Dosages of antibiotics and various other therapeutic agents are presented in the box "Drugs for Reptiles and Amphibians."

Most reptile parasites are easily treated. Ivermectin, fenbendazole, levamisole, metronidazole, and praziquantel are the most common antiparasitic agents. Ivermectin is very toxic in turtles and tortoises. Levamisole or fenbendazole is effective in treating nematode parasites in these reptiles. Ivermectin may cause skin discoloration if injected subcutaneously in chameleons and other thin-skinned species. Oral treatment is apparently effective in most cases. In treating small specimens, the stock solution is diluted 1:10 or 1:100 in propylene glycol.

Establishing and maintaining hydration is important, especially if potentially nephrotoxic antibiotics are administered. I have successfully used lactated Ringer's solution for several years. The use of hypotonic solutions, to more closely replace intracellular fluids, is arguably more appropriate.[6] Because intravenous administration is impractical in most cases, a large volume of fluid is typically given intracoelomically.

Turtles and tortoises, especially those with lower respiratory disease, benefit from the administration of fluids into the epicoelomic space. The epicoelomic technique involves passing a 1- or 1.5-inch needle through the pectoral musculature at a point ventral to the pectoral girdle and just dorsal to the plastron. The needle is directed toward the contralateral hindleg.[6] If placement is correct, there is no resistance to the injection of the fluids.

ANESTHESIA

Procedures that require chemical restraint or surgery are relatively common in reptile practice. Even the physical

Drugs for Reptiles and Amphibians (continued)

Levamisole phosphate Dosage: 10 to 20 mg/kg subcutaneously or intramuscularly, repeated in 10 to 14 days. Used to treat nematode infestation.

Metronidazole Dosage: 40 to 125 mg/kg, repeated in 10 to 14 days for most protozoan parasites. Lower doses are recommended for tricolor king snakes, indigo snakes, and uracoan rattlers. A dosage interval of 72 hours for five to seven doses is recommended in treating *Entamoeba invadens*. 50 to 100 mg/kg given orally may stimulate appetite.

Praziquantel Dosage: 8 mg/kg intramuscularly or orally, repeated in 14 days. Used to treat cestode infestation.

Chemical Restraint and Anesthesia

Benzocaine Dosage: By absorption. Used for anesthesia in amphibians. A bath is prepared using 50 to 100 mg/L water dissolved in ethyl alcohol or acetone.

Isoflurane and halothane Dosage: Induce at 3% to 5%, and maintain at 1% to 3%. Induction may be prolonged (30 to 60 minutes) if mask or chamber induction is used. Some patients can be intubated while conscious. Succinylcholine chloride and ketamine hydrochloride may be used for immobilization.

Ketamine hydrochloride Dosage: 20 to 60 mg/kg intramuscularly or 5 to 15 mg/kg intravenously. Muscle relaxation is marginal in many cases. Analgesia may be marginal. Recovery is slow with high doses.

Lidocaine hydrochloride Dosage: In local analgesia, the minimum volume necessary for analgesia is used. Immobilization with succinylcholine chloride or ketamine hydrochloride is often required.

Succinylcholine chloride Dosage: 0.25 to 1.0 mg/kg intramuscularly. Effects occur in 20 to 60 minutes and last one to four hours. Used for immobilization only, not anesthesia or analgesia. Respiration must be assisted if respiratory muscles are paralyzed. The practitioner should begin with the lowest dose in unfamiliar species. The dose is titrated to the minimum required for the procedure to be performed.

Tiletamine hydrochloride and zolazepam Dosage: 20 to 40 mg/kg of the combined drug intramuscularly in lizards and snakes and 5 to 15 mg/kg in turtles and tortoises. The low dose is used for restraint or immobilization. Recovery is prolonged with the high dose.

Fluids

Hypotonic parenteral fluids Dosage: 1% to 3% of body weight intracoelomically or epicoelomically every 24 hours. One part lactated Ringer's solution is mixed with two parts 2.5% dextrose in 0.45% sodium chloride solution.

Lactated Ringer's solution Dosage: 1% to 3% of body weight intracoelomically or epicoelomically every 24 hours.

Miscellaneous

Atropine Dosage for organophosphate toxicity: 0.1 to 0.2 mg/kg, repeated as needed to control signs. Dosage for bradycardia: 0.04 to 0.10 mg/kg; the cause of the bradycardia should be corrected.

Calcium glubionate Dosage: 10 ml/kg orally every 12 to 24 hours. Used to treat calcium deficiency in debilitated reptiles.

Calcium gluconate Dosage: 10 to 50 mg/kg intramuscularly. Used before oxytocin to treat hypocalcemia or egg binding.

Calcium glycerophosphate and lactate Dosage: 1.0 to 2.5 ml/kg intramuscularly or subcutaneously. Used before oxytocin to treat hypocalcemia or egg binding.

Oxytocin Dosage: 1 to 10 IU/kg intramuscularly. Should be administered in conjunction with calcium. Aids egg expulsion in turtles and tortoises and helps stop uterine bleeding.

Vitamins A, D, E Dosage: 0.15 ml/kg intramuscularly, repeated in 21 days. Used to treat hypovitaminosis D_3 and hypovitaminosis A.

Vitamin B complex Dosage: 0.25 ml/kg intramuscularly. Used to stimulate appetite.

Vitamin C Dosage: 100 to 250 mg/kg intramuscularly. May aid in treating mouth rot and the splitting-skin syndrome of some large constrictors.

Vitamin K Dosage: 0.25 to 0.50 mg/kg intramuscularly. Aids the formation of coagulation factors.

examination of many tortoises and of large, dangerous specimens may require chemical restraint. Once the practitioner gains experience with the drug, succinylcholine chloride is an excellent tool for simple immobilization. The dose should be titrated to a level at which the patient does not resist yet does not lose control of respiration. If this dose is exceeded, respiration must be assisted until the patient can breathe on its own.

Anesthesia is simplified if the patient can be induced and maintained using an inhalation agent. A face mask or chamber can be used to induce anesthesia in most species of snakes and lizards (Figure 5). Intubation is usually possible when the righting reflex is lost. With isoflurane anesthesia, the patient can be induced at 5% and maintained at 1.5% to 3%.

Some species, notably turtles and tortoises, can remain apneic for extended periods; induction with an inhalation agent is thus impractical. These patients can be induced with ketamine hydrochloride or tiletamine and zolazepam; or they can be immobilized with succinylcholine chloride, intubated, and manually ventilated with oxygen and isoflurane. Anesthesia is monitored via the presence of the righting reflex and the response to painful stimuli (toe pinch or pinprick). In some snakes and lizards, the heart rate may be palpated or visualized through the abdomen. Large specimens may be monitored via electrocardiogram.

The information presented on pages 986 and 987 consists of the doses used in my practice. Many were extrapolated from mammalian doses, estimated using metabolic scaling or trial and error. When possible, doses were based on pharmacokinetic studies. The few studies that have es-

tablished proper dose regimens for reptile patients have been performed in optimum conditions. Although these doses have proven to be safe and efficacious in my practice, there is no guarantee of safety or efficacy; the doses are applied at the risk of the user.

About the Author
Dr. Jenkins, who is a Diplomate of the American Board of Veterinary Practitioners (Avian Practice), is affiliated with the Avian & Exotic Animal Hospital, San Diego, California.

REFERENCES
1. Jacobson ER: Evaluation of the reptile patient, in Jacobson ER, Kollias GV (eds): *Contemporary Issues in Small Animal Practice, Exotic Animals.* New York, Churchill Livingstone, 1988, pp 1–18.
2. Frye FL: *Biomedical and Surgical Aspects of Captive Reptile Husbandry.* Bonner Springs, KS, Veterinary Medical Publishing Co, 1981, pp 134–174.
3. Rubel GA, Isenbugel E, Wolvekamp P: *Atlas of Diagnostic Radiology of Exotic Pets.* Philadelphia, WB Saunders Co, 1991, pp 176–221.
4. Jacobson ER: Use of chemotherapeutics in reptile medicine, in Jacobson ER, Kollias GV (eds): *Contemporary Issues in Small Animal Practice, Exotic Animals.* New York, Churchill Livingstone, 1988, pp 35–48.
5. Jacobson ER, Kollias GV, Peters LS: Dosages for antibiotics and parasiticides used in exotic animals. *Compend Contin Educ Pract Vet* 5(4):315–324, 1983.
6. Jarchow JL: Hospital care of the reptile patient, in Jacobson ER, Kollias GV (eds): *Contemporary Issues in Small Animal Practice, Exotic Animals.* New York, Churchill Livingstone, 1988, pp 19–34.
7. Jarchow JL: Diagnosis and management of the reptile patient. *Proc Annu Avian/Exotic Anim Med Symp*:73–77, 1988.
8. Ross RA: *The Bacterial Diseases of Reptiles.* Stanford, CA, Institute for Herpetological Research, 1984, pp 5–105.
9. Beehler BA, Sauro AM: Aerobic bacterial isolates and antibiotic sensitivities in a captive reptile collection. *Annu Proc Am Assoc Zoo Vet*:198–201, 1983.

Husbandry and Clinical Evaluation of *Iguana iguana*

KEY FACTS

- Poor husbandry is the leading cause of disease in iguanas.
- The history often is the most informative part of the clinical evaluation.
- A thorough physical examination and diagnostic workup are necessary steps for successful treatment of sick iguanas.
- Iguanas require an external heat source to maintain body temperature and digest food.
- Young iguanas should be fed one part protein food to two parts plant food; older iguanas should be fed approximately 90% vegetable food one to two times weekly.

The Ohio State University
Nancy L. Anderson, DVM

THIS ARTICLE consolidates and organizes information on the green iguana (*Iguana iguana*) into a useful guide for veterinarians who treat reptiles. Basic biostatistics, significant anatomic considerations, husbandry, physical examination, and diagnostic procedures are covered.

BASIC BIOSTATISTICS

The green iguana is a diurnal, herbivorous, arboreal lizard that is native to Central and South America. Wild iguanas spend a large portion of the day thermoregulating and absorbing ultraviolet light by basking along forest edges. Adult males can be differentiated from females by larger dewlaps and body size as well as by highly developed femoral pores on the caudoventral portion of the thighs. Breeding usually occurs in January or February. Oviposition takes place approximately 47 to 49 days postcopulation; females dig extensive tunnels into loose soil before laying clutches of 25 to 40 eggs. Incubation takes approximately 73 to 90 days at a suggested temperature of 29° to 31°C (84° to 88°F) and humidity of –150 kPa. In newly hatched iguanas, the average length from snout to vent is 6.6 centimeters, and weights range from 10.5 to 13.8 grams. Young iguanas should grow approximately 30 to 60 cm/yr and reach sexual maturity in three years.[1-4]

With appropriate care, most captive iguanas can live 13 to 15 years, grow as much as 1.8 meters in length, and weigh up to 6.8 kilograms.[5] Because of its large body size and pleasant-tasting flesh, the green iguana is overhunted by humans and has become endangered over much of its range.[6]

ANATOMIC CONSIDERATIONS

The gross anatomy of the iguana is similar to that of mammals, but there are a few significant differences. Iguanas have no diaphragm. Their lungs are saccular with many divisions. Because respiration is accomplished by movement of the rib cage,[7] restraint techniques must allow for excursion of the chest wall.

Iguanas have a three-chambered heart. The ventricle is not completely divided into two parts. The thyroid gland is located just cranial to the heart.[8] A swell mechanism, by which the circulatory system can increase blood pressure in the head region, is believed to aid in ecdysis (skin shedding).[7] Of special note is the large vein that runs down the ventral midline of the body wall. Because of the position of this vein, laparotomy incisions must be made off the midline. Another large blood vessel is located on the ventral surface of the tail vertebrae. This vessel is useful when blood samples must be obtained.

Updated from original publication in Volume 13, Number 8, August 1991

In the iguana, with the exception of the intestines, blood from tissues caudal to the kidneys can drain directly back to the kidneys. This capability is referred to as a renal portal system. Most injections should be given cranial to the kidneys to avoid renal toxicities and rapid clearance problems.

Because they excrete uric acid instead of urea, the kidneys of reptiles are inherently different from those of mammals. The cranial pole of each kidney in male iguanas is structurally unique and is referred to as the sexual segment.[7] The epithelial cells lining the tubules in this portion of the kidney become hypertrophic during the breeding season. The adrenal glands of reptiles also are different from those of mammals because of the unusual location of the glands; that is, the adrenal glands are close to the gonads rather than the kidneys.

The reproductive system of the iguana is similar to that of birds with one exception: both right and left halves of the reproductive system are developed. Oviducts enter the cloaca cranial to their respective ureters. The ovaries are closely attached to the dorsal body wall, which makes surgical excision difficult. Male iguanas have two copulatory organs, which are referred to as hemipenes. These organs, when not in use, lie in recesses that exit the caudal wall of the cloaca and run parallel to the tail. The presence or absence of these recesses can be determined with a blunt probe. This technique can be used to determine the sex of young iguanas.

IN THE IGUANA, the digestive system is monogastric and the cecum is large. Newly hatched iguanas require intestinal inoculation of adult iguana bacteria and protozoa. This is done by providing them with a stool from a healthy, parasite-free adult iguana.[9]

The teeth of the iguana are ankylosed to their respective jawbones. Each tooth has a pulp cavity that is covered by enamel.[7] Broken teeth are extremely painful and may cause anorexia until the tooth is shed and replaced. Oral examinations should be performed as gently as possible by using cotton-tipped applicators, which should always be moved in a rostral to caudal direction to avoid entanglement on the caudally curved teeth.

The skin of reptiles is covered with epidermal scales and has only a few glands. Healing occurs most rapidly when incisions are placed between scales. Damage to scales can cause shedding difficulties. Typically, iguanas shed their skin in large patches. A rough surface should be available to the iguana because this will aid in removing dead skin.

HUSBANDRY

The leading cause of death in reptiles is failure to adapt to captivity.[10] Inappropriate environments are so alien to reptiles that the resultant stress from being placed in such environments leads to starvation and fatal secondary disease. Proper housing and nutrition are of paramount importance in keeping reptiles healthy.

Young iguanas can be temporarily housed in aquariums. Because of the fast growth of iguanas, a custom-made cage will quickly be required. Polyurethane-sealed wood and glass cages are very popular because they are well-insulated, inexpensive, nonabrasive, and easy to clean and customize.[5]

Iguanas are ectotherms. They require an external heat source to maintain body temperature and to digest food. Cage ambient air temperatures should be maintained between 29.5° and 32°C (85° to 90°F) during the day and between 24° and 26.5°C (75° to 80°F) at night. A focal source of heat (37.5° to 43.5°C [100° to 110°F]) should be provided so that a temperature gradient that allows the reptile to thermoregulate its body temperature is available.

The preferred optimum temperature for iguanas, that is, the temperature that ensures proper digestive and reproductive processes, is between 29.5° and 39.5°C (85° to 103°F). Iguanas should be exposed to temperatures at the higher end of this range. Care must be taken, however, to make available a time at which temperatures within the cage are at the lower end of the range; otherwise, thyroid dysfunction or possibly death can result. Iguanas cannot tolerate temperatures higher than 46.1°C (114.8°F).[11]

Heat may be provided by placing a heater under one end of the cage. Heating pads and heat tape work well. Hot rocks or shielded heat lamps can be placed inside cages. All heating elements that can attain temperatures higher than 43.5°C (110°F) should be shielded from direct contact. Because all heating appliances can fatally burn a reptile, these appliances should be controlled by reliable thermostats that are tested periodically for accuracy.

In addition to allowing the iguana to thermoregulate its body temperature, basking provides ultraviolet light. The iguana should have access to approximately 10 hours of unfiltered sunshine daily and at least 12 hours of darkness in order to create the necessary light cycle. Indoor specimens need an artificial light source (Vitalites®—Durotest; Sylvania Design 50®—General Telecommunications and Electronics; Chroma lamps®—General Electric) with a chromatic index greater than 88. Ultraviolet light should be provided at a rate of 20 watts/91 to 182 cm³ (3 to 6 cubic feet) of cage space for a maximum time span of 8 to 10 hours daily. A basking area should be placed 45 to 61 cm (18 to 24 inches) from the light source. Black light tubes from bug zappers also work well, but the potential for damage to human as well as reptile vision has not been evaluated.[12,13]

Cages must be kept extremely clean. Wild iguanas defecate from trees and rarely contact their own feces. Daily cleaning and weekly disinfecting of cages are essential. Phenolic cleaners, such as Lysol® pine cleaner, are toxic to reptiles. Sodium hypochlorite mixed with water (one part bleach to 30 parts water) is safe, effective, and inexpensive.[14]

The ideal cage liner is newspaper. It is nontoxic, inexpensive, and disposable. Cage papers should be changed at least once daily. Artificial turf is second in choice to newspaper. Although more aesthetically pleasing, the use of turf requires more work. At least three pieces of turf must be available (one to be used inside the cage; one to be cleaned and dried, which takes 48 hours; and one to replace the piece of turf inside the cage that will become soiled after 24 hours). Only clean, dry turf should be placed in the cage. Loose strings should be removed to prevent potential foreign bodies.

Additional forms of cage substrate are large stone gravel and bark chips; these are not preferred because they can be ingested and because they harbor bacteria, parasites, and moisture. Kitty litter, small stone gravel, and corncobs should never be used. These materials are often ingested, thereby causing impactions, and are associated with skin infections.

The ideal humidity for caged iguanas is 33% to 66%.[11] Low humidity can cause dehydration and shedding difficulties. High humidity predisposes iguanas to bacterial disease.

Cage wall surfaces should be smooth to prevent abrasions, particularly to the nose. A rough branch or stone is needed to aid in shedding. Additional branches and a space in which the iguana can climb should be provided to stimulate activity. Reptiles should also be given places to hide; boxes, clay pots, and plastic plants serve this need well. Insecure iguanas often pace in their cages and can abrade their noses and mouths, which can lead to fatal infections.

IGUANAS are primarily solitary animals. Cagemates are not recommended. Newly acquired animals must be strictly quarantined for at least 60 days before being introduced into a collection. Some iguanas can be affectionate toward their owners; but in general, iguanas become stressed during handling. Handling should be frequent enough so that the iguana becomes used to and therefore calm with the procedure, but handling should never be done for an extended time.

NUTRITION

Water is an extremely important nutrient. Not only do iguanas need a constant source of fresh, clean drinking water, but small iguanas need a place to soak. Large, shallow dishes are ideal for this purpose. Larger iguanas also like to soak; but because of space limitations, misting is often done as an alternative three to four times weekly.

An iguana's diet varies with age. Young, rapidly growing iguanas generally require two feedings daily, which consist of one part protein food to two parts plant food.

Older iguanas eat approximately 90% vegetable food one to two times weekly. Adult iguanas can be offered, on occasion, a neonatal mouse.[9] Excess protein should be restricted in obese lizards and may predispose a healthy animal to nutrition-related problems.

Protein foods consist of a combination of Purina Trout Chow® (Purina Mills), cooked egg and shell, cooked white meats, earthworms, and soft mealworms. Live foods can transmit diseases. Locating a reliable, high-calcium, disease-free source is essential. Vegetable foods should *not* include iceberg lettuce or canned fruit cocktail, both of which are very palatable but have low nutritional value. Dark green and yellow vegetables, such as chard, romaine, broccoli, and carrots, as well as peas, corn, squash, berries, apples, dandelions, alfalfa sprouts, and rabbit pellets are high in nutritional value.[9,12,15]

Both protein and vegetable foods should be chopped into small pieces and mixed thoroughly to ensure that finicky eaters still receive all nutrients. The mixture should be tightly sealed and refrigerated. It can be fed for one to three days without spoilage. Just before feeding, the food should be sprinkled with a calcium source (Nekton-MSA®—Nekton-Produkte, Pforzheim, Germany; D-Ca-Phos®—Fort Dodge Laboratories) and an appropriate reptile vitamin (Nekton-rep®—Nekton-Produkte; VitaLife®—Terrafauna). Food should be removed from the cage before it spoils.

RESTRAINT

Small iguanas are easily restrained by using the thumb and forefinger to grasp the caudal mandibular area from behind the head. The dorsal body is cradled in the palm of the same hand. The abdomen, chest, and pelvis are controlled with the remaining fingers, while allowing for respiration.

Larger iguanas may be grasped over the head with one hand, while the second hand grabs the base of the tail. The back legs can then be taped to the tail to avoid scratches. Large iguanas can inflict serious bites and often use their powerful tails as whips. Unruly specimens may require the use of thin leather gloves.[16] Some larger iguanas can be restrained on their backs by stroking the ventral midline; this can produce a trancelike state.

CLINICAL EVALUATION

The history is often the most informative part of the clinical evaluation. For many animals, improper husbandry is the predisposing factor for many diseases. Unless the diet and environment are improved, the best treatment plan will fail.

The owner should be asked for information about the following[17-19]:

- Species, age, sex
- Origin—initially, wild caught or captive bred; recently, pet shop or supply house

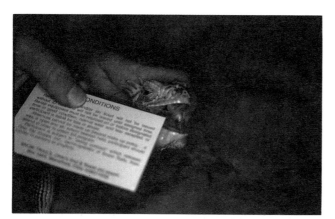

Figure 1—A thin plastic card can be used as leverage to open the mouth of an iguana. The thin edge fits between the jaws, thereby minimizing soft tissue damage and the incidence of broken teeth.

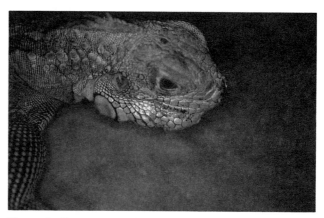

Figure 2—The mandibles of this iguana are markedly swollen and rubbery as a result of secondary hyperparathyroidism attributed to diet.

- Length of ownership, previous experience
- Environment, caging, cleaning, temperature, humidity, photoperiod
- Diet, supplements, appetite, last meal, last stool
- Dates of unusual activity, breeding, egg laying, shedding
- Cagemates, quarantine history, aggressive behavior
- Medical history, weight
- Purpose of ownership—pet, breeder, display, education.

The physical examination of an iguana follows the same pattern as that for mammals or birds. A current, accurate weight in grams is extremely important. Inexperienced clinicians should obtain healthy specimens so that they can become familiar with the characteristics of the iguana, such as normal behavior, locomotion, weight, skin tone, and color. Healthy young iguanas should be very active except when hiding. They should vigorously resent capture. Head tilts are abnormal. Older iguanas that are used to being handled may be more difficult to assess. All iguanas should have a filled-out appearance. The tail and leg muscles should be plump and resilient. A healthy iguana can lift its body off the floor and run rapidly. The skin should be a luminescent green. There should be no moist, black ulcerations or subcutaneous swellings. The presence of patches of skin that appear almost ready to be shed is normal, but large areas may indicate a problem. The nose should be examined for abrasions, and the remaining areas of skin should be checked for parasites.

A THOROUGH ophthalmic, tympanic membrane, nasal, and oral examination should be performed. No exudate should be present. The mouth can be opened by gently but firmly pulling on the dewlap while holding the maxilla. With resistant patients, a thin plastic card can be used as a wedge to open the mouth gently (Figure 1). Normal mucous membranes of the mouth and fleshy tongue are bright pink. Clear viscous saliva is normal. Ulcers, purulent or caseous exudate, parasites, or plaques are indications of disease. Broken teeth and rubbery, swollen mandibles (Figure 2) are additional signs of disease.

Although Gram stains of the pharynx and choanae are recommended, care must be taken not to place too much emphasis on the results. The normal flora in this region are gram-negative. Intracellular or large, monomorphic populations of bacteria suggest pathogenic organisms; but confirmation of pathogenicity can be made only by (1) evidence of increased numbers of inflammatory cells on cytologic stains, (2) clinical signs of disease, or (3) cultures showing at least moderate growth or resistance to many antibiotics.

With experience, the heart and lungs can be auscultated by using a towel held between the body wall of the iguana and the stethoscope. The heart rate can be palpated or observed through the chest wall. Respirations are easily counted from excursions of the chest wall. There should be no signs of dyspnea.

The abdomen can be palpated for masses, eggs, or gas in all except obese animals. The cloaca should be swabbed. Gram stains and cytologic stains, fecal smears, and cultures provide useful information. There should be good cloacal tone. Stools should be examined for consistency and color. Stools have two parts: the urates and urine from the renal system and fecal matter from the digestive tract. Polyuria can be differentiated from diarrhea by the presence of the liquid part of the stool in the urate rather than the fecal portion. Urinalyses can be performed when polyuria is present, but reference values are difficult to obtain.

Fecal examinations should be performed on all iguanas. Most infections can be diagnosed by a fresh saline smear and flotation test. Centrifugation and Baermann tests are rarely needed. With the aid of an appropriate guide, most cysts, eggs, and larvae can be identified to taxonomic family; thus, the proper anthelmintic treatment can be selected. When an animal does not respond to treatment, fecal samples should be shipped to a parasitologist for further analysis. Most infections are the result of poor husbandry or contaminated foodstuffs, or they originated from an unidentifiable source in the wild. Often, small numbers of parasites are incorrectly blamed for signs of disease; however, further investigation will reveal the true cause of the infection.[20]

If the sex of an iguana cannot be determined by visual examination, a lubricated tomcat catheter can be gently slipped into the caudolateral vent area. In males, the catheter will slip in past 1.25 centimeters (one-half inch). This technique, however, may lead to perforation and resultant abscess formation.[19] A second technique described in the literature involves injecting saline into the hemipenes, which causes them to evert. As fluid is resorbed, the hemipenes return to their sulci.[21]

All extremities should be palpated for swelling or fractures. Fractures as sequelae to secondary hyperparathyroidism are very common in green iguanas.

About the Author
Dr. Anderson is affiliated with the Department of Veterinary Clinical Sciences, College of Veterinary Medicine, The Ohio State University, Columbus, Ohio.

REFERENCES

1. Mendelssohn H: Observations on a captive colony of *Iguana iguana*, in Murphy JB, Collins JT (eds): *Reproductive Biology and Diseases of Captive Reptiles.* Lawrence, KS, Meseravil Printing, Inc, Society for the Study of Amphibians and Reptiles, 1980, pp 119–123.
2. Phillips JA, Garel A, Packard GC, Packard MJ: Influence of moisture and temperature on eggs and embryos of green iguanas. *Herpetologica* 46(2):238–245, 1990.
3. Licht P, Moherly WR: Thermal requirements for embryonic development for the tropical lizard *Iguana iguana. Copeia* 4:515–517, 1965.
4. Rand AS: The temperatures of iguana nests and their relation to incubation optima and to nesting sites and season. *Herpetologica* 28:252–253, 1972.
5. Corcoran JH: A quality cage for *Iguana iguana.* Informational handout. Palm Harbor, FL, 1988.
6. Allen ME, Oftedal OT, Werner DI: Management of the green iguana (*Iguana iguana*) in Central America. *Proc Am Assoc Zoo Vet*:19–22, 1990.
7. Evans HE: Introduction and anatomy, in Fowler ME (ed): *Zoo and Wild Animal Medicine,* ed 2. Philadelphia, WB Saunders Co, 1986, pp 118–125.
8. Dolensek EP: Necropsy techniques in reptiles. *JAVMA* 159:1616–1617, 1971.
9. Woerpel RW, Rosskopf WJ: *Avian-Exotic Animal Care Guides.* Goleta, CA, American Veterinary Publications, Inc, 1988.
10. Cowan DF: Diseases of captive reptiles. *JAVMA* 153:848–859, 1968.
11. Wallach JD: Environmental and nutritional diseases of captive reptiles. *JAVMA* 159:1632–1644, 1971.
12. Barten SL: The care of reptiles in captivity, in *Chicago Herpetological Society Members Handbook.* Chicago, Chicago Herpetological Society, 1989.
13. Corcoran JH: The importance of ultraviolet light and raising iguanas in captivity. Informational handout. Palm Harbor, FL, 1988.
14. Fowler ME: Disinfectant and insecticide usage around birds and reptiles, in Kirk RW (ed): *Current Veterinary Therapy. Small Animal Practice,* ed 8. Philadelphia, WB Saunders Co, 1983, pp 606–611.
15. King FW: Housing, sanitation, and nutrition of reptiles. *JAVMA* 159:1612–1615, 1971.
16. Fowler ME: *Restraint and Handling of Wild and Domestic Animals.* Ames, IA, Iowa State University Press, 1978.
17. Jacobsen ER: Evaluation of the reptile patient, in Jacobsen ER, Kollias GV (eds): *Contemporary Issues in Small Animal Practice: Exotic Animals.* New York, Churchill Livingstone, 1988, pp 1–18.
18. Jackson OF: *The Clinical Examination of Reptiles.* London, British Herpetological Society (c/o Zoological Society of London), 1985, pp 91–97.
19. Jackson OF: Clinical aspects of diagnosis and treatment, in Cooper JE, Jackson OF (eds): *Diseases of the Reptilia,* vol 2. New York, Academic Press, 1981, pp 507–534.
20. Jacobson ER: Parasitic diseases of reptiles, in Kirk RW (ed): *Current Veterinary Therapy. Small Animal Practice,* ed 8. Philadelphia, WB Saunders Co, 1983, pp 599–606.
21. Frye FL: Sexual dimorphism and identification in reptiles, in Kirk RW (ed): *Current Veterinary Therapy. Small Animal Practice,* ed 10. Philadelphia, WB Saunders Co, 1989, pp 796–803.

Editor's Note: Several of the references are from sources that will be difficult to locate by the reader. We therefore suggest that the author be contacted directly. Dr. Anderson will be glad to supply readers with information on how to obtain the obscure references cited in her text.

UPDATE

HEAT SOURCES

Heat for green iguanas can be efficiently provided through a combination of an infrared or ceramic heat lamp, placed outside of the cage to minimize the risk of thermal burns, and a heating pad, placed under ⅓ to ½ of the cage. The undercage heating pad usually will provide an ambient temperature of 85°F in the cage, with the surface temperature being slightly higher. The lamp should be positioned over a favorite basking location for at least three to four hours a day, at a temperature of 100–110°F. Infrared and ceramic heating elements may be used 24 hours a day as they do not affect circadian rhythms like incandescent bulbs. These types of radiant heat sources are extremely important for large iguanas: Ventral heat, such as from heating pads and hot rocks, is not capable of warming the core body temperature enough to allow adequate digestion in large iguanas.

NUTRITION

An iguana's diet should vary with its age. Young, rapidly growing iguanas require diets that consist of 70% to 80% dark, leafy greens; 10% to 20% fruits and vegetables; and 5% to 10% protein. Older iguanas should eat 80% to 90% dark leafy greens; 10% to 15% fruits and vegetables; and no more than 5% from protein sources. Dark leafy greens can be derived from a variety of chard, parsley, endive, romaine lettuce, dandelions, broccoli, carrot tops, turnip greens, spinach, etc. Fruits and vegetables should consist of squash, berries, apples, citrus fruits, peas, corn, green beans, etc. Protein sources can include alfalfa sprouts, rabbit or guinea pig pellets, and most commercial iguana foods. Several sources have expressed concern that an increased incidence of renal disease is associated with feeding animal source protein to iguanas. In this author's experience, animal proteins such as trout chow, hard boiled eggs, meal worms, and dog food have NOT been associated with renal disease if fed as described above.

If a well-balanced, varied diet and adequate ultraviolet light are provided, the need for supplements should be minimal. Excessive supplementation of vitamins and minerals, especially vitamin D and phosphorus, has been associated with renal failure in conjunction with metastatic calcification and gout in middle-aged iguanas. Growing iguanas fed good diets may be supplemented with reptile vitamins sprinkled on their food two to three times a week. Well-maintained adult iguanas should only be supplemented once every week to two weeks. While young iguanas should receive calcium daily to every other day and older iguanas only once a week, calcium supplements should NOT contain additional vitamin D or phosphorus, such as calcium glubionate (Neocalglucon®) and calcium carbonate (crushed egg or oyster shell).

Diseases of *Iguana iguana*

KEY FACTS

- Isoflurane is the anesthetic agent of choice for iguanas.
- Before the animals are returned to their regular diet, isotonic fluids followed by hypertonic enteral fluids should be administered to iguanas that have been anorectic for more than one week.
- Many respiratory infections in iguanas begin as oral infections.
- Surgical techniques developed for mammals work well in iguanas when compensations for differences in metabolism and anatomy are made.
- Dystocia is common and often is related to poor nutrition; surgical intervention often is necessary.

The Ohio State University
Nancy L. Anderson, DVM

THIS ARTICLE offers information on diseases affecting *Iguana iguana* (the green iguana). Diagnostic procedures and specific disorders are discussed.

DIAGNOSTIC PROCEDURES

The minimum data base for the health check of an iguana comprises a thorough history and physical examination, cloacal and choanal Gram's stains, fecal testing, and weighing of the animal. Depending on the owner's wishes and the condition of the iguana, further diagnostic procedures may be done. Although blood reference values for reptiles are incompletely documented, serial complete blood counts and chemistry profiles are extremely useful (Tables I and II), especially in evaluating the animal's response to therapy. Blood samples are most frequently taken from the tail vein that runs immediately ventral to the spine (Figure 1). Until the clinician or technician has received special training and is comfortable in dealing with these samples, they should be sent to a laboratory familiar with reptilian blood.

Heterophils are the reptile analogue to mammalian neutrophils. Although the total white blood cell count is normally lower in iguanas than in most mammals, changes in white blood cell numbers and maturity represent disease processes similar to those that affect mammals. Although blood parasites are fairly common, they rarely cause overt disease in iguanas.[1]

Profile values of iguanas are more difficult to interpret because of differences in such parameters as body temperature and diet. Determination of creatinine and blood urea nitrogen does not adequately allow assessment of kidney function; however, levels of these substances rise rapidly with dehydration. Uric acid rises with marked reduction in kidney function or high-protein diets. A concurrent drop in packed cell volume also occurs with renal disease. Alkaline phosphatase can rise with severe renal disease. Alanine transaminase and lactate dehydrogenase are not liver specific in reptiles; values should thus be interpreted with caution. Low glucose often indicates starvation or septicemia. Calcium levels must be interpreted in light of clinical presentation. Female reptiles can produce a marked periovulatory hypercalcemia that has no pathologic significance. Males or reproductively inactive females with high calcium levels should be evaluated for excess calcium and vitamin D supplementation before other causes are investigated. If the calcium level of an iguana is low, the diet should be evaluated. Hyper- and hypovitaminosis D are extremely common problems in pet iguanas. Other electrolytes in iguanas may be interpreted in the same manner as for mammals.[2]

Radiography is very useful in evaluating skeletal and soft tissues. High detail and short exposures are necessary, especially for small specimens. Rare earth screens, such as DuPont® Quanta Detail with DuPont® Cronex 7 or 10 x-ray film (DuPont), have been suggested. The x-ray machine

TABLE I
Hematology and Biochemistry Values

Test	Value
White Blood Cells (10^3)	3–10
Packed Cell Volume (%)	30–42
Heterophils (10^3)	42–68
Lymphocytes (10^3)	29–54
Azurophils (10^3)	0–8
Basophils (10^3)	0–2
Eosinophils (10^3)	0–1
Total protein (g/dl)	5–7.8
Alanine aminotransferase (IU/L)	10–70
Lactate dehydrogenase (IU/L)	10–70
Creatinine phosphate kinase (IU/L)	50–500
Uric Acid (mg/dl)	2–8
Calcium (mg/dl)	9–15
Glucose (mg/dl)	90–145
Phosphorus (mg/dl)	4.5–8
Cholesterol (mg/dl)	202

From Dr. Alan Fudge, California Avian Laboratory, Citrus Heights, CA.

should have a 200 mA capability. Exposure time should not exceed 1/60th second. Kilovolt settings lower than 40 allow better imaging of small lizards.[3] Immobilization for positioning of radiographs is achieved with masking tape (Figure 2), manual restraint, or general anesthesia. Practitioners may wish to make their own atlas of normal animals as a reference. Both lateral and dorsoventral projections are diagnostically beneficial. Barium preparations can be used to diagnose intestinal obstructions but may precipitate in the intestines and cause impaction in severely dehydrated animals.

RED BRUNSWICK feeding catheters may be gently passed into the stomach to obtain samples for culture, cytology, or Gram's stain. Small amounts of physiologic saline may be used to enhance recovery of material when necessary.[4] The distance from the nose to the last rib is measured and marked on the tube. The mouth is opened, and the trachea is located and avoided. A larger hard plastic tube may be placed in the mouth in a manner similar to placement of a Frick tube in cattle to prevent loss of the softer feeding tube as a result of chewing. The end of the feeding tube is placed through the stiff tube, over the larynx, and down the esophagus. This route also is an accurate and efficient method for administering drugs and fluids.

Other diagnostic techniques used in mammals should be considered for reptiles. Such techniques include biopsy, ophthalmic examination, and endoscopy. Injectables that are not caustic or voluminous should be given in the front leg or epaxial muscles cranial to the kidneys. Small amounts of nonirritating drugs or isotonic fluids can be given subcutaneously. Intracoelomic injections are not recommended but may be necessary to rehydrate animals unable to tolerate enteral fluids. Aseptic technique is important to prevent peritonitis. Intracoelomic injections must be given laterally away from the ventral midline.

ANESTHESIA

Quality and duration of anesthesia in reptiles depend on the temperature of the animal. External heat sources are needed during anesthesia and recovery. Isoflurane inhalation anesthesia is preferred.[5] In my experience, induction at 2% to 4% isoflurane through a mask followed by intubation and maintenance at 1% to 2% of isoflurane per one liter of oxygen flow has been successful. Isoflurane has allowed recoveries as rapid as 20 minutes after 90 minutes of surgery, and recovery is extremely rapid when isoflurane is used for short diagnostic procedures. Heart and respiratory rates must be carefully monitored. If either of these rates is markedly decreased, the percentage of isoflurane being administered must be reduced. In my experience, positive-pressure ventilation at a rate of one to two breaths/min has allowed for smoother anesthesia and quicker recoveries. Halothane anesthesia has also been used successfully, but methoxyflurane has caused deaths in a group of reptiles.[6]

Injectable anesthetics can be used, but recovery may be prolonged (greater than two days). Tiletamine zolazepam (Telazol®—A.H. Robins) has been used intramuscularly in iguanas at a range of 10.0 to 26.5 mg/kg. Induction usually is less than 30 minutes.[7] Ketamine hydrochloride can be used at doses of 50 to 130 mg/kg intramuscularly with similar results.[8] Calderwood warns against possible fatalities.[9]

The first sign of induction is excitement, after which voluntary motor control is lost. Loss of righting reflex is followed by muscle relaxation, which signifies attainment of surgical anesthesia. Most iguanas retain a slight third eyelid reflex even when no pain response is elicited. In these animals, loss of the blink reflex can indicate a need to lessen anesthesia.

DISEASES

Proper husbandry and nutrition are critical in prevention of reptilian disease. Calcium, phosphorus, and vitamin D_3 imbalances are extremely common in iguanas. The most frequent manifestation of low levels of calcium, vitamin D, and ultraviolet light is secondary hyperparathyroidism. Young iguanas frequently are presented for caudal paresis. The history of a diseased iguana reveals inadequate housing and diet. Physical examination reveals poor body and skin condition, including such disorders as oral ulcers (from other vitamin deficiencies or secondary infections); swollen, rubbery mandibles; hard, swollen muscles; and unhealed fractures of the ribs and extremities. Tetanic paresis results from low serum calcium. Flaccid paralysis most often results from fractured vertebrae. Vitamin B_1 deficiency has also been cited.[10] Gravid females may be presented for dystocia.[11]

Radiographs are helpful in locating all fractures (especially those involving the vertebrae) and assessing the prognosis for recovery (Figure 3). Treatment must correct prob-

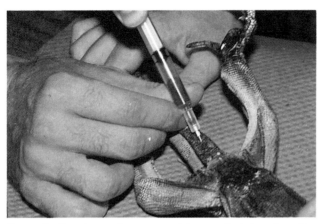

Figure 1—Blood samples are most frequently taken from the tail vein that runs immediately ventral to the spine. The needle should be inserted in a cranial direction at a 45° angle. The needle should meet the vertebral body and then be withdrawn one to two millimeters until blood is seen in the hub of the needle.

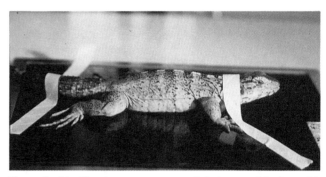

Figure 2—Masking tape can successfully be used for immobilizing depressed iguanas for radiography.

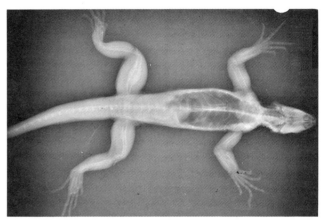

Figure 3—Typical radiograph of an iguana with secondary hyperparathyroidism. Note the lack of bone density and presence of fibrous metaplasia at fracture sites.

lems with the diet and husbandry techniques, provide parenteral calcium and vitamin D_3, and correct secondary problems. Most fractures of the extremities are relatively stable and heal rapidly as soon as problems with the diet are corrected. Unstable, vertebral, and mandibular fractures can be immobilized in the same manner as that used for cats and birds.[12,13] Oral ulcers usually improve with parenteral vitamin A, vitamin C, and topical diluted povidone-iodine. Cytology and culture are indicated if the ulcer is extensive or is healing slowly.

OVERSUPPLEMENTATION of vitamin D and/or ultraviolet light in conjunction with an adequate supply of calcium already provided in the diet causes metastatic calcification of soft tissue. Large arteries, the kidneys, and the stomach are most commonly affected. The history reveals a diet consisting of 60% to 90% protein foods and liberal use of vitamin supplements. Owners are frequently attempting to expedite growth of their pets. Clinical signs include anorexia and weakness. Diagnosis is made by the history, evaluation of radiographs, and measurement of blood calcium and phosphorus. Treatment is supportive and often unsuccessful.

Failure to adapt to captivity frequently causes an anorexia-constipation-regurgitation syndrome. The history may reveal that the iguana has had a recent change in owner, diet, or environment. The lizard may not have eaten for a period ranging from one week to several months and, as a result, may be in poor health with concurrent bacterial and nutritional disorders. Treatment should first be geared toward assessing husbandry deficits. Secondary diseases should be evaluated using appropriate diagnostic tests;

treatment must be started promptly. Reptiles that have not eaten within one week should not be force-fed solid food—the gut of the iguana must become acclimated to receiving and digesting food. Hydration can be improved and maintained with warmed lactated Ringer's solution given orally. The isotonic quality of the solution is ideal for stimulating the intestines. Vomiting of lactated Ringer's solution indicates severe disease and a grave prognosis. Later, an oral glucose-electrolyte powder may be added to lactated Ringer's solution to increase osmolality.

After the strength is increased to one part glucose-electrolyte powder to three parts lactated Ringer's solution, the formula may be changed to an avian hand-feeding formula. These formulas should initially be given at 1:6 dilutions and then increased to label strength. After the iguana can tolerate the formula at label strength, vegetable or fruit baby food can be added to the formula and the regular diet of the iguana can be left in the cage. As soon as the iguana starts feeding on its own, supplementation can gradually be discontinued. Addition of natural flora from the feces of a healthy iguana or lactobacillus products (i.e., yogurt) may also be beneficial.

For animals with an adequate environment, the anorexia-

Miniformulary for Treatment of Iguanas

Antibiotics

Amikacin sulfate	2.0 mg/kg intramuscularly every 72 hours × 5 treatments; potential nephrotoxin; adequate hydration essential[a]
Carbenicillin	100 mg/kg intramuscularly or orally once daily for two weeks or 400 mg/kg intramuscularly every other day[a]; synergistic effect with amikacin sulfate
Ceftozidine	20 mg/kg intramuscularly every 72 hours[b]
Cephalothin	40–80 mg/kg divided twice daily[b]
Chloramphenicol	20 mg/kg intramuscularly twice daily for nine days[a]
Enrofloxacin	2.5 mg/kg intramuscularly every 24 hours for three days, then every 48 hours
Metronidazole	275 mg/kg orally[a] repeated in two weeks or 40–125 mg/kg[c] orally in untried species for anaerobes and protozoa as well as for appetite stimulation
Oxytetracycline HCL	10 mg/kg orally once daily for one week[a]
Trimethoprim/sulfadiazine	15 mg/kg orally once daily for two weeks[a]
Tylosin	5 mg/kg intramuscularly once daily for 10 days[a]

Antifungals

Ketoconazole	25 mg/kg orally every other day[b]
Nystatin	100,000 IU/kg orally once daily[b]

Anthelmintics

Fenbendazole	50–100 mg/kg orally repeated in two weeks for nematodes[b]
Ivermectin	0.2 mg/kg intramuscularly or orally repeated in two weeks for nematodes and sensitive external parasites
Levamisole	10 mg/kg intraperitoneally repeated in two weeks for nematodes[a]
Praziquantel	3.5 mg/kg subcutaneously or 20 mg/kg orally repeated in two weeks for cestodes[b]

Sulfadiazine, sulfamerazine, sulfamethazine	25 mg/kg orally once daily for Coccidia[a]

Miscellaneous

Aminophylline USP	2–4 mg/kg intramuscularly as needed[d]
Arginine vasotocin	0.01–1.0 μm/kg intravenously or intraperitoneally; 0.2–0.5 ml/kg of calcium glycerophosphate/calcium lactate intramuscularly or subcutaneously before vasotocin for dystocia is recommended[e]
Atropine sulfate	0.04 mg/kg intramuscularly, intravenously, or subcutaneously as needed[d]
Calphosan® (Glenwood)	0.5–1.0 ml/kg intramuscularly weekly[b]
Dexamethasone	0.0625–0.125 mg/kg intravenously or intramuscularly only in cases of great need[d]
Neoglucagon® (Sandoz Pharmaceuticals)	1 ml/30 ml drinking water[b]
Furosemide	5 mg/kg intravenously or intramuscularly once to twice daily; watch hydration[d]
Oxytocin	1–10 IU/kg intramuscularly after calcium supplementation for dystocia[b]
Vitamin A	1000–5000 IU intramuscularly every 10 days for 4 treatments[a]
Vitamin B complex	0.5 ml/kg intramuscularly, intravenously, or subcutaneously[d]
Vitamin C	10–20 mg/kg intramuscularly once daily[d]

[a]Jacobson ER, Kollias GH, Peter LJ: Dosages for antibiotics and parasitides used in exotic animals, in *The Compendium Collection: Exotic Animal Medicine in Practice.* Lawrenceville, NJ, Veterinary Learning Systems Co, 1986, pp 317–318.
[b]Anderson NL: Unpublished data, The Ohio State University, 1990.
[c]Wack R: Personal Communication, The Columbus Zoo, Columbus, Ohio, 1991.
[d]Frye FL: *Biomedical and Surgical Aspects of Captive Reptile Husbandry.* Edwardsville, KS, Veterinary Medicine Publishing Co, 1981.
[e]Lloyd ML: Reptilian dystoclas review—Causes, prevention, management, and comments on the synthetic hormone vasotocin. *Proc Am Assoc Zoo Vet:* 290–294, 1990.

constipation-regurgitation syndrome can be a sign of parasites, infectious enteritis, hepatitis (bacterial, viral, fungal, or mycobacterial), obstruction, or metabolic derangement (e.g., gout or organ failure). A thorough diagnostic workup, including complete blood count, chemistry profile, radio-graphs, stomach gavage and cytology, and fecal examination, should be done immediately.

Hypovitaminosis A in the diet can lead to squamous metaplasia of oral epithelium and predisposition to oral, dermal, and ophthalmic infections. Hypovitaminosis C causes weakening of the skin and a predisposition to oral bacterial (i.e., *Aeromonas hydrophila*) infections, better known as infectious stomatitis or mouth rot.

Obesity may indicate hypervitaminosis D and gout. Gout is the pathologic deposition of uric acid in soft tissue and most often affects the kidneys. Gout is associated with high-protein diets; water deprivation; and the presence of renal toxins, especially gentamycin. Diagnosis of gout is made by the presence of high levels of serum uric acid, palpation of mineralized masses in the abdomen, increased radiodensity of the kidneys, and positive histopathology. Special tissue fixatives are necessary to preserve uric acid crystals. Treatment is supportive and is aimed at minimizing the effects of renal failure. Use of allopurinol and colchicine has been reported with poor success.[14] Uric acid can be deposited in any soft tissue and can, although less frequently, cause any sign.

In addition to vitamin deficiencies, the skin is susceptible to a number of disorders. Ticks and mites are extremely common in iguanas taken from the wild. Ticks should be stunned with a water-soluble pyrethrin flea spray safe for kittens and then removed with forceps 10 minutes later. The area should be cleaned thoroughly with topical povidone-iodine solution. If the area is inflamed, parenteral antibiotics for gram-negative bacteria are advised. Abscesses resulting from ticks or other causes should be surgically removed and cultured. Hydrotherapy using warm water is useful in removing caseous debris and reducing swelling. Ointments containing fibrolysin, deoxyribonuclease, and elastase (Elase®—Parke-Davis) designed to break down caseous exudate can be used to stimulate drainage.

Moist bedding also predisposes iguanas to skin abscesses and blister disease. Abscesses and blisters may appear as soft, dark, or red areas. Treatment involves improving sanitation, surgical debridement (if indicated), topical antiseptics, and parenteral antibiotics. Sebaceous inclusion cysts, which resemble abscesses, have been reported on tails of iguanas. The cysts should be removed.

MITES CAN BE CONTROLLED by cleaning and disinfecting of the cage daily during treatment. Only disposable cage liners should be used if the iguana is infested with mites. I have been successful in using the pyrethrin spray that is safe for kittens in caging and on adult lizards with no recognizable signs of toxicity. Owners are cautioned to spray only the cage at first. The cage and tail are sprayed three days later. If no signs of toxicity are noted, the entire lizard and cage are sprayed every three days for three weeks.

Dysecdysis is seen less commonly in iguanas than in other reptiles. Underlying causes, such as mites or abscesses, should be eliminated. For treatment, the iguana is placed in a tub of 29°C (85°F) water. The water should be just deep enough to touch the mandible of the iguana when it is resting. A wet towel placed over the iguana keeps the back moist and provides an abrasive surface. Soaking time ranges between 20 and 60 minutes, depending on the size and condition of the iguana. The iguana is then placed in a warmed cage with branches and rocks available. Loose pieces of dead skin may be gently teased off with forceps.[15]

If not treated promptly, injuries to distal extremities often result in dry gangrene. For a solitary animal with inactive lesions and owners who will follow through with scheduled reevaluations, the clinician can let nature take its course. For most injuries to the distal extremities that have resulted in gangrene, surgical amputation proximal to the gangrenous site is recommended. The removed tissue should be cultured aerobically and anaerobically. Ligations are best made with polydioxanone or polyglactin 910. Skin sutures may be nylon, polydioxanone, or steel.[16,17]

OPHTHALMIC DISORDERS of iguanas may be approached in a manner similar to ophthalmic disorders in small animals. In lizards, the lower lid is more mobile than the upper lid. The third eyelid reflex is brisk. The harderian gland is in a ventromedial direction to the eye, and the lacrimal glands are dorsotemporal to the eye. Dacryosialitis is fairly common.

Because the iris is composed of striated muscle, common mydriatic agents are ineffective. General anesthetic agents or intraocular curare is necessary to dilate the pupil. The vitreous fluid contains the conus papillaris, which projects from the optic nerve. Although its purpose is not known, the conus papillaris seems to be similar to the pectin in birds. Ophthalmic conditions are similar to those seen in mammals and birds. Many infections spread to the eyes from the oral cavity through the nasolacrimal ducts.[18,19]

Respiratory infections can start as oral infections. Respiratory disorders are commonly caused by bacteria, fungi, viruses, and parasites. Clinical signs include bubbling and wheezing, anorexia, lethargy, gasping, and uveitis. Diagnosis is made by physical examination, radiography, complete blood count, and tracheal swabbing or washing. Tracheal washing can be done with 0.3 to 2.0 milliliters of warmed, sterile physiologic saline solution using a sterile tomcat catheter placed through a sterile endotracheal tube. If general anesthesia is inappropriate or for small patients, small diameter swabs (Calgiswab®—Spectrum Laboratories) are useful for obtaining direct tracheal samples. Although more common in snakes, oral flukes can stimulate openmouthed breathing in iguanas. The flukes can easily be removed from the glottis area with forceps.

Digestive tract disease is very common in iguanas. Once again, most problems originate from poor husbandry. Other common causes of diarrhea in lizards can be attributed to

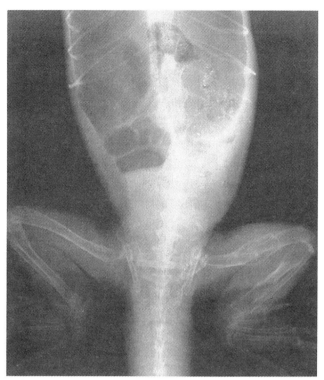

Figure 4—Dorsoventral radiograph indicating gaseous distention of the cecum and large intestinal obstruction.

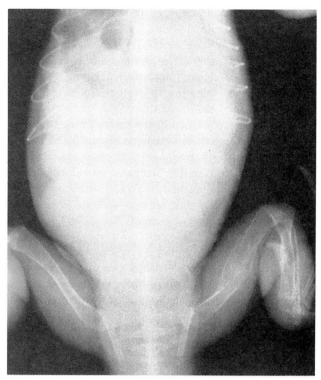

Figure 5—The abdominal densities shown in this dorsoventral radiograph are noncalcified eggs. The iguana was in dystocia as a result of being fed a calcium-deficient diet. Note the healing fractures of the right rear leg.

protozoa, such as *Entamoeba*, *Cryptosporidium*, *Trichomonas*, Coccidia, and *Giardia*. Fresh saline smears are very helpful but sometimes reveal false-negative results. Treatment with metronidazole is often curative.[8,19] Bacterial enteritis in iguanas is usually gram-negative, but *Clostridium*, *Staphylococcus*, and *Mycobacterium* must also be considered as causative factors. Fungal enteropathy evidently is more common in reptiles than in mammals, possibly because of ectothermy.[19] Gastrointestinal obstruction resulting from foreign bodies is common in young iguanas (Figure 4). Gastrotomy and enterotomy may be done in the same manner as for birds and mammals.[20] Metabolic, toxic, and neoplastic disorders of the gastrointestinal system of iguanas have also been described.[10,21,22] Diagnosis of these disorders is often made after death.

Cloacal prolapse occurring by itself is uncommon, but it is seen fairly regularly in association with cloacal inflammation, infection, or dystocia. Repair of cloacal prolapse can usually be done under light sedation. The cloaca is cleaned, lubricated, and gently repositioned using blunt instruments. A pursestring suture is not usually needed but can be placed with some difficulty in the event of recurrence. Amputation may be required if tissue is devitalized. Chronic recurrence requires an abdominal approach and cloacopexy.[17,23–25] Male iguanas may have prolapsed hemipenes, which may be treated similarly to prolapsed cloacas. Replacing a prolapsed hemipene may also be facili-

tated by the use of an ointment containing 3% shark oil, live yeast cell derivative, and phenolmercuric nitrate (Preparation H®—Whitehall Laboratories), which will reduce edema.

DYSTOCIA is a common reproductive disorder in iguanas and is frequently linked to a poor diet. Initial assessment involves determining whether dystocia is actually present. Many female iguanas hold partially mature eggs for several weeks. Indications for intervention include a partial lay, nesting behavior but no eggs produced, anorexia, prolonged laying intervals compared with previous clutches, and calcified eggs in the oviducts (Figure 5). Initial treatment involves administration of parenteral calcium and oxytocin or vasotocin. If oviposition is noted with the first treatment, large clutches may require the hormone to be repeated one time per week until all eggs are laid. *Gentle* manual expression may be attempted but is usually unsuccessful unless only a few eggs remain in the oviducts. Oviductectomy or cesarean section is required; 4-0 or smaller polydioxanone is recommended. A double-layer, inverting, continuous suture pattern is recommended. The thinness and friability of the oviducts very often necessitate use of a single layer of simple, continuous sutures.[17,26–28] If dystocia recurs or if infection is present, an ovario-oviductectomy may be elected. Because of the vasculature of the ovaries, the surgeon may choose to leave them in place and, if necessary, remove them during a subsequent procedure after they have atrophied. Although the ovaries may ovulate into the abdomen, my experience with many pet birds and a few reptiles suggests that this does not occur regularly.

Dystocia may be accompanied by rents in the oviducts. When this occurs, yolk leaks into the abdomen and creates severe inflammation. Egg yolk peritonitis is associated with a poor prognosis for survival. Treatment should include copious lavage and debridement of necrotic tissue. In severe cases, flushing an open abdomen with warmed, diluted heparinized saline may increase chances of survival.

CONCLUSION

In general, less is known about specific reptilian diseases than those that affect mammals. Although a herpesvirus of disputed pathogenicity and an oncovirus have been isolated from iguanas, most viral disorders are never diagnosed.[29]

About the Author
Dr. Anderson is affiliated with the Department of Veterinary Clinical Sciences, College of Veterinary Medicine, The Ohio State University, Columbus, Ohio.

REFERENCES
1. Telford S: Parasitic diseases of reptiles. *JAVMA* 159:1644–1652, 1971.
2. Dressauer HC: Blood chemistry of reptiles: Physiological and evolutionary aspects, in Gans C (ed): *Biology of the Reptilia*, vol 3. New York, Academic Press, 1970, pp. 1–54.
3. Silverman S: Advances in avian and reptilian imaging, in Kirk RW (ed): *Current Veterinary Therapy. Small Animal Practice*, ed 10. Philadelphia, WB Saunders Co, 1989, pp 786–789.
4. Jackson OF: Clinical aspects of diagnosis and treatment, in Cooper JE, Jackson OF (eds): *Diseases of the Reptilia*, vol. 2. New York, Academic Press, 1981, pp 507–534.
5. Werner RE: Isoflurane anesthesia: A guide for practitioners. *Compend Contin Educ Pract Vet* 9(6):603–606, 1987.
6. Calderwood HW: Anesthesia for reptiles. *JAVMA* 159:1618–1625, 1971.
7. Schobert E: Telazol® use in wild and exotic animals. *Vet Med* 82:1080–1088, 1987.
8. Cooper JE, Jackson OF: Anesthesia and surgery, in Cooper JE, Jackson OF (eds): *Diseases of the Reptilia*. New York, Academic Press, 1981, pp 535–549.
9. Calderwood HW: Anesthesia for reptiles. *JAVMA* 159:1618–1625, 1971.
10. Woerpel RW, Rosskopf WJ, in Pratt PW (ed): *Avian-Exotic Animal Care Guides*. Goleta, CA, American Veterinary Publications, 1988.
11. Wallach JD, Hoessle AA: Fibrous osteodystrophy in green iguanas. *JAVMA* 153:863–865, 1968.
12. Redisch RI: Repair of a fractured femur in an iguana. *VM SAC* 73:1547, 1978.
13. Hartman RA: Use of an IM pin in repair of a midshaft humeral fracture in a green iguana. *VM SAC* 71:1634, 1976.
14. Jackson OF, Cooper JE: Nutritional diseases, in Cooper JE, Jackson OF (eds): *Diseases of the Reptilia*, vol. 2. New York, Academic Press, 1981, pp 415–416.
15. Frye FL: Epidermal shedding problems in reptiles, in Kirk RW (ed): *Current Veterinary Therapy. Small Animal Practice*, ed 8. Philadelphia, WB Saunders Co, 1983, pp 596–599.
16. Bennett RA, Yaeger MJ, Trapp A, Cambre RC: Tissue reaction to sutures in rock doves (*Columbia livia*). *Proc Am Assoc Zoo Vet*:165–167, 1990.
17. Bennett RA: Surgery of reptiles. *Proc Am Assoc Zoo Vet*:168–171, 1990.
18. Millichamp NJ: Diseases of the eye and ocular adnexae in reptiles. *JAVMA* 183:1205–1212, 1983.
19. Marcus L: Infectious diseases of reptiles. *JAVMA* 159:1626–1632, 1971.
20. Hartman RA: Gastrotomy for removal of foreign bodies in a crocodile. *Vet Med* 71:1634, 1976.
21. Jacobson ER: Neoplastic diseases, in Cooper JE, Jackson ER (eds): *Diseases of the Reptilia*, vol. 2. New York, Academic Press, 1981, pp 429–468.
22. Schlumberger HG: Tumors of fishes, amphibians, and reptiles. *Cancer Res* 8:657–754, 1948.
23. Leash AM: Amputation prolapsed rectum of an African Rock Python. *JAVMA* 171:980, 1977.
24. Shalev M: Rectal prolapse in an adult chameleon. *JAVMA* 171:872–874, 1977.
25. Bodri MS, Sadanaga KK: Circumcostal cloacapexy in a python. *JAVMA* 198:297, 1991.
26. Kaufman AF: Granulomatous oophoritis in a turtle. *JAVMA* 153:860–862, 1968.
27. Frye FL: Clinical obstetric and gynecologic disorders in reptiles. *Proc AAHA*:497–499, 1974.
28. Lloyd ML: Reptilian dystocias review—Causes, prevention, management, and comments on the synthetic hormone vasotocin. *Proc Am Assoc Zoo Vet*:290–296, 1990.
29. Clark HF, Lunger PD: Viruses, in Cooper JE, Jackson OF (eds): *Diseases of the Reptilia*. New York, Academic Press, 1981, pp 135–161.

UPDATE

HEMATOLOGIC AND CHEMISTRY VALUES

Since the publication of the 1992 article, National Development and Research Laboratory in Redmond, Washington, the laboratory that provided the normal values, was prosecuted for alleged fraud. A current literature search has not provided a published reference for blood values in *Iguana iguana*. The tables for both the blood values and the chemistry values have been removed from the article and replaced with a table that provides newer data.

Blood urea nitrogen and creatinine do not have clinical applications for *Iguana iguana*. Current research has not been able to document elevations in BUN or creatinine in iguanas with dehydration. Uric acid only rises with marked reduction in kidney function. An increase in the calcium:phosphorus ratio (> 1:1) is often the first indication of renal disease in iguanas.

Available literature indicates that iguanas cannot orally absorb vitamin D, and that hypervitaminosis D may only result from iatrogenic parenteral administration of vitamin D.

RADIOLOGY

Standing lateral radiographs using a horizontal beam have more clinical value than lateral films taken with the lizard in lateral recumbency. It is essential to pull the front legs forward and the rear legs backward to ensure adequate visualization of the celomic cavity.

ANESTHESIA

Spinal needles can be used to place intraosseous catheters into the distal femur or proximal tibia of most

(continues on page 34)

Diagnosis and Treatment of Lumps and Bumps in Snakes

ABVP Diplomate-Avian Practice
Avian and Exotic Pet Service
The Animal Medical Center
New York, New York
Karen Rosenthal, DVM, MS

Diplomate, ACVIM
Elizabeth Russo, DVM

The presence of an unusual swelling is a common problem in the captive or pet snake. This article discusses an approach to the diagnosis and treatment of such lumps and bumps. A thorough history precedes the physical examination of any reptile. The history should concentrate not only on the current problem but also on where the snake was obtained, husbandry, and nutrition. Questions include whether the snake was wild-caught or domestically bred, the size and type of enclosure in which the animal is housed, the cage substrate, and the temperature range in the enclosure and the heat source. For example, is there an under-the-cage heating pad, a "hot rock," or an overhead light bulb? In addition, ask about other cage accessories, such as a water bowl, a "hide box," and branches or rocks.

Examine cleaning and sanitation. Poor husbandry is a potential factor for some types of lumps and bumps, and improvement in husbandry is an essential part of treatment. Proper ambient temperature is very important for the well-being of reptiles. Since they are poikliotherms, their physiologic processes, including their immune response, depend on an adequate ambient temperature. If this is not provided, especially for tropical species, infectious processes, such as stomatitis, pneumonia, or septicemia, are more likely to occur. Heat is best provided by an overhead source located outside and at one end of the enclosure or by an undercage heating pad. Such an arrangement provides a temperature gradient within the cage and allows the reptile to thermoregulate itself to a certain extent. Thermometers are located at each end of the cage. Knowledge of the size, type, and source of food items offered and the frequency of feeding are essential, as anorexia may be associated with some causes of swellings. Determine if there are other reptiles in the collection, their source and time of acquisition, and whether they have had close contact with the patient. Finally, questions about the snake's shedding history are pertinent.

Advise owners to bring their snake into the clinic in a cage or a pillowcase rather than wrapped around their shoulder, which can alarm clients in the waiting room or injure the snake. Before you pick up the snake, ask whether

Updated from original publication in Volume 9, Number 8, August 1987

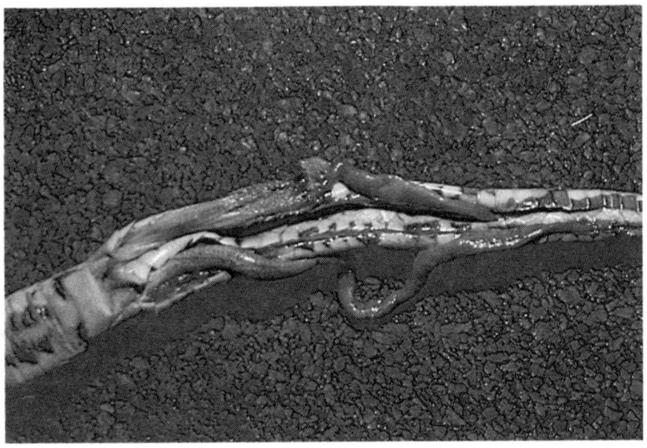

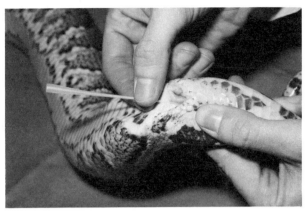

Figure 1A

Figure 1B

Figure 1—(**A**) Dissection of the ventral tail of a snake demonstrating the hemipenes. One of the hemipenes *(left)* has been incised along its length. Spines are visible within: these become external when the hemipene is everted during copulation. (**B**) A closed-end feline urinary catheter may be used to gently probe the hemipene to determine the sex of a snake.

the animal is accustomed to being handled. Even then, it is safest to initially grasp just behind the snake's head before lifting the rest of the animal. Most pet snakes are used to being handled by their owners and are no more dangerous to the veterinarian than a dog or cat. For some aggressive snakes, a clipboard is held above and behind the head so that it will not see the approaching hand and strike. While holding the snake's head, it is important to support the rest of its body rather than allowing it to hang toward the floor or writhe on the examination table. This may require the assistance of a veterinary technician, or, if the snake is very large, several people. For personal safety and for legal reasons, the owner should not assist with holding the snake.

THE PHYSICAL EXAMINATION

A physical examination on a snake is not difficult, although this procedure may seem alien to many veterinarians. Begin the complete physical examination of a snake at the head. Examine the head for symmetry and the skin around the head for abnormalities, such as discolorations, displaced scales, or scars. Discolored areas may represent burns or past ectoparasite attachments and may be associated with localized bacterial infections. Vesicles in the skin also may be associated with systemic bacterial infections. Cutaneous lesions in conjunction with an internal swelling suggest that the swelling may be an abscess causing septicemia. Scars indicate the past existence of a wound and the possible introduction of infection. Wounds or scars on the rostrum are usually the result of poor husbandry. A snake in a small cage or one that is trying to escape from its enclosure can develop a wound when it rubs its nose while "pacing" its cage or striking repeatedly at something outside its cage, hitting the glass. Such a wound is an initiating factor in rostral infections. Increasing

the enclosure space or providing a hiding spot in the cage prevents or stops such behavior. Closely examine the scales, particularly of the ventral head and neck, for the presence of mites. Snake mites can carry blood parasites or pathogenic bacteria, such as *Aeromonas hydrophila*, which causes pneumonia, infectious stomatitis ("mouth rot"), or septicemia.[1] Snake mites are also implicated as carriers of the virus that causes inclusion body disease.[2] Examine the eyes with a penlight. Protrusion of the conjunctiva can indicate the presence of snake mites around the edges of the eye.

Open the mouth and examine it for petechiae, exudates, and swellings, which can indicate infectious stomatitis. If there is bubbling mucus, pneumonia is possible. These conditions may accompany or lead to septicemia and may be associated with abscesses or granulomas elsewhere in the body. Open the mouth carefully to avoid trauma to the mucosa, which can predispose this area to infection. Insert a plastic pen cap with a tapered end into the center of the anterior aspect of the mouth between the gaps in the teeth. As the snake opens its mouth, gently turn the pen transversely to act as a gag. An alternative method is to use a rubber cooking spatula and insert it between the teeth.

Palpate the entire length of the snake for signs of weight loss (i.e., loose skin), muscle tone, and swellings. Healthy snakes have firm musculature that is difficult to indent by palpation. A flaccid snake is a sick snake. Excessive intestinal fluid and gas may be associated with enteritis or intestinal obstruction. Auscultation is not as useful in snakes as it may be in other species.

Sex determination is not performed routinely as part of the physical examination except in snakes destined for breeding. Sex determination is a diagnostic procedure, however, when gravidity is ruled out for coelomic swelling. Determine the sex by probing the hemipene

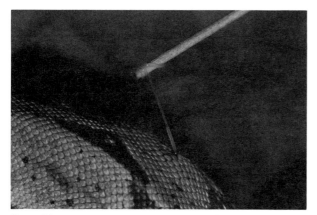

Figure 2A

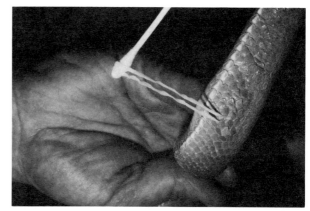

Figure 2B

Figure 2—(**A** and **B**) A sterile applicator stick may be used to remove subcutaneous parasites.

sac (Figure 1).[3] Males have two hemipenes that lie ventrolaterally distal to the cloacal opening. Normally, the hemipenes are in an inverted position and not apparent externally. During copulation, hemipenes are everted. Hemipenes are present externally if they prolapse. Although a set of metal sexing probes of varying sizes is commercially available from numerous sources, the lubricated rounded end of a red latex feeding tube or a feline urinary catheter also can be used for probing. Slightly flex the snake dorsally and direct the probe caudally from the cloacal opening. In a male, the probe enters the hemipene "pocket" and passes to a distance extending 8 to 16 subcaudal scales. In a female, the probe does not go beyond two to three subcaudal scales.

If a fresh fecal sample is not available, obtain one by performing a colonic wash. Do a direct smear to diagnose protozoan endoparasites. Perform a cloacal wash by passing a lubricated, firm rubber feeding tube (Sovereign™ Sterile Disposable Feeding Tube and Urethral Catheter—Sherwood Medical) through the cloacal opening, guiding it through the ventral cloaca into the colon. Hold the snake with its tail upward and firmly "pinch off" the ventral part of the cloaca between the fingers as the tube is passed anteriorly toward the colonic opening. When the tube enters the colon, it should continue to pass easily; if it meets resistance, it is pressing against the dead-end dorsal pouch of the cloaca. Once in the colon, flush saline through the catheter and aspirate the fluid to examine on a wet mount. Perform a cloacal wash if a colonic wash is not obtained, but this may provide less than satisfactory results.

SKIN AND SUBCUTANEOUS SWELLINGS

The differential diagnosis for subcutaneous swellings in snakes includes parasites, abscesses, granulomas, neoplasia, blister disease, and steatitis. Masquerading as subcutaneous masses are such internal swellings as recently ingested food, enlarged kidneys, or gravidity in females.

Subcutaneous Parasites

Many parasitic stages invade the subcutaneous tissues of various reptiles. Pleurocercoids of various pseudophyllidean tapeworms[4,5] may infect the subcutaneous tissues, muscles, or coelomic cavity of reptiles. The definitive host is a mammal. The pleurocercoids, known as spargana, may be as long as 30 cm and are difficult to identify without development in the definitive host.[6] Other subcutaneous parasites include larval dracunculids, acanthocephalans,[4,7] and spiruroids.[8] Such subcutaneous parasites rarely cause illness but the small, 1-cm to 5-cm diameter, soft, raised areas are noticed by the observant owner. These areas may be single or multiple swellings and can appear even after several years in captivity.[4] There is usually no break in the skin until larval release occurs.[4] The parasites are easily removed during an office visit. Prepare the skin over the swelling with a surgical scrub. Make a small nick with a scalpel blade over the swelling through the skin between scales. Use a sterile applicator stick as a probe. Remove the parasite by winding it slowly around the stick (like spaghetti on a fork) (Figure 2). Fill the remaining hole daily with antibiotic ointment for a few days.

Abscesses/Granulomas

Abscesses are common in reptiles and result from infection with numerous microorganisms, including gram-negative aerobes, anaerobes, and mycobacteria.[1,9,10] Abscesses are single or multiple firm swellings and usually are well encapsulated. The material in the abscess is inspissated and typically laminated. Fine-needle aspiration reveals leukocytes and microorganisms. Gram stains and acid-fast stains are valuable diagnostic aids. Causes of abscesses include local penetrating wounds and hematogenous spread of an infection. Multiple abscesses are suggestive of septicemia. It is best to excise abscesses with their capsules and to culture and biopsy the removed tissue. Administer systemic antibiotics for several weeks. Recommended dosages of antibiotics are reported.[11,12] Pending culture and MIC results, there are a number of antibiotics to choose from based on their broad gram negative spectrum. These include piperacillin, amikacin, and enrofloxacin. Prolonged use of amikacin should be accompanied by use of parenteral or oral fluids.

Granulomas result from invasion by bacteria, fungi, actinomycetes, foreign bodies, or algae into underlying tissue.[9,13] Like abscesses, granulomas can be an external manifestation of a more widespread systemic infection.[10] Infections by opportunistic organisms, such as saprophytic soil fungi, are often the result of decreased immunity due to suboptimal environmental conditions.[10] Diagnosis is by fine-needle aspiration or excisional biopsy with histopathology. Treat bacterial granulomas with excision and antibiotics. Fungal and algal granulomatous diseases are only cured if the infection is localized to the skin and complete surgical excision is possible.

Neoplasia

Neoplasia is less common in reptiles than it is in mammals, but tumors should be included in any differential diagnosis of cutaneous and subcutaneous lumps and bumps. The neoplastic diseases of reptiles have been thoroughly reviewed.[14,15] Both benign and malignant tumors of connective tissue (e.g., fibroma, fibrosarcoma, melanoma) and epithelial origin (e.g., carcinoma) are described.[15] In general, the biologic behavior and response to treatment (i.e., radiation and chemotherapy) of most neoplasms in snakes is not known. Fine-needle aspiration cytology of reptilian tumors is a useful diagnostic tool, but biopsy is recommended.

Blisters

Another cause of cutaneous and subcutaneous swellings is a syndrome called blister disease.[9] It is characterized by fluid-filled blisters within the skin or under the skin and is caused by poor husbandry. These blisters usually are the result of exposure to environmental filth and moisture with secondary bacterial infection. These infections can disseminate and are sometimes fatal. Similar vesicular lesions also may be the *outcome* of a septicemia. Immune-mediated or virus-associated vesicular skin diseases have not yet been documented in snakes. Culture and biopsy the vesicles, and treat the snake with systemic antibiotics. The snake should be removed to a clean, dry environment for improved husbandry conditions.

Steatitis

Steatitis is rare in snakes but can cause either diffuse or localized subcutaneous swellings.[9] The pathogenesis is due to prolonged ingestion of unsaturated fatty acids. Peroxidation of these fatty acids results in the production of ceroid and a subsequent granulomatous inflammatory reaction. Steatitis is reported in snakes fed obese laboratory rats or certain fish.[16] In affected animals, fat appears yellow to brown and nodular or indurated. Use vitamin E as a preventive because of its antioxidant properties. The vitamin E dose recommended is 1 IU/kg BW.[17]

SWELLINGS OF THE HEAD

Several conditions cause swellings of the head and are unique to this area of the body. They are discussed below.

Infectious Stomatitis

Infectious stomatitis or "mouth rot" causes swelling of the gums and lips and gaping of the mouth. Other clinical findings include oral mucus and gingival petechiation, as well as ulceration, accumulation of caseous or necrotic debris, bleeding, and, eventually, osteomyelitis in severe cases. The causative organisms are usually gram-negative bacteria, but fungi are occasionally found. The microorganisms usually are secondary, opportunistic invaders.[10] In almost all cases of infectious stomatitis, improper husbandry is to blame. Inciting factors include inadequate environmental temperature, unclean enclosure, or any poor condition that leads to rostral rubbing. Diagnostics include cytology, culture (aerobic, anaerobic, and fungal) and sensitivity, and radiography if bony disease is suspected. Treat with gentle debridement, which is best performed under general anesthesia to avoid further trauma to the mouth, flushing with antiseptic solutions, and parenteral antibiotics as indicated by culture and MIC results.

Pharyngeal Edema/Cellulitis

Pharyngeal edema/cellulitis may be associated with infectious stomatitis (Figure 3) or occur as an isolated finding.[18] It may appear as a subcutaneous accumulation of fluid similar to that which occurs in blister disease.[18] The exact pathogenesis is unknown, but pharyngeal swelling is often associated with gram-negative bacterial infections, both local and systemic. Treat these snakes with antibiotics as indicated by culture and by sensitivity of the fluid aspirated from the swellings.

Pseudobuphthalmos[5]

Swelling around the eye also has been associated with infectious stomatitis. Another cause is a blocked lacrimal duct, usually due to an abscess or infectious stomatitis. This is characterized by an accumulation of fluid and pus in the corneospectacular space. Aspirate the

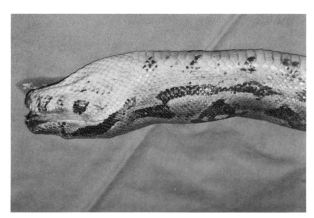

Figure 3—Pharyngeal edema accompanying severe infectious stomatitis in a boa constrictor.

fluid for culture and to relieve the swelling, and treat the cause of the blocked lacrimal duct. It may be necessary to incise the spectacle if the lacrimal duct cannot be unblocked.

LUMPS IN THE COELOMIC CAVITY

Causes of lumps and bumps in the coelomic cavity include abscesses, granulomas, reproductive disease, and tumors. Plain radiographs often are not diagnostic because they may reveal only a nonspecific, soft tissue density in the area of the swelling. A knowledge of the anatomic location of various organs, however, will narrow the diagnostic possibilities. Simplistically, consider the snake as having four anatomical areas along its length from the head to the cloacal opening (Figure 4).

First Quarter

The major structures in this area include the esophagus and trachea, although the lungs also extend anterior to the heart in some viperids and elapids. The heart lies approximately one quarter to one third of the way down the body. Swellings anterior to the heart might involve the esophagus, trachea, or coelomic space and include abscesses, granulomas, and tumors or even a meal still in the esophagus. Cardiomyopathy may cause an enlarged heart.[19,20] Enlargement also may be caused by accumulation of fluid or pus in the pericardial sac.[9]

Second Quarter

The second quarter of the body contains the continuation of the esophagus, the liver, and the lung(s). Most snakes, with the exception of the boids (and amphisbaenians), have only a right lung; the left lung is vestigial. The air sac continues posteriorly from the lung for a variable distance. The stomach is located at about the midbody. Recently ingested food items may create a visible or palpable swelling in this area. Swellings in the second quarter of the body also include abscesses and granulomas of the liver or coelomic cavity and tumors of the liver, esophagus, or stomach.

A hypertrophic gastritis resulting from *Cryptosporidium* infection is reported.[21] This infection can cause a firm, midbody swelling along with postprandial regurgitation. A gastric wash may show coccidial oocysts, but biopsy is a more definitive way to diagnose this disease. Infection with *Monocercomonas*, a flagellate, also has been associated with gastritis and midbody swelling.[22] Confirm the diagnosis by finding typical flagellates on direct fecal examination.

Third Quarter

The cranial part of the third quarter contains the gall bladder, pancreas, and spleen. The small intestine runs the length of the third quarter. The gonads, adrenal glands, and proximal part of the oviducts in females are present in this quarter. The pancreas and spleen are commonly involved with abscesses or granulomatous processes. Abscesses and granulomas may be located in the coelomic cavity. Palpable enlargement of the gall-

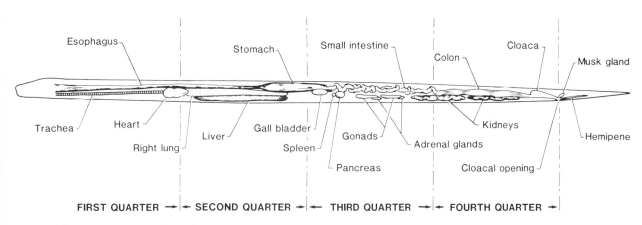

Figure 4—Schematic anatomy of a snake.

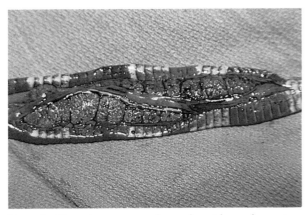

Figure 5—Granulomatous nephropathy with renal gout in a gray-banded kingsnake. The enlarged kidneys caused a swelling in the fourth quarter of the body.

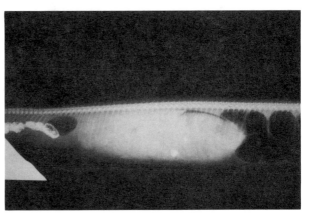

Figure 6—Lateral radiograph of an obstipated Burmese python. There is gaseous distention of the small intestine, and a barium enema did not pass anterior to the obstruction. A mass of hair and feces was removed by colotomy.

bladder caused by *Monocercomonas* infection is reported.[23] Cholecystectomy followed by metronidazole was curative in that case.

Fourth Quarter

The last quarter of the body contains the termination of the small intestine, the colon and cloaca, the distal oviducts in females, and the kidneys. Swellings in the fourth quadrant can be caused by granulomatous nephritis and renal gout (Figure 5). In addition to inflammatory renal disease, renal neoplasia also may produce visible or palpable swellings in this area. Unilateral nephrectomy has been performed successfully in cases of renal gout, in which at least half of the contralateral kidney was normal.[24]

Either the small intestine or the colon may be obstructed by ingested material, such as hair or feathers (Figure 6), and this may give the appearance of a subcutaneous mass. Apparent discomfort resulting from obstruction in either area may be manifested by the snake arching a segment of its body; such a clinical sign may be an indication that surgical treatment is necessary. Anorexia and/or the lack of feces also indicates obstruction. Perform an enterotomy or colotomy to remove the obstruction. Snakes with mild constipation should be induced (Figure 7) to defecate by soaking them in shallow water or by administration of warm water or mineral oil enemas.

Eggs or fetal snakes cause a swelling in the third and fourth quarters of female snakes. Eggs of oviparous species, for example, elapids and pythons, are poorly calcified but still appear radiopaque. Eggs of viviparous species, such as boas and viperids, do not contain calcium in the shell membrane; radiography may not confirm gravidity in these species until the skeletons of the young are mineralized. Egg retention may occur but is difficult to assess based on the duration of gestation

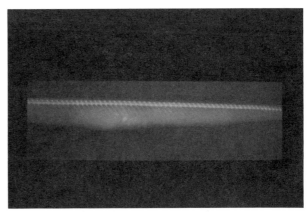

Figure 7—Lateral radiograph of an Arizona mountain kingsnake that had a caudal coelomic swelling but no other clinical signs. The radiographic appearance of the swelling was diagnostic of feces. In this case, the fecal mass was passed after soaking the snake in shallow water for a few hours.

alone, due to inadequate owner observation, multiple breeding times, sperm retention, and delayed fertilization in some species.[25,26] Suspect retained eggs when a snake lays eggs and abdominal swelling is still present.[25] "Dud eggs," "duds," or "slugs," as they are called, are unfertilized yolks in viviparous snakes.[27] Retained eggs and duds may be associated with anorexia, regurgitation, and septicemia. Ultrasound may identify ova and duds within the oviduct. Oxytocin, arginine vasotocin, manipulation, and celiotomy-salpingotomy are possible modes of therapy.[26] The success of the various methods depends on the number of ova, the physical condition of the snake, and the cause of the retention.

Cloacitis is reported to cause swelling in the area just proximal to the cloacal opening sometimes without abnormality of the opening itself. It may be caused by

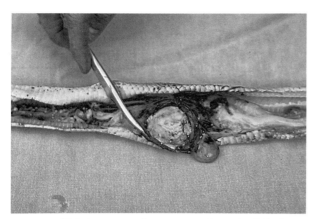

Figure 8—This boa constrictor was euthanatized during a celiotomy to identify its midbody swelling. A large abscess was present in the coelomic cavity, but multiple small granulomas were also visible in the liver adjacent to it. At necropsy, the granulomas were found to involve many organs.

gram-negative or gram-positive bacteria.[8,28] Reported neoplasms of the cloaca include transitional cell carcinoma, squamous cell carcinoma, and hemangioma.[14]

DIAGNOSIS OF INTRACOELOMIC MASSES

The diagnostic approach for intracoelomic masses is based on the knowledge of the organs present and the conditions that may affect those organs. It is important to remember that abscesses, granulomas, and tumors can occur anywhere in the coelomic cavity, both within organs and external to them. Steatitis may occur wherever there are coelomic fat bodies. Plain radiographs may not be diagnostic and further imaging techniques may be required for a diagnosis. A contrast study of the gastrointestinal tract will reveal whether the mass involves the stomach, small intestine, or colon. Contrast studies of the oviducts will reveal retained eggs or duds. An elevated serum uric acid level supports a diagnosis of nephropathy in the case of a caudal intracoelomic swelling.

An exploratory celiotomy (Figure 8) may be the only means or the most cost-effective means to make a diagnosis and simultaneously offer a mode of treatment for coelomic masses. It is important to remember, however, that although an abscess or granuloma causes a lump in one area, its removal may not "cure" the animal if it has disseminated disease. Similarly, retained eggs, intestinal obstruction, and other conditions may be accompanied by septicemia.

Lumps Caudal to the Cloacal Opening

Swellings in the tail may reflect iatrogenic damage to the hemipenes during attempted sex determination. The scent, musk, or cloacal glands also lie in this area and can produce a swelling if impacted. (The ducts of these sacs open at the cloaca, medial to the opening of the inverted hemipene in the male; the sacs lie dorsal to the hemipene.) Abscesses, granulomas, and neoplasia also can occur in this area.

REFERENCES

1. Cooper JE: Bacteria, in Cooper JE, Jackson OF (eds): *Diseases of the Reptila*. London, Academic Press, 1981, pp 165–191.
2. Schumacher J, Jacobson ER, Homer BL, Gaskin JM: Inclusion body disease in boid snakes. *JZWM* 25(4):511–524.
3. Laszlo J: Probing as a practical method of sex recognition in snakes. *Int Zoo Yrbk* 15:178–179, 1975.
4. Frank W: Endoparasites, in Cooper JE, Jackson OF (eds): *Diseases of the Reptila*. London, Academic Press, 1981, pp 291–358.
5. Marcus LC: *Veterinary Biology and Medicine of Captive Amphibians and Reptiles*. Philadelphia, Lea & Febiger, 1981.
6. Rossi JV: Dermatology, in Mader DR (ed): *Reptile Medicine and Surgery*. Philadelphia, WB Saunders Co, 1985, pp 104–117.
7. Lane TJ, Mader DR: Parasitology, in Mader DR (ed): *Reptile Medicine and Surgery*. Philadelphia, WB Saunders Co, 1985, pp 185–203.
8. Lichtenfels JR, Lavies B: Mortality in red-sided garter snakes, *Thamnophis sirtalis parietalis*, due to larval nematode, *Eustrongylides* sp. *Lab Anim Sci* 26:465–467, 1976.
9. Frye FL: *Biomedical and Surgical Aspects of Captive Reptile Husbandry*. Edwardsville, KS, Veterinary Medicine Publishing Co, 1981.
10. Rosenthal KR, Mader DR: Microbiology, in Mader DR (ed): *Reptile Medicine and Surgery*. Philadelphia, WB Saunders Co, 1985, pp 117–125.
11. Jacobson ER, Kollias GV, Peters IJ: Dosages for antibiotics and parasiticides used in exotic animals. *Compend Contin Educ Pract Vet* 5(4):315–318, 1983.
12. Klingenberg RJ: Therapeutics, in Mader DR (ed): *Reptile Medicine and Surgery*. Philadelphia, WB Saunders Co, 1985, pp 299–321.
13. Austwick PKC, Keymer IF: Fungi and actinomycetes, in Cooper JE, Jackson OF (eds): *Diseases of the Reptila*. London, Academic Press, 1981, pp 193–231.
14. Jacobson ER: Neoplastic diseases, in Cooper JE, Jackson OF (eds): *Diseases of the Reptila*. London, Academic Press, 1981, pp 429–468.
15. Done LB: Neoplasia, in Mader DR (ed): *Reptile Medicine and Surgery*. Philadelphia, WB Saunders Co, 1985, pp 125–141.
16. Langham RF, Zydeck FA, Bennett RR: Steatitis in a captive Marcy garter snake. *JAVMA* 159:640–641, 1971.
17. Donoghue S, Langenberg J: Nutrition, in Mader DR (ed): *Reptile Medicine and Surgery*. Philadelphia, WB Saunders Co, 1985, pp 148–175.
18. Kiel JL: A synopsis of some bacterial diseases in snakes. *Southwest Vet* 27:33–36,1974.
19. Barten SL: Cardiomyopathy in a kingsnake (*Lampropeltis calligaster rhombomaculata*). *VM SAC* 75:125–129,1980.
20. Jacobson ER, Seely JC, Novilla MN, Davidson JP: Heart failure associated with unusual hepatic inclusions in a Deckert's rat snake. *J Wildlife Dis* 15:75–81,1979.
21. Brownstein DC, Strandberg JD, Montali RJ, et al: *Cryptosporidium* in snakes with hypertrophic gastritis. *Vet Pathol* 14:606–617,1977.

22. Zwart P, Teunis SFM, Cornelissen JMM: Monocercomoniasis in reptiles. *J Zoo Anim Med* 15:129–134,1984.
23. Page CD, Jacobson ER: Cholecystectomy in a diamond python (*Morelia spilotes spilotes*). *Proc Annu Meet Am Assoc Zoo Vet* 15–16, 1981.
24. Raphael BL: Diagnosis and management of renal gout in captive snakes. *Proc Annu Meet Am Assoc Zoo Vet*. 53,1984.
25. Millichamp NJ, Lawrence K, Jacobson ER, et al: Egg retention in snakes. *JAVMA* 183:1213–1218, 1983.
26. DeNardo D: Reproductive biology, in Mader DR (ed): *Reptile Medicine and Surgery*. Philadelphia, WB Saunders Co, 1985, pp 212–224.
27. Jacobson ER, Spencer CP: Colono-uterine fistula in a rhinoceros viper. *JAVMA* 183:1309–1310,1983.
28. Cooper JE: A fatal case of cloacitis in a gray-beaked snake (*Scapphiophis albopunctalus albopunctalus*). *J Herpetol* 7:316–317, 1973.

Diseases of *Iguana iguana* (continued from page 26)

iguanas. These catheters provide the equivalent of intravenous access in an animal otherwise requiring a cut-down procedure.

DISEASES

The administration of calcitonin to NORMOCALCEMIC iguanas (application to iguanas not normocalcemic may prove fatal) with metabolic bone disease may speed recovery.

THERAPEUTICS

Neocalglucon	0.1–0.25 ml/100 g orally every 12 to 24 hours for hypocalcemia 0.1 ml/100 g orally one to four times per week.
Calcitonin	50 IU/kg intramuscularly in front legs twice at a seven-day interval. Serum/plasma calcium levels MUST be within the normal range.
Ivermectin	treatment for mites: 0.2–0.3 mg/kg intramuscularly or orally every two weeks for three to four treatments. The environment must be cleaned.

ADDITIONAL REFERENCES

Barten SL: Lizards, in Mader DR (ed): *Reptile Medicine and Surgery*. Philadelphia, WB Saunders, 1996, pp 324–331.
Boyer TH: Metabolic bone disease, in Mader DR (ed): *Reptile Medicine and Surgery*. Philadelphia, WB Saunders, 1996, pp 385–392.

Reptilian Surgery Part I. Basic Principles

KEY FACTS

- A basic knowledge of the variation in reptilian anatomy among orders, families, and species is essential for surgery.
- Reptilian skin wounds heal in phases similar to those in mammals.
- It is essential that aseptic technique be used; cutaneous infections can result in septicemia and can lead to visceral granuloma formation.
- Anesthetic recovery can be monitored by righting reflex, response to noxious stimuli, tongue withdrawal, and opening of the glottis to breathe.

University of Florida
R. Avery Bennett, DVM, MS

REPTILES are susceptible to a variety of conditions that require surgical management. Combining basic surgical principles with a grasp of the unique aspects of reptilian anatomy and physiology allows veterinarians to manage reptilian surgical patients successfully. Part I of this two-part presentation addresses the basic anatomy of and surgical principles applicable to reptiles. The second part will discuss the management of key surgical diseases.

ANATOMY

The anatomy of reptiles varies among orders, families, and even species.[1-3] A knowledge of the basic features of reptilian anatomy is therefore vital to surgeons.

Cardiovascular System

Chelonians (turtles and tortoises) and squamate reptiles (lizards and snakes) are considered to have a three-chambered heart because the ventricular septum is incomplete. Reptiles have two aortic arches that spiral on each other and are called right and left based on the position each occupies in the coelomic cavity before they join to become the abdominal aorta. This position is opposite to the site of origin. The left aortic arch receives part of its blood from the oxygen-poor right ventricle; the right aortic arch mainly receives oxygenated blood from the left ventricle.

Crocodilians are considered to have a four-chambered heart, although the foramen of Panizza is present within the septum and allows some mixing of ventricular blood. The right aortic arch receives blood from the left ventricle; the left aortic arch receives blood from the right ventricle. Some oxygenated blood from the left ventricle passes through the foramen of Panizza and exits through the left aortic arch.

Reptiles have a renal portal system that receives venous blood from the pelvis, the rear legs, and the caudal part of the abdomen. The system carries blood to the renal arterial circulation.

Lymphatic System

Most reptiles do not have lymph nodes but do have lymphatic vessels. Lymph is propelled into the venous system by so-called lymph hearts, which are muscular dilations in the major lymphatic channels. Lymph follicles are present within the spleen and the gastrointestinal tract, and some reptiles (e.g., alligators) have tonsils. The spleen can be closely associated with the pancreas or separate from it. Thymic tissue is present in most reptiles, but its location and form vary.

Respiratory System

The lungs of reptiles are simple sacs with internal ridges for increased surface area. Crocodilian lungs are more complex and have chambers supplied by parabronchi. Some lizards have air sacs similar to those of birds. In most snakes, the left lung is small or absent. In boids (boas and pythons), both lungs are present but the left lung is smaller.

Reptiles lack a diaphragm; the combined thoracic and abdominal cavity is called the pleuroperitoneal, or coelomic, cavity. Most turtles have a membranous structure that partially separates the thorax and the abdomen.

The glottis of most reptiles is located in the rostral portion of the mouth just caudal to the base of the tongue (Figure 1). This rostral location makes intubation and tube feeding easy. Chelonians can retract the head into the shell, which makes tube feeding difficult. In some species of chelonians and in crocodilians, the glottis is located more caudally.

Digestive System

The reptilian digestive organs and divisions of the gastrointestinal tract are similar to those of mammals. Except for most snakes, reptiles have a cecum. The stomach of crocodilians has two compartments. The first compartment is very muscular, like that of the avian gizzard, and frequently contains stones to aid in grinding ingesta. The second compartment is similar to the glandular stomach of mammals.[2]

All reptiles have a gallbladder. The liver of many reptiles contains melanin and can have black spots or streaks. Reptiles generally have scant subcutaneous fat and store fat in discrete masses (called fat bodies) in the caudal abdominal cavity.

Urinary System

The metanephric kidneys of reptiles are lobulated. Crocodilians have two lobules; each empties into a separate branch of the ureter. One or more renal arteries can be present to receive blood from the renal portal system.

The nitrogenous wastes of reptiles are in the form of ammonia, urea, uric acid, or a combination of these depending on the natural environment. Crocodilians, snakes, and some lizards do not have a urinary bladder. In chelonians and lizards that do have a bladder, it is connected to the cloaca by a short urethra.[4] Urine passes into the cloaca and from there refluxes into the urinary bladder, if present, or into the distal colon where water resorption occurs.

Cloaca

The cloaca typically consists of three chambers. The coprodaeum is positioned most cranially and receives fecal material from the colon and urinary wastes from the urinary bladder. The urodeum is the middle section and receives genital secretions and urinary wastes from the urogenital ducts. The caudal proctodeum acts as a reservoir for fecal and urinary wastes before they are excreted; this is also the location of the openings of the scent (musk) glands.

Integument

The skin of reptiles is dry and virtually devoid of glands. Many lizards have femoral glands, which open on the me-

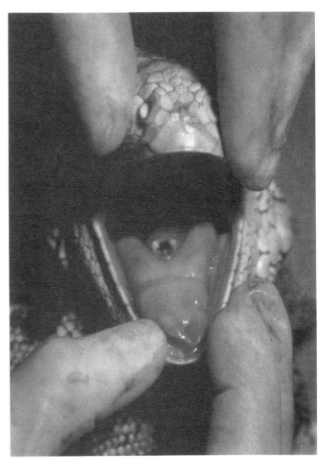

Figure 1—The glottis of this green iguana (*Iguana iguana*) can easily be visualized at the base of the tongue. (Courtesy of Peter D. Schwarz, DVM, Colorado State University)

dial aspects of the thighs. The openings, called femoral pores, appear radiographically as a line of radiodense dots along the femur (Figure 2). The holocrine secretion from these glands is believed to be involved in chemosensory recognition between individuals. Crocodilians have a pair of scent glands in the medial aspect of the lower jaw and another pair within the cloaca. In proposing sites for surgical incisions, these glandular areas should be avoided.

The skin of most reptiles is made up of scales and scutes. Scutes are the large scales that are usually along the ventral surface of the animal. Scales are arranged in distinct patterns that are species specific and useful for identification. Soft-shelled turtles and some lizards do not have scales and scutes but instead have leathery, smooth skin. Crocodilians and some lizards have calcific plates, called osteoderms, located within the dermis and designed for protection. Incisions can usually be made between osteoderms.

The shells of chelonians are composed of bony dermal plates covered with keratinized epidermal shields (Figure 3). In most chelonians, there are 54 epidermal shields: 38 on the carapace (the top of the shell) and 16 on the plastron (the bottom of the shell). The carapace contains 10 fused thoracic, lumbar, and sacral vertebrae as well as the ribs. The plastron and the carapace are joined at the so-called

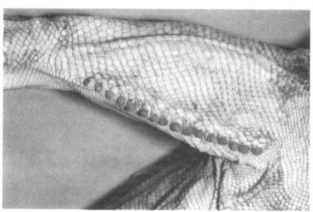

Figure 2A

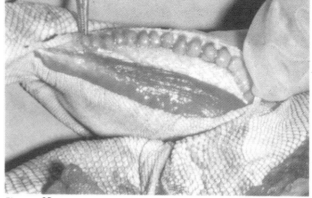

Figure 2B

Figure 2—(A) The femoral pores and (B) the femoral glands are located along the medial aspect of the thigh on this 13-year-old male green iguana. The glands are usually larger in males.

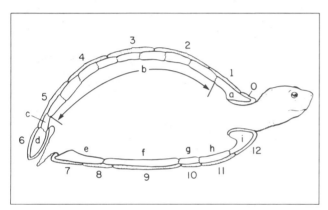

Figure 3—In chelonians, epidermal shields cover the bony dermal plates of the carapace and the plastron. Celiotomy is usually performed through the femoral and abdominal shields. Bony dermal plates: (*a*) nuchal, (*b*) neurals, (*c*) suprapygal, (*d*) pygal, (*e*) xiphiplastron, (*f*) hypoplastron, (*g*) hyoplastron, (*h*) entoplastron, and (*i*) epiplastron. Epidermal shields: (*O*) precentral, (*1* through *5*) centrals, (*6*) postcentral, (*7*) anal, (*8*) femoral, (*9*) abdominal, (*10*) pectoral, (*11*) humeral, and (*12*) gular.

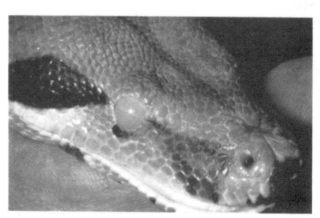

Figure 4—The spectacle of this common boa (*Constrictor constrictor*) is opaque, which indicates that the skin will be shed soon.

bridge. The shell normally accounts for approximately 30% of the total body weight.

Histologically, the epidermis of reptiles has three layers. The outer layer (stratum corneum) is heavily keratinized, is acellular, and has a serrated external surface. The inner layer (stratum germinativum) is a single layer of cuboidal cells that produces the cells of the other layers. The middle layer (intermediate zone) is composed of daughter cells of the stratum germinativum in various stages of differentiation. These three layers are present during the skin's resting phase after shedding (ecdysis). As ecdysis begins (the renewal phase), the cells of the stratum germinativum undergo synchronous mitosis to form a new intermediate zone and stratum corneum under the old generation.[2,5] The action of enzymes breaks down the cells of the base of the old intermediate zone, and the subsequent influx of lymph causes separation between the old intermediate zone and

the new stratum corneum.[2] Blood vessels and sinuses in the head become engorged and cause it to swell, and the old skin splits.[6] Ecdysis is completed by the animal rubbing off the old skin.

In squamate reptiles, this process occurs simultaneously over the entire body. In chelonians and crocodilians, proliferation and keratinization are continuous (similar to mammalian skin) and shedding occurs only at the flexible regions of the body (the neck and the joints of the limbs) while keratin is retained over the large scales. This produces growth rings between these scales as they grow and the previous, smaller layers are not lost.

DURING ECDYSIS, reptiles often become intractable and anorectic. Their skin becomes cloudy or opaque but clears again before shedding (Figure 4). Handling during this period can result in permanent damage to the epidermis. The frequency of ecdysis is proportional to the growth and metabolic rates of the animal. Age, environmental temperature, availability of food, and space can in-

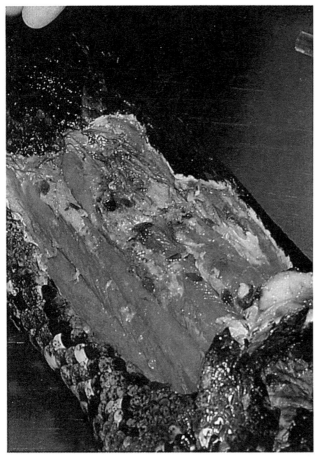

Figure 5A

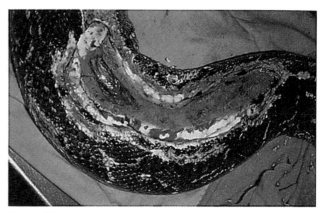

Figure 5B

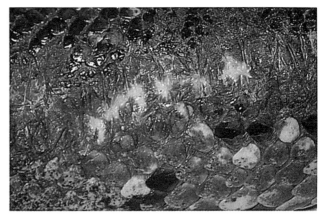

Figure 5C

Figure 5—(A) This female Burmese python (*Pythona molurus bivittatus*) received a severe burn along the dorsum from a heating lamp. (**B**) The wounds were treated by debridement, irrigation, and application of topical dressings. The wounds were allowed to heal by second intention. The epithelium that covered these areas did not contain scales and cracked when the snake ate a large prey item. (**C**) The cracks healed quickly, and the snake remained in good condition.

fluence the frequency of ecdysis.[5] In squamate reptiles, the epidermis is active only during ecdysis; this activity apparently promotes healing.[6]

The dermis of reptilian skin is made up of connective tissue, blood vessels, lymphatics, smooth muscle, and nerves. The bony dermal plates that compose the shell of chelonians and the osteoderms and chromatophores in squamate reptiles and crocodilians are located within the dermis. Chromatophores are responsible for color and the ability to change color.

WOUND HEALING

Skin wounds of reptiles undergo phases of healing similar to those observed in mammals. The healing of cutaneous defects in snakes has been studied.[6] A scab of exuded fibrin and proteinaceous fluid forms over the defect. A thin layer of epithelial cells migrates under the scab, and epithelial proliferation occurs in order to restore epithelial thickness. Below the scab, heterophils and macrophages move in to clean up tissue debris and bacteria. Fibroblasts migrate into the area and begin producing a transversely oriented fibrous scar. Fibroplasia occurs slowly, and het-

erophils remain until the scar tissue matures. Consequently, wounds strengthen slowly and skin sutures are generally not removed until at least three to four weeks after placement.[2,6]

Because the mitotic activity that occurs during ecdysis apparently promotes healing, suture removal should be delayed until after the subsequent ecdysis. Induction of ecdysis with hormone therapy might prove useful for promoting skin wound healing in squamate reptiles.[6] Thyroidectomy prevents ecdysis in lizards but increases its frequency in snakes.[1,5]

MANY FACTORS influence wound healing in reptiles.[6] Maintenance of environmental temperature at the high end of the optimum range (30° to 36°C; 85° to 95°F) can promote healing. In snakes, cranial-to-caudal–oriented wounds heal faster than dorsal-to-ventral wounds. Open wounds heal well by second intention at optimum temperatures with a low incidence of secondary bacterial infections[6] (Figure 5). Good environmental hygiene is important in preventing contamination with enteric organisms.

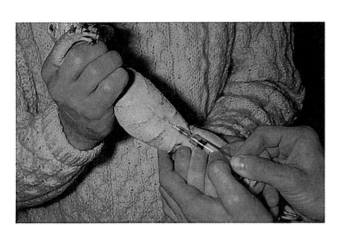

Figure 6—The ventral abdominal vein lies along the ventral midline just inside the body wall and can be used for venipuncture.

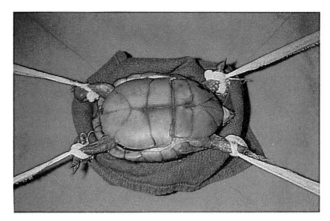

Figure 7—A towel is used to prevent the dome of the carapace of a three-toed box turtle (*Terrapene carolina triunguis*) from rolling during surgery.

PREPARATION OF PATIENTS FOR SURGERY

Ideally, laboratory data should be obtained before induction of anesthesia. Because of the small size of many patients and the inaccessibility of most peripheral veins, however, blood samples are often difficult to obtain. Normal ranges for laboratory parameters for many reptilian species are unknown. Environmental conditions, time of day, and laboratory variations can influence blood cell counts and biochemistry data and can make interpretation difficult even when normal ranges are reported.[7] If blood samples can be obtained repeatedly, trends might provide valuable information.

The hydration and nutritional status of patients is assessed as it would be for mammalian patients. Dehydrated, malnourished patients are thin and have an abundance of loose skin; skin turgor decreases with dehydration. Balanced electrolyte solutions can be given intravenously by bolus, subcutaneously, or intracoelomically to improve the preoperative hydration status.[8] Fluids that contain dextrose can be beneficial in nutritionally compromised patients. The ventral abdominal vein is a large vein situated along the ventral midline just inside the body wall[3]; the vein is accessible for venipuncture in some reptiles, especially lizards (Figure 6). Other sites for venipuncture have been described.[7]

Reptiles are susceptible to various microbial infections; it is imperative that aseptic technique be used. Many cutaneous infections result in septicemia and lead to visceral granuloma formation.[2,9,10] A warm postoperative environment should be provided to speed healing, but such an environment also can potentiate bacterial growth. There are numerous reports of the use of postoperative antibiotic therapy in reptiles.[11-18] Perioperative antibiotic therapy is more appropriate if intraoperative contamination with bacteria is anticipated. At the Colorado State University Veterinary Teaching Hospital, most bacteria isolated from reptiles are gram-negative and susceptible to aminoglycoside antibiotics.

Pharmacokinetic studies conducted with amikacin sulfate in gopher snakes (*Pituophils melanoleucus catenifer*) and with gentamicin in gopher snakes and red-eared slider turtles (*Pseudemys scripta elegans*) indicate that the plasma half-life of these antibiotic agents is quite long.[19-21] Based on these results, it has been suggested that amikacin sulfate be used in snakes at a loading dose of 5 mg/kg followed by 2.5 mg/kg every 72 hours. Gentamicin at 2.5 mg/kg every 72 hours maintains adequate therapeutic plasma concentrations. In red-eared sliders, a dose of 6 mg/kg maintains therapeutic plasma concentrations for two to five days.

In view of the long plasma half-life of these aminoglycoside antibiotics, one dose before surgery should be sufficient to inhibit the development of infection or septicemia by susceptible organisms. The antibiotics should be given in the cranial half of the reptilian body because drugs injected into the caudal half are rapidly presented to the kidneys via the renal portal system. This presentation can result in more rapid excretion of the drug and potentially in more renal damage.

PATIENT POSITIONING is a challenge, especially for small and legless reptiles. If the patient has legs, they can be tied or taped to the operating table. For snakes, a sterile stockinette can be rolled over the surgically prepared patient. The snake with its sterile covering can then be placed on a sterile drape that provides an aseptic field for surgery. The dome shape of the carapace of chelonians makes it difficult to position a patient in dorsal recumbency. A towel can be rolled into a ring and placed on the operating table; the carapace will fit into the ring to prevent the patient from rolling (Figure 7). Tires and inner tubes can be used in a similar manner for large chelonians.[22]

Because reptilian patients can function at low body temperatures, no supplemental heat is recommended during surgery. The lowered metabolic rate can even reduce the amount of anesthetic required for maintenance. When surgery is completed, raising the environmental temperature to 30° to 36°C (85° to 95°F) increases the metabolism of anesthetics and can decrease recovery time.[1,7]

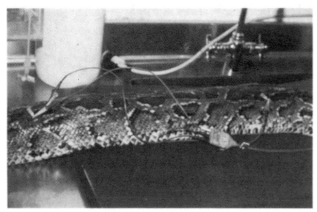

Figure 8—A two-lead electrocardiograph can be used in snakes by connecting one lead cranial and the other caudal to the heart.

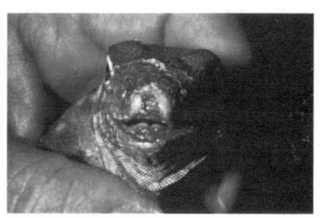

Figure 9A

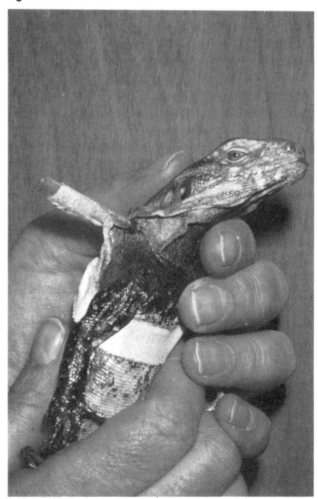

Figure 9B

Figure 9—(**A**) This spiny-tailed iguana (*Ctenosaurus pectinata*) became anorectic after severely traumatizing its face on the front of a cage. (**B**) A feeding pharyngostomy tube was placed to provide alimentation until healing occurred and the lizard began eating on its own.

Alcohol and povidone-iodine scrub solutions are used for reptilian skin preparation.[7,11,12,15,18,22-29] Chlorhexidine has also been used.[14] The shell of chelonians must be clean and dry in order for patching materials to adhere. Acetone and ether have been recommended as cleansers.[7] Trichlorotrifluoroethane (Freon® Skin Degreaser—Miller-Stephenson Chemical) is used as a skin cleanser and degreaser in human surgery and can be used for shell preparation in chelonians.

Clear plastic adhesive drapes (Barrier™ Incise Drape—Surgikos) are very useful for reptiles. The entire patient remains visible under the sterile drape; this allows proper anesthetic monitoring. Sterile spray adhesives (Vi-Drape® Adhesive—Deseret Medical) can also be used to allow paper or cloth drapes to stick to the patient and thus avoid the use of towel clamps. This is especially helpful with chelonians. Some reptiles are small and have delicate skin that can be damaged or torn when adhesive drapes are removed.

INSTRUMENTATION

With a few exceptions, the instruments needed for surgery on reptiles are found in a general surgical pack. Most abscesses in reptiles contain caseous, inspissated pus, which might indicate that the heterophils lack many of the lysosomal enzymes necessary to liquefy cellular debris. Dental curettes or cerumen loops help in removing this material from abscesses. Eyelid retractors work well as abdominal retractors for small reptilian patients. With most chelonians, some type of saw or drill is needed to approach the coelomic cavity. An orthopedic burr is ideal because it can be autoclaved. A woodworking rotary tool also can be used; the tool is covered with a sterile stockinette, and autoclaved tool bits are utilized. A restorative material should be available for repair of shell defects (e.g., Technovet®—Jorgensen Laboratories). These materials will be discussed in Part II of this presentation.

SUTURE MATERIALS AND PATTERNS

The edges of incised reptilian skin have a tendency to invert.[23] An everting suture pattern, such as horizontal mattress, achieves accurate skin edge apposition. A simple interrupted or continuous pattern can be used, but sutures should be placed close to the skin edges to prevent inversion. The tough skin and scales help prevent sutures from tearing through the skin. Most reptiles are not able to traumatize their incisions by chewing or scratching at them. The use of an interrupted pattern in anatomic areas subject to environmental stress has been advocated.[7] In my experience, continuous patterns do not allow wound dehiscence even in areas of stress.

The use of stainless-steel suture material has been recommended because a very strong suture was believed to be needed to withstand abrasion by the environmental substrate as the patient crawled or slithered.[7] There are reports of the use of chromic gut,[30] polyglycolic acid,[13] silk,[12,28] and nylon[11,12,27] in the skin of reptiles without complications. I have used polyglactin 910, nylon, and polypropylene in the skin of reptiles with no suture failure. These materials might be more comfortable for patients than stainless steel is. Although polyglactin 910 is absorbed fairly rapidly in mammals, it remains for long periods in reptilian skin; I have observed it intact in the skin of a Burmese python two months after placement. Removal of skin sutures, even those of absorbable materials, is recommended.

B URIED SUTURES of synthetic absorbable materials work well. Absorption is probably prolonged, although no studies have reported this. Chromic gut has been used frequently in reptilian patients.[11-13,24-28,30-32] Because reptilian heterophils might lack many proteolytic enzymes and because the absorption of chromic gut depends on proteolysis, this absorption is uncertain in reptiles. Chromic gut was still present in a rhinoceros viper (*Bitis nasicornis*) 12 weeks after the material was used to close the patient's pleuroperitoneum and subcutaneous tissue.[33] Other suture materials not dependent on proteolysis (such as polyglycolic acid, polyglactin 910, polypropylene, and polydioxanone) therefore should be used.

Skin healing should be strong enough to allow suture removal in three to four weeks.[1,2,11,23,34] In squamate reptiles with intermittent shedding, suture removal should be performed after the ecdysis subsequent to surgery. The shed skin usually sticks in the sutured area but can be gently peeled away. After suture removal, one or two more shed skins might stick along the incision site; usually normal ecdysis resumes soon.

POSTOPERATIVE CARE

Anesthetic recovery in reptiles can be prolonged and difficult to monitor. Righting reflex, response to noxious stimuli, tongue withdrawal, and opening of the glottis as evidence of breathing can be used to monitor recovery. Increasing environmental temperature to 30° to 36°C will increase the rate of metabolism of anesthetic agents.[1,7] Balanced electrolyte solutions (20 to 40 ml/kg/day) can be given intracoelomically or subcutaneously to promote renal excretion of some agents and to aid in maintaining adequate hydration.[7,18,27] Fluids also can be left in the coelomic cavity before closure of a celiotomy. Doxapram hy-

drochloride is an effective respiratory stimulant in reptiles and can be used in apneic patients.[7]

T HE HEARTBEAT of most reptiles is not auscultated easily; however, in snakes the heart can usually be palpated while in lizards this is much more difficult. Because of the protective plastron, the heart of turtles cannot be auscultated or palpated. As a result, if a patient is not breathing spontaneously and a heartbeat is not detectable, it can be difficult to determine whether the patient is alive. An electrocardiogram monitor is useful in such patients. In snakes, a two-lead system is sufficient[11] (Figure 8). In patients with legs, conventional three- or four-lead systems work well. Leads can be attached to needles inserted between scales or to stainless-steel sutures placed into the skin.

Once the patient is awake and responsive, it should be placed in a warm, dark, quiet place to complete its recovery. Clean paper should be provided in the recovery area to prevent contamination of the incision. Hibernation should be delayed for at least six months because it delays healing.[16,18] Many reptiles spend much time in water, which also can delay wound healing. Swimming therefore should be prevented for 7 to 14 days after surgery.[1,18,23] Intracoelomic or subcutaneous fluids can be given to maintain hydration if necessary. Many reptiles become anorectic after surgery. Force feeding or tube feeding might be necessary; the technique has been described in the literature.[1,2,7,18] A pharyngostomy tube can be placed for long-term alimentation of reptiles (Figure 9). Because the larynx is located far rostrally in most reptiles, the tube can easily be positioned to exit the pharynx caudal to the larynx, thus preventing interference with laryngeal function.

DEDICATION

The author dedicates this article to the late Dr. Elizabeth A. Russo, College of Veterinary Medicine, Texas A&M University, and acknowledges her help in the preparation of the manuscript.

About the Author
Dr. Bennett, a Diplomate of the American College of Veterinary Surgeons, is affiliated with the College of Veterinary Medicine at the University of Florida, Gainesville, Florida.

REFERENCES

1. Marcus LC: *Veterinary Biology and Medicine of Captive Amphibians and Reptiles*. Philadelphia, Lea & Febiger, 1981, pp 12–50, 68–79.
2. Cooper JE, Jackson OF: *Diseases of the Reptilia*. London, Academic Press, 1981, pp 10–73, 542–549.
3. Porter KR: *Herpetology*. Philadelphia, WB Saunders Co, 1972.
4. Ottaviani G, Tazzi A: *Biology of the Reptilia*, vol 6. New York, Academic Press, 1977, p 437.
5. Jacobson ER: Histology, endocrinology, and husbandry of ecdysis in snakes. A review. *VM SAC* 72(2):275–280, 1977.
6. Smith DA, Barker IK: Preliminary observations on the effects of am-

bient temperature on cutaneous wound healing in snakes. *AAZV Annu Proc*:210–211, 1983.

7. Frye FL: *Biomedical and Surgical Aspects of Captive Reptile Husbandry*. Edwardsville, KS, Veterinary Medicine Publishing Co, 1981, pp 247–278.
8. Rosskopf WJ, Woerpel RW: Egg yolk peritonitis in a California desert tortoise. *California Vet* 36(3):13–15, 1982.
9. Boever WJ, Williams J: *Arisona* septicemia in three boa constrictors. *VM SAC* 70(11):1357–1359, 1975.
10. Cooper JE: Use of a surgical adhesive drape in reptiles. *Vet Rec* 108(3):56, 1981.
11. Jacobson ER, Ingling AL: Pyloroduodenal resection in a Burmese python. *JAVMA* 169(9):985–986, 1976.
12. Millichamp NJ, Lawrence K, Jacobson ER, et al: Egg retention in snakes. *JAVMA* 183:1213–1218, 1983.
13. Patterson RW, Smith A: Surgical intervention to relieve dystocia in a python. *Vet Rec* 104(24):551–552, 1979.
14. Peters AR, Coote J: Dystocia in a snake. *Vet Rec* 100(20):423, 1977.
15. Robinson PT, Sedgwick CJ, Meier JE, et al: Internal fixation of a humeral fracture in a Komodo dragon lizard. *VM SAC* 73(5):645–649, 1978.
16. Rosskopf WJ, Woerpel RW: Repair of shell damage in tortoises. *Mod Vet Pract* 62(12):938–939, 1981.
17. Rosskopf WJ, Woerpel R: Treatment of an egg-bound turtle. *Mod Vet Pract* 64(8):644–645, 1983.
18. Rosskopf WJ, Woerpel RW, Pitts BJ, Rosskopf GA: Abdominal surgery in turtles and tortoises. *Anim Health Tech* 4(6):326–330, 1983.
19. Bush M, Smeller JM, Charache P, Arthur R: Biological half-life of gentamicin in gopher snakes. *Am J Vet Res* 39:171–173, 1978.
20. Mader DR, Conzelman GM, Baggot JD: Effects of ambient temperature on the half-life and dosage regimen of amikacin in the gopher snake. *JAVMA* 187:1134–1136, 1985.
21. Raphael B, Clark CH, Hudson R: Plasma concentration of gentamicin in turtles. *J Zoo Anim Med* 16:136–139, 1985.
22. Crane S, Curtis M, Jacobson ER, Webb A: Neutralization bone plating repair of a fractured humerus in an Aldabra tortoise. *JAVMA* 177(9):945–948, 1980.
23. Frye FL: Surgery in captive reptiles, in Kirk RW (ed): *Current Veterinary Therapy V*. Philadelphia, WB Saunders Co, 1974, pp 640–641.
24. Frye FL, Schuchman S: Salpingotomy and cesarian delivery of impacted ova in a tortoise. *VM SAC* 69(4):454–457, 1974.
25. Holt PE: Obstetrical problems in two tortoises. *J Small Anim Pract* 20(6):353–359, 1979.
26. Isenbugel E, Barandum G: Surgical removal of a foreign body in a bastard turtle. *VM SAC* 76(12):1766–1768, 1981.
27. Millichamp NJ: Surgical management of an ovarian neoplasm. *Vet Med* 80(11):54–55, 1985.
28. Mulder JB, Hauser JJ, Perry JJ: Surgical removal of retained eggs from a king snake. *J Zoo Anim Med* 10(1):21–22, 1979.
29. Zwart P, Dorrestein GM, Stades FC, Broer BH: Vasectomy in the garter snake. *J Zoo Anim Med* 10(1):17–18, 1979.
30. Redisch RI: Repair of a fractured femur in an iguana. *VM SAC* 73(12):1547–1548, 1978.
31. Frye FL: Surgical removal of a cystic calculus from a desert tortoise. *JAVMA* 161(6):600–602, 1972.
32. Jordan RD, Kyzar CT: Intra-abdominal removal of eggs from a gopher tortoise. *VM SAC* 73(8):1051–1054, 1978.
33. Jacobson ER, Millichamp NJ, Gaskin JM: Use of a polyvalent autogenous bacterin for treatment of mixed gram-negative bacterial osteomyelitis in a rhinoceros viper. *JAVMA* 187(11):1224–1225, 1985.
34. Wallach JD, Boever WJ: *Diseases of Exotic Animals*. Philadelphia, WB Saunders Co, 1983, pp 1027–1043.

UPDATE

Since this article was published, enrofloxacin, a broad spectrum fluoroquinolone antibiotic with activity against most species of *Pseudomonas*, has become available to veterinarians. Many of the pathogens infecting reptile patients are susceptible to this antibiotic. Enrofloxacin may be administered to most species of reptiles at 5 to 10 mg/kg/24 hours orally, intramuscularly, subcutaneously, or intra-coelomic,[1] and in pythons every 48 hours.[2] As a surgical prophylaxis, it is best administered intra-coelomic, as it will have a more rapid onset of action.

Intravenous catheters and intraosseous catheters are commonly used to provide fluid support and maintain venous access for reptile surgical patients. Techniques for catheter placement in veins, such as the right jugular vein in many species of chelonians, and for intraosseous catheter placement are described.[3] The ventral abdominal vein may be used for placement of an intravenous catheter in most lizards but requires a cutdown procedure.

The article indicates that supplemental heat is not required and may increase the amount of anesthetic required to maintain the patient. Currently, it is generally accepted that maintenance of body functions is of utmost importance for reptile patients. Supplemental heat, therefore, is considered beneficial because most body functions, including the immune system, operate best in warm conditions. Efforts should be made during anesthesia and surgery to keep the patient within the preferred optimum temperature zone for its species.

A Doppler flow probe is very valuable to monitor the patient's heart rate and function. The probe, which senses blood flow and produces an audible sound confirming that blood is flowing through the heart or artery, is placed over the heart or peripheral artery if accessible. Peripheral arteries are difficult to locate, although the carotid arteries may be identified in some species. The heart, generally located in the cranial quarter of the body, is easily identified by visual inspection. In lizards, the heart is usually located on midline between the shoulders much farther cranial than might be expected. In chelonians, since sound waves do not penetrate bone, the probe must be placed in the thoracic inlet with the ultrasound waves directed toward the midline, which is the location of the heart. Similarly, in lizards with an ossified sternal plate, the probe must be placed in the thoracic inlet and directed toward midline.

A new plastic drape has become available that can be applied to reptile patients. This drape (Surgical Drape™; Veterinary Specialty Products, Inc., Boca Raton, FL) is 24" × 24" with a 3.5" × 5" central adhesive surface and is a thicker plastic than most transparent drapes. Another valuable tool for reptile surgery is the hemostatic clip (Hemoclip™; Solvay Animal Health, Mendota Heights, MN). The clips, made of surgical stainless steel and biologically inert, are invaluable for surgery of the reproductive system. They allow control of hemorrhage from vessels in locations that are difficult to access.

Suture removal is usually performed four to six weeks postoperatively in reptiles. In most cases, every other suture is removed at four weeks. The incision is evaluated by gently spreading the tissue. If further healing time is required, the remaining sutures are removed after an additional two weeks. With this technique, incisional dehiscence is less likely to occur following suture removal.

(continues on page 91)

Reptilian Surgery Part II. Management of Surgical Diseases

KEY FACTS

- Superficial bacterial infections can result in septicemia and major organ involvement; antibiotics are indicated for contaminated wounds.
- Celiotomy indications include egg binding, egg peritonitis, gastrointestinal obstruction, ovariohysterectomy for uterine prolapse, colopexy for colon prolapse, cystotomy for urolithiasis, and exploration for obtaining biopsies.
- Clinical signs of gastrointestinal abnormalities include regurgitation, anorexia, lack of stool production, weight loss, and abdominal distention.

University of Florida
R. Avery Bennett, DVM, MS

P ET REPTILES are susceptible to various conditions necessitating surgical management. A range of surgical procedures can be performed on reptiles when indicated. The first part of this two-part presentation dealt with the basic principles of surgery in reptiles. Part II discusses some common surgical diseases of reptiles. Many anatomic and physiologic distinctions between analogous conditions in mammalian and reptilian patients must be considered.

LACERATIONS

Reptiles can present with lacerations caused by various traumatic events, such as being bitten by a dog or a cat, hit by a vehicle, cut by nails used for cage construction, or attacked by prey. Local anesthetics are effective for purposes of suturing superficial lacerations (Figure 1). General principles of wound debridement and suturing apply to reptiles. Povidone-iodine (1%) is an effective irrigation solution. Severely comtaminated wounds or wounds with extensive tissue damage should be managed as open wounds; periodic debridement to remove caseous material and necrotic tissue before surgical closure is essential. Open wounds will heal by second intention.[1]

A clinical trial on dermal lesions in reptiles involved the use of a surgical adhesive polyurethane dressing (Opsite®—Smith and Nephew) designed to exclude bacteria but to allow oxygen and water-vapor penetration.[2] The researchers reported that wounds treated with this dressing were cleaner and apparently healed more quickly. Patients were able to swim without adversely affecting healing while the wound was covered. The dressing evidently is useful for protecting open wounds, burns, and surgical incisions.

Superficial bacterial infections in reptiles can lead to septicemia and major organ involvement.[2,3] When dealing with contaminated wounds, antibiotics are indicated. Antibiotic therapy should be based on the results of culture and sensitivity testing when possible. At the Colorado State University Veterinary Teaching Hospital, most bacterial isolates from reptiles are gram-negative and are susceptible to aminoglycoside antibiotics.

Based on pharmacokinetic studies conducted in gopher snakes (*Pituophis melanoleucus catenifer*) and red-eared slider turtles (*Pseudemys scripta elegans*), gentamicin at a dosage of 2.5 mg/kg given every 72 hours is expected to maintain therapeutic plasma concentrations.[4,5] Because of

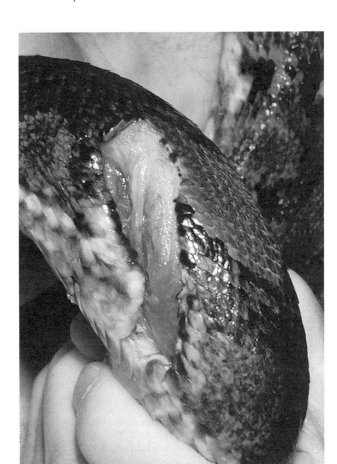

Figure 1A

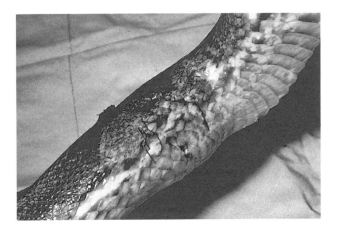

Figure 1B

Figure 1—(**A**) This Burmese python (*Pythona molurus bivittatus*) received several lacerations from a nail protruding into its cage. (**B**) The lacerations were sutured with polyglactin 910 while the patient was under local anesthesia.

the results of a study conducted with gopher snakes, it has been recommended that amikacin sulfate be given at a 5 mg/kg loading dose followed by 2.5 mg/kg every 72 hours.[6] Bacteria were twice as sensitive to amikacin sulfate at 37°C (98.6°F) compared with 25°C (77°F); it is there-

fore recommended that reptiles treated with this antibiotic be maintained at the upper end of their preferred optimum ambient temperatures.[6]

Because of the renal portal system of reptiles, these antibiotics should be given in the cranial half of the patient's body. From 20 to 40 ml/kg/day of a balanced electrolyte solution given intracoelomically or subcutaneously can help to prevent renal damage, especially in dehydrated patients. If therapy is continued beyond five treatments, the risk of renal injury apparently increases.

CELIOTOMY

Indications for celiotomy in reptiles include egg binding, egg peritonitis, gastrointestinal obstruction, ovariohysterectomy for uterine prolapse, colopexy for colon prolapse, cystotomy for urolithiasis, and exploration for obtaining biopsies. The technique of celiotomy varies depending on the family to which the patient belongs.

Snakes

In snakes, abdominal incisions can be made at the lateral margin of the scutes (where they join the scales of the lateral body wall) or between the first and second rows of lateral scales.[7-12] Incisions should be made between rather than through scales if possible because this approach is believed to enhance healing.[7,8] The surgeon must avoid the tips of the patient's ribs at the junction of the scutes and the scales. One pair of ribs attaches to each scute. There is reportedly no difference in exposure between midline and lateral approaches, but the lateral approach is easier to keep clean after surgery because the suture line is not in direct contact with the substrate and is not stressed by rectilinear motion as the snake crawls.[11,13]

SOME SURGEONS use a ventral midline incision with care to avoid the large ventral abdominal vein present just inside the body wall along the ventral midline of the caudal aspect of the body.[13-15] This approach has the advantage of providing good exposure to both sides of the coelomic cavity. Adverse effects or delayed healing have not been observed with the use of ventral midline incisions.[13,14]

Three layers are encountered: skin, muscle, and pleuroperitoneum.[8,9] In large reptiles, three layers can be identified; in many of the small reptiles commonly kept as pets, however, the layers are not discernible. Closure of the muscle layer and the skin should be performed separately if possible. When separate layers are not identifiable, a single-layer closure is adequate. The great tensile strength of the skin of most reptiles apparently provides sufficient holding power to prevent dehiscence.

Lizards and Crocodilians

Paralumbar and midline incisions have been recommended for approaching the coelomic cavity of lizards and crocodilians.[8] The ventral abdominal vein is a very large vein located inside the body wall on the ventral midline. This vein receives blood from the body wall[16]; if the vein is damaged during the approach to the coelom, serious hemorrhage can occur. Because the effects of ligating the vein are unknown, the vein should be avoided during celiotomy by using a paramedian incision.

Chelonians

The bony shell of chelonians provides a challenge in performing celiotomy. In chelonians with a small plastron (sea turtles and snapping turtles), the majority of abdominal structures can be approached through an incision between the plastron and the femur in the flank region.[17-19] In other chelonians, it is necessary to perform an osteotomy of the plastron. The pelvic bones should be avoided. Radiographs help to determine the location of the pelvic bones in relation to the shields of the plastron.

Usually the femoral and abdominal shields are osteotomized for the approach. The bone of the plastron is cut in a rectangle across the midline or on one side of the midline (paramedian)[20] for the proposed celiotomy. A high-speed burr or an orthopedic saw is used (Figure 2). Irrigating fluids are used to dissipate heat and to remove bone dust during the osteotomy. When the osteotomy is complete, the rectangle of bone is elevated from the underlying abdominal musculature by using a periosteal elevator or the back of a scalpel handle. The incision into the abdominal wall can be performed using a flap technique or a ventral midline incision. The flap, however, might provide better exposure of the viscera. The flap incision should be made several millimeters from the osteotomy to allow closure. By incising only three sides, vascular supply to the muscle flap is maintained.

It has been recommended that the pleuroperitoneum be incised as a separate layer from the muscles,[8,18] but it is usually impossible to separate these layers. There are venous sinuses on each side of the midline approximately midway between the midline and the bridge. These sinuses should be avoided if possible but can be ligated if necessary without adverse effect.[8]

Closure is accomplished with a simple continuous pattern of an absorbable suture material in the pleuroperitoneum and the muscle. The bone is replaced using restorative material as is described for repair of large shell defects with replacement of a fragment.

SHELL FRACTURE REPAIR

Shell fractures are most commonly presented after chelonians are hit by lawn mowers, bicycles, automobiles, or human feet. Such fractures are also observed after encounters with dogs and cats. Because reptiles do not have a functional diaphragm and respiration therefore does not require negative intrapleuroperitoneal pressure, respiratory distress does not occur with shell fracture. Intrapulmonary smooth muscle and extrapulmonary skeletal muscle are responsible for lung inflation.[8] Pneumopleuroperitoneum occurs as a result of celiotomy and many instances of shell fracture but is not a life-threatening condition.

Principles of wound lavage and debridement should be observed when treating chelonians with shell fractures. Most such fractures are contaminated and can be left open until conditions are appropriate for delayed closure. This usually takes at least one week of appropriate antibiotic therapy and daily debridement.

Small defects or cracks in the shell can be maintained by reduction with wires, external bandages, or acrylic materials.[12,18,21] Interfragmentary orthopedic wires are used to appose the separated portions of shell. The wires are passed through holes drilled into the shell with a Kirschner wire. Acrylic materials, such as those used for hoof reconstruction and dental repairs, can be used to hold fragments in apposition. The fracture should be maintained in reduction for three to seven days without exposure to water so that a seal can form; after this, the patient can be allowed to swim.[18,21] The fixation should not be removed until there is radiographic evidence of union.

Large defects should be repaired by prosthesis. Various restorative materials have been used, including hoof or dental acrylics, boat or autobody fiberglass, and epoxy resin.[22] Epoxy resin has the advantages of being clear, producing good cosmesis, and being inexpensive and readily available; in addition, curing times can be accurately predicted.

Patches of fiberglass cloth of various sizes can be autoclaved for sterile application. Fiberglass provides a matrix to enable the resin to bridge the defect. The patch should be large enough to extend beyond the margin of the defect. The shell around the defect should be cleaned with acetone, ether, or trichlorotrifluoroethane (Freon® Skin Degreaser—Miller-Stephenson Chemical) for proper bonding of the resin to occur. The resin is applied to the shell around the defect circumferentially. Care must be taken to keep the epoxy from the edge of the defect because the presence of the resin over the edge will delay fracture healing.[8] A sterile gauze dressing can be placed over the defect to protect it from the epoxy.

The tissues will heal deeply to superficially, and the dressing and the epoxy will be external to the shell. The fiberglass patch is stretched over the defect and held in place, allowing the resin to penetrate the cloth and to bond it to the shell surface.

When this layer has cured, a light coat of epoxy is applied to the fiberglass cloth. The resin must not be allowed to saturate the cloth and drip into the coelomic cavity. After this layer has cured, several more thin layers of epoxy should be applied to strengthen and seal the defect completely (Figure 3). For very large defects in large turtles, one layer of fiberglass might not provide enough strength; additional layers impregnated with resin can be applied for

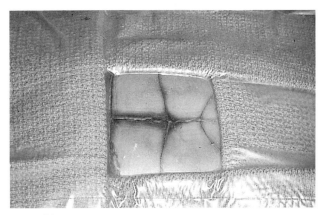

Figure 2A

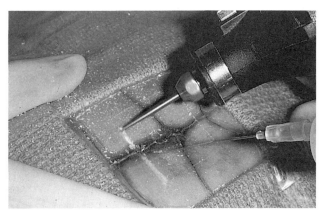

Figure 2B

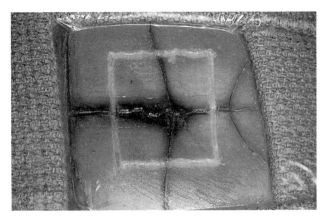

Figure 2C

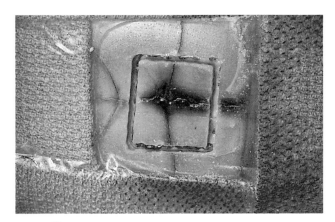

Figure 2D

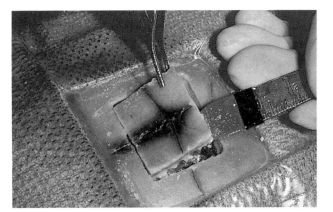

Figure 2E

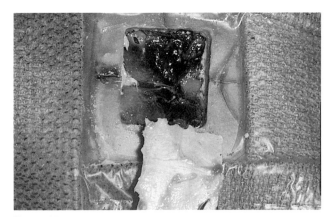

Figure 2F

reinforcement.

If a large fragment is to be replaced, as in the case of closing a celiotomy, the piece should be bonded to the center of the cloth patch with epoxy before the patch is applied to the defect (Figure 2). It is again important not to allow the resin to run down the edges of the fragment to be reattached.

HEALING of bone in reptiles takes at least 6 to 18 months.[8,21-23] In a growing chelonian, the patch should be

removed from the growth rings after healing is complete to allow the shell to continue to grow.[8,18,22,24,25] This removal can be accomplished with any type of burr drill. Epoxy dust can be toxic and carcinogenic to humans; copious irrigation therefore should be used to prevent aerosolization, and a face mask must be worn by the clinician.[8]

DYSTOCIA

Reproductive physiology in reptiles varies considerably among species. Some species produce brittle, hard-shelled eggs (most chelonians); some produce pliant, leathery

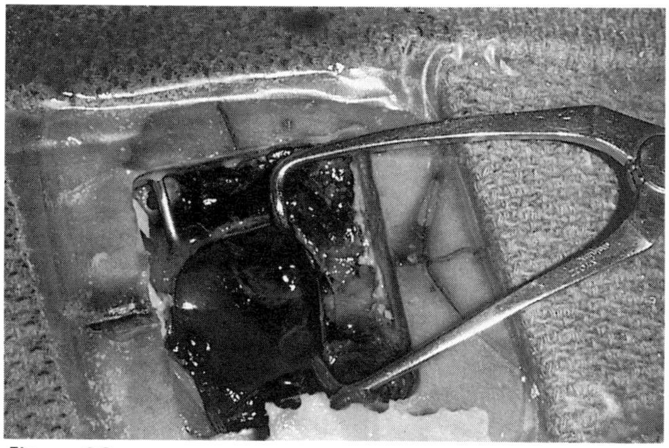

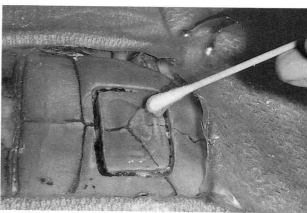

Figure 2G

Figure 2H

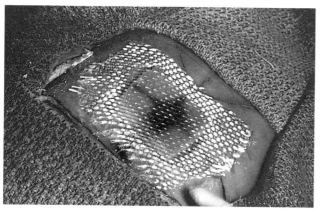

Figure 2I

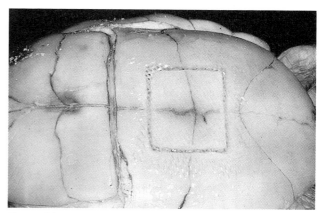

Figure 2J

Figure 2—(**A**) A clear plastic adhesive drape was used for a laparotomy in this three-toed box turtle (*Terrapene carolina triunguis*). (**B** through **D**) A burr was used to perform an osteotomy of the femoral and abdominal shields. (**E** and **F**) The segment was elevated with the back of a scalpel handle. (**G**) Eyelid retractors were used to retract the body wall. The defect was repaired with fiberglass and epoxy. The patch was applied (**H**) to the removed section of bone first and then (**I**) to the plastron using epoxy. (**J**) Several more layers of epoxy were applied, allowing the epoxy to cure between layers.

shelled eggs (some lizards and snakes); and others produce live young (some lizards and snakes).[26] Dystocia can occur in any species of reptile, but the highest incidence is reported in chelonians.[26,27] Very large eggs, misshapen eggs, more than one egg attempting to pass simultaneously, dead fetuses, trauma, and bacterial salpingitis are some of the reported causes.[8,13,14,22,28,29] In some cases, the cause of egg retention is not easily determined. Endocrine abnormalities and such environmental factors as low temperature, improper diet, lack of exercise leading to poor muscle tone, an unclean cage, lack of seclusion, and an abnormal photoperiod are potential causes of egg or fetus retention.[13,14]

CLINICAL SIGNS of dystocia include anorexia, regurgitation, almost constant straining, cloacal discharge that is often malodorous, paresis, respiratory distress, and edema of the cranial extremities.[8,12-14,26,27,30] Many patients

have histories of passing several eggs before the onset of clinical signs. In squamate reptiles, the eggs are often palpable; in chelonians, radiographs might be necessary to determine the presence and number of remaining eggs. In some chelonians, it might be possible to palpate eggs cranial to the hindlegs. The soft, leathery shells of the eggs of some species are not very radiopaque.

Noninvasive procedures to relieve dystocia should be attempted before surgical intervention. Manipulation of the eggs or fetuses with lubrication of the cloacal and uterine openings can be successful in relieving the dystocia.[13,14,26] Intramuscular oxytocin at a dose of 1 to 10 units/kg and intramuscular or subcutaneous 1% calcium borogluconate solution at 10 ml/kg have been successfully used to relieve dystocia in snakes that could not be relieved by manipulation.[14] Similar therapeutic regimens have been used in chelonians.[22,27,29] Manipulation should not be performed after oxytocin has been given because uterine contraction prevents movement of the eggs or fetuses during manipulation.[14] Reptiles treated with oxytocin and calcium boroglu-

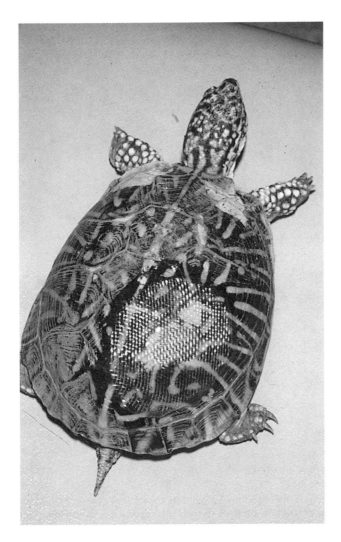

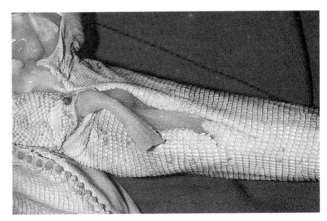

Figure 4—This cadaver specimen of a male green iguana (*Iguana iguana*) demonstrates an everted hemipene.

Figure 3—This western box turtle (*Terrapene ornata*) sustained a shell defect after being hit by a lawn mower. The wound was debrided and lavaged, and the surrounding shell was cleaned and degreased. A fiberglass and epoxy patch was applied.

conate should be placed in a dark, warm (30° to 36°C; 85° to 95°F), quiet environment to allow patients to attempt to pass the eggs.[13-15]

In species that produce soft and leathery eggs, percutaneous ovocentesis using a needle and syringe can collapse the eggs and thus allow them to pass more easily.[14,15,29] Because of embryonal death and decomposition, the eggs will often swell and become too large to pass.[14,15] In such cases, ovocentesis can be very helpful.

SALPINGOTOMY is indicated if noninvasive techniques fail to relieve dystocia or if there is radiographic evidence that natural passage is impossible. In chelonians, the oviduct and the uterus are mobile within the coelomic cavity and can be exteriorized and packed off after celiotomy.[18] In squamate reptiles, the oviduct and the uterus are not very mobile. It might be necessary to make more than

one incision into the skin, body wall, and uterus of long snakes in order to remove all eggs or fetuses.[13,15] Frequently, the eggs have begun to deteriorate and are adherent to the uterus, which is very thin and friable.[11,13,15]

The incision in the salpinx and the uterus should be repaired with an inverting suture pattern of an absorbable material, such as polyglactin 910 or polydioxanone. Salpingohysterectomy should be considered if dystocia recurs, if the patient is not being maintained for breeding, or if bacterial salpingitis is present.

It has been suggested that the entire ovary must be removed to prevent release of eggs into the peritoneal cavity.[25,26] The ovaries of many reptiles are not pedunculated and therefore are difficult to remove.[8] Other clinicians have indicated that removal of the ovaries might be unnecessary.[8,14] In birds, it is unnecessary to remove the ovary along with the uterus to prevent egg peritonitis. Birds in which hysterectomy has been performed demonstrate maternal behavior yet do not lay eggs or release yolks into the peritoneal cavity.[31] The mechanism for these behaviors is unknown. During salpingohysterectomy in a reptile, the oviduct should be pulled free from the ovary and the uterus should be ligated as close to the cloaca as possible.[8] Future egg laying also can be suppressed by the use of medroxyprogesterone acetate (20 mg/kg).[32]

Occasionally, eggs or yolks are lost from the reproductive tract into the pleuroperitoneal cavity. Two of the reported causes of this loss in chelonians are turning the animal on its back while it is producing eggs and the presence of cystic calculi that result in trauma to developing eggs.[32] The presence of egg yolk within the coelomic cavity of reptiles produces a severe inflammatory reaction. Fibrin deposition and serosal thickening are typical. Surgical removal of the yolk material and coelomic lavage are indicated; the prognosis is grave.[8,26,32]

CLOACAL ORGAN PROLAPSE

The cloaca has openings from the colon, the ureters, the urinary bladder (if present), and the reproductive tract. Ureteral prolapse has not been reported in reptiles; prolapse of the colon, the reproductive tract, and the urinary bladder do occur.[8,33]

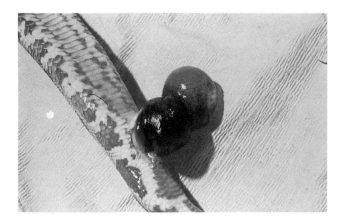

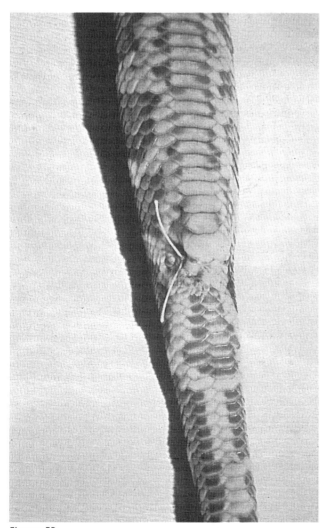

Figure 5B

Figure 5—(A) This young Burmese python (*Pythona molurus bivittatus*) had colonic prolapse, which (**B**) was reduced and maintained with a purse-string suture. (Courtesy of Dr. E. A. Russo, Texas A&M University)

Copulatory Organ Prolapse

The male copulatory organ varies anatomically according to the reptilian order. Squamate reptiles have paired copulatory organs, called hemipenes, which lie in an inverted position within the tail (Figure 4). One of the hemipenes is everted during copulation. Chelonians have a single penis, which is everted during copulation. This organ is quite large compared with the smaller, single copulatory organ of crocodilians, which is palpable within the cloaca by digital examination.

Although prolapse of the penis or the hemipenes has been reported as a sequela to constipation and neurologic dysfunction,[8,34] such prolapse is most frequently the result of infection, forced separation during copulation, or swelling secondary to probing by a clinician to determine gender. Medical management is based on identification and treatment of the primary cause. The organ should be cleaned, gently lubricated with an ophthalmic antibiotic ointment, and gently replaced with a cotton swab. A purse-string suture is placed in the cloaca tight enough to prevent prolapse but to allow voiding. The suture is left in place for three to four weeks.[10] Glycerin and concentrated sugar solutions can help to decrease edema within the organ.[34] If the prolapse cannot be reduced, the cloacal opening can be enlarged by incising to accommodate the swollen gland.[8]

SURGERY is indicated in cases in which the organ has been everted for an extended period and is severely swollen and damaged. Amputation is performed after mattress sutures are placed at the base of the organ to prevent postoperative hemorrhage. The organ is amputated 2 mm distal to the sutures, and the stump is replaced into the cloaca. Snakes and lizards with one hemipene are considered fertile.[8]

Prolapse of the uterus is rare but does occur in reptiles.[8,26] Replacement should be attempted by the use of the techniques described for penis or hemipene prolapse. If reduction is impossible, a celiotomy to prepare for salpingo-hysterectomy should be performed. Amputation of the exposed tissue using transfixing mattress sutures has also been recommended.[26]

Colon Prolapse

Colon prolapse can result from straining because of constipation or bacterial or parasitic enteritis. Constipation can be caused by confinement in an environment too small to allow sufficient exercise.[12] The primary cause of the straining must be determined and appropriate therapy instituted. Conservative management should be attempted before surgical therapy. Often colon prolapses are reducible and can be successfully managed by treating the primary cause while maintaining a purse-string suture in the cloaca[8,12] (Figure 5).

Frequently, the venous return from the prolapsed colon is severely compromised; the organ rapidly becomes engorged and friable. If it is impossible to reduce the pro-

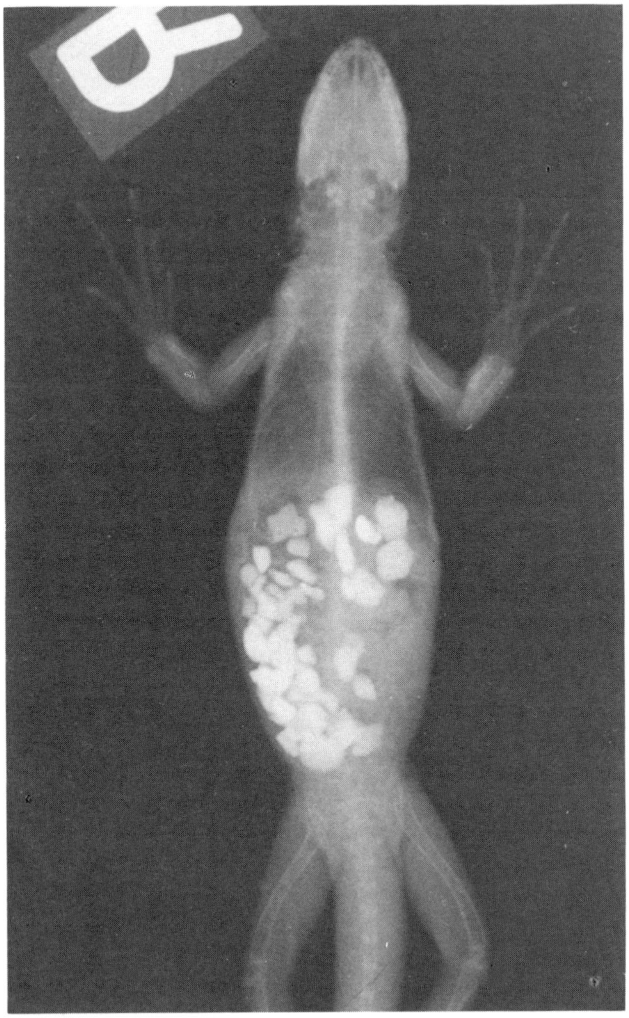

Figure 6A

lapse, celiotomy and colopexy are the recommended treatments.[8] An area of healthy colon should be selected and sutured to the body wall. Because the colon wall is usually very thin, care must be taken to prevent penetration into the intestinal lumen. If the colon is severely compromised, it can be resected and anastomosis can be performed.[12]

GASTROINTESTINAL PROCEDURES

A variety of gastrointestinal surgical procedures have been performed on reptiles, including gastrotomy, intestinal resection-anastomosis, and enterotomy.[9,17] Foreign body ingestion occurs with some frequency in captive reptiles[8,17] (Figure 6). Sharp objects or obstructing foreign bodies should be surgically removed. Parasitic and bacterial enteritides have been associated with intussusception.[12]

Clinical signs of gastrointestinal abnormalities include regurgitation, anorexia, lack of stool production, weight loss, and abdominal distention. Loss of the stratum corneum of the skin can be a sign of toxic peritonitis.[9] A patient's history can help in making a diagnosis, especially with foreign body ingestion.

PRINCIPLES of gastrointestinal surgery in reptiles are similar to those in mammals. The intestines of most reptiles are thin walled, and the use of fine suture material and an atraumatic needle (5-0 or 6-0) is recommended. In small patients, ophthalmic instruments are appropriate for such delicate work. Because of the questionable absorption of chromic gut, it should be avoided when performing gastrointestinal procedures. Such sutures as polydioxanone are strong and maintain their tensile strength for several

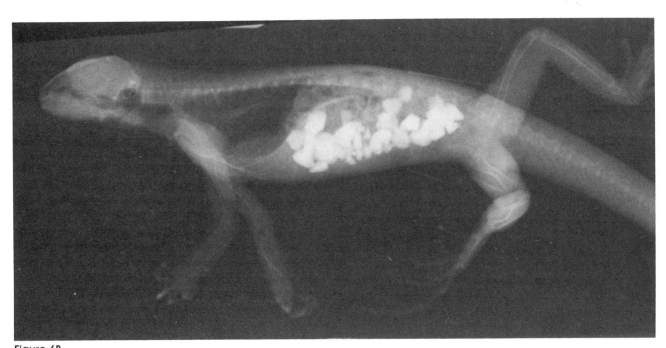

Figure 6B

Figure 6—(A and **B)** Gravel ingestion is common in captive reptiles maintained on a gravel substrate. Such ingestion can cause gastrointestinal obstruction.

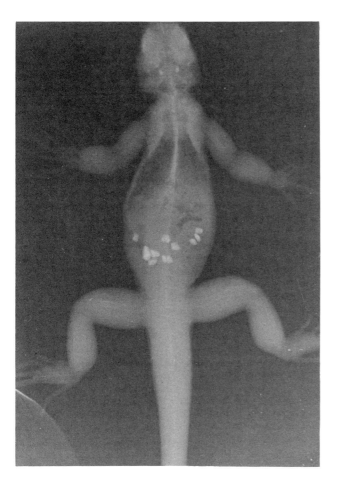

Figure 7—The soft, demineralized bones of reptiles with metabolic bone disease fracture easily. Such bones do not hold internal fixation devices well.

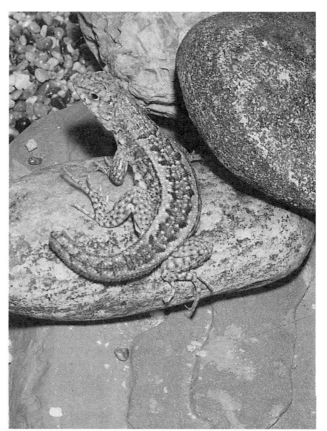

Figure 8A

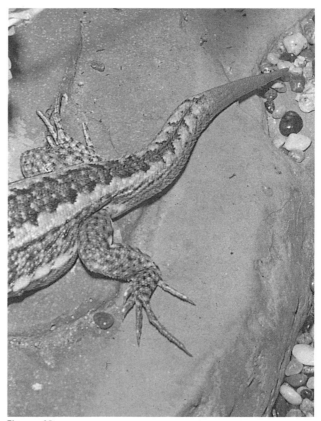

Figure 8B

Figure 8—(**A**) After the tail of this curled-tail lizard (*Leiocephalus carinatus*) broke off, the end sealed with a fibrinous scab. (**B**) One month after injury, the tail had completely regenerated.

months in mammals; this can be advantageous in slow-healing reptiles.

The length of the mesentery is variable in reptiles.[17,18] If the affected section cannot be adequately exteriorized, it should be well packed off before enterotomy. Copious coelomic lavage with saline should be performed before closure.

CYSTOTOMY

Crocodilians, snakes, and some lizards do not have a urinary bladder.[25] In species that do have urinary bladders, cystic calculi can occur. Desert tortoises evidently have the highest incidence of cystic calculi among reptile species. In a case of dystocia in a spur-thighed tortoise (*Testudo graeca*), two eggs were located within the urinary bladder. The eggs were believed to be unable to pass from the cloaca, and they subsequently migrated into the urinary bladder.[22]

Clinical signs associated with cystic calculi are non-specific and include anorexia, lethargy, and depression. Radiographs establish the diagnosis because the calculi are usually radiodense. Cystotomy is easily performed in reptiles. The urinary bladder is very mobile within the coelomic cavity and is easily isolated during surgery.[20] A two-layer closure using an inverting pattern of an absorbable suture material is preferred.[18,20] Analysis of one stone demonstrated the presence of urates and magnesium.[20]

FRACTURE REPAIR

General principles of fracture repair—anatomic reduction and stable fixation—apply to reptiles. Reptilian bones apparently heal much slower than mammalian bones do and require at least 6 to 18 months for complete healing.[8,23,25] Many fractures in reptiles result from trauma.

Various splinting techniques and casts can be used in reptiles. Modified Schroeder-Thomas splints, soda-straw splints, ball bandages for foot fractures, plaster casts, taping of the affected limb to the body, and folding the limb into the space between the carapace and the plastron (in chelonians) have been recommended.[8,12,23,25,35,36]

Internal fixation by means of orthopedic wires, intramedullary pins, or bone plates has been used with considerable success.[7,23,35,37,38] During the surgical approach, muscles should be separated rather than divided; blood vessels and nerves should be preserved.

PATHOLOGIC fractures resulting from nutritional secondary hyperparathyroidism also are common. Fractures resulting from metabolic bone disease are difficult to stabilize because the bone is too soft to hold internal fixation devices (Figure 7). It is therefore best to correct the metabolic cause of the osteomalacia and to treat the fracture with an external coaptation splint. The patient should be on a diet with a proper calcium-to-phosphorus ratio and should be provided with exogenous vitamin D_3 or an ultraviolet light source so that vitamin D_3 can be synthesized. Because death from hypervitaminosis D_3 has been reported as a result of oversupplementation in green iguanas (*Iguana iguana*),[8] an ultraviolet light source is the preferred treatment method.

Tail defects pose a special problem in lizards. In some reptiles, tails that have been traumatized can be amputated back to healthy tissue. Lizards, however, have the ability to regenerate lost portions of their tails (Figure 8). These lizards are able to break off their tails by a process called autotomy.[25] Some small lizards have so-called fracture planes in the tail; these are uncalcified areas in the caudal vertebrae at which the tail can easily break through the vertebral body in an escape maneuver.[25] The regenerated segment contains a cartilaginous rod but no vertebrae.[25] Primary closure of the exposed end will prevent regeneration of the tail.[8]

IF THE SURGEON is uncertain as to whether a particular patient will regrow its tail, the best approach is to wait and see. If there is no evidence of regeneration after four to six weeks, it is unlikely to occur. Reptilian wounds heal by second intention; unless bone is exposed, a surgical procedure might be unnecessary for the tail end to heal.

OTHER PROCEDURES

A variety of technically difficult procedures can be performed on reptiles, including laminectomy for spinal cord decompression, enucleation in snakes (which lack eyelids for closure), blepharoplasty and rhinoplasty for reconstruction after traumatic or burn wounds, vasectomy, and cryotherapy for neoplasms.[8,39] A knowledge of the basic principles of surgery as well as the anatomic and physiologic differences between reptiles and mammals permits a wide range of surgical procedures to be performed on reptiles when indicated.

DEDICATION

The author dedicates this article to the late Dr. Elizabeth A. Russo, College of Veterinary Medicine, Texas A&M University, and acknowledges her help in the preparation of the manuscript.

About the Author

Dr. Bennett, a Diplomate of the American College of Veterinary Surgeons, is affiliated with the College of Veterinary Medicine at the University of Florida, Gainesville, Florida.

REFERENCES

1. Smith DA, Barker IK: Preliminary observations on the effects of ambient temperature on cutaneous wound healing in snakes. *AAZV Annu Proc*:210–211, 1983.
2. Cooper JE: Use of a surgical adhesive drape in reptiles. *Vet Rec* 108(3):56, 1981.
3. Boever WJ, Williams J: *Arisona* septicemia in 3 boa constrictors. *VM SAC* 70(11):1357–1359, 1975.
4. Bush M, Smeller JM, Charache P, Arthur R: Biological half-life of gentamicin in gopher snakes. *Am J Vet Res* 39:171–173,1978.
5. Raphael B, Clark CH, Hudson R: Plasma concentrations of gentamicin in turtles. *J Zoo Anim Med* 16:136–139, 1985.
6. Mader DR, Conzelman GM, Baggot JD: Effects of ambient temperature on the half-life and dosage regimen of amikacin in the gopher snake. *JAVMA* 187:1134–1136, 1985.
7. Cooper JE, Jackson OF: *Diseases of the Reptilia*. London, Academic Press, 1981, pp 542–549.
8. Frye FL: *Biomedical and Surgical Aspects of Captive Reptile Husbandry*. Edwardsville, KS, Veterinary Medicine Publishing Co, 1981, pp 247–278.
9. Jacobson ER, Ingling AL: Pyloroduodenal resection in a Burmese python. *JAVMA* 169(9):985–986, 1976.
10. Millichamp NJ: Surgical management of an ovarian neoplasm. *Vet Med* 80(11):54–55, 1985.
11. Patterson RW, Smith A: Surgical intervention to relieve dystocia in a python. *Vet Rec* 104(24):551–552, 1979.
12. Wallach JD, Boever WJ: *Diseases of Exotic Animals*. Philadelphia, WB Saunders Co, 1983, pp 1027–1043.
13. Millichamp NJ, Lawrence K, Jacobson ER, et al: Egg retention in snakes. *JAVMA* 183:1213–1218, 1983.
14. Grain E, Evans JE: Egg retention in 4 snakes. *JAVMA* 185(6):679–681, 1984.
15. Peters AR, Coote J: Dystocia in a snake. *Vet Rec* 100(20):423, 1977.
16. Porter KR: *Herpetology*. Philadelphia, WB Saunders Co, 1972, p 167.
17. Isenbugel E, Barandum G: Surgical removal of a foreign body in a bastard turtle. *VM SAC* 76(12):1766–1768, 1981.
18. Rosskopf WJ, Woerpel RW, Pitts BJ, et al: Abdominal surgery in turtles and tortoises. *Anim Health Tech* 4(6):326–329, 1983.

19. Brannian RE: A soft tissue laparotomy technique in turtles. *JAVMA* 185:1416-1417, 1984.
20. Frye FL: Surgical removal of a cystic calculus from a desert tortoise. *JAVMA* 161(6):600-602, 1972.
21. Rosskopf WJ, Woerpel RW: Repair of shell damage in tortoises. *Mod Vet Pract* 62(12):938-939, 1981.
22. Holt PE: Obstetrical problems in two tortoises. *J Small Anim Pract* 20(6):353-359, 1979.
23. Crane S, Curtis M, Jacobson ER, Webb A: Neutralization bone plating repair of a fractured humerus in an Aldabra tortoise. *JAVMA* 177(9):945-948, 1980.
24. Frye FL: Surgery in captive reptiles, in Kirk RW (ed): *Current Veterinary Therapy. V.* Philadelphia, WB Saunders Co, 1974, pp 640-641.
25. Marcus LC: *Veterinary Biology and Medicine of Captive Amphibians and Reptiles.* Philadelphia, Lea & Febiger, 1981, pp 77-79, 196.
26. Frye FL: Clinical obstetric and gynecologic disorders in reptiles. *Proc AAHA* 41:497-499, 1974.
27. Glassford JF, Brown K: Treatment of egg retention in a turtle. *VM SAC* 72(10):1641-1645, 1977.
28. Mulder JB, Hauser JJ, Perry JJ: Surgical removal of retained eggs from a king snake. *J Zoo Anim Med* 10(1):21-22, 1979.
29. Rosskopf WJ, Woerpel R: Treatment of an egg-bound turtle. *Mod Vet Pract* 64(8):644-645, 1983.
30. Frye FL, Schuchman S: Salpingotomy and cesarian delivery of impacted ova in a tortoise. *VM SAC* 69(4):454-457, 1974.
31. Harrison GJ: Selected surgical procedures, in Harrison GJ, Harrison LR (eds): *Clinical Avian Medicine and Surgery.* Philadelphia, WB Saunders Co, 1986, pp 592-593.
32. Rosskopf WJ, Woerpel RW: Egg yolk peritonitis in a California desert tortoise. *California Vet* 36(3):13-15, 1982.
33. Rosskopf WJ, Woerpel RW: Bladder prolapse and diabetes mellitus in a California desert tortoise (*Gopherus agassizi*). *Centers for Disease Control Newsletter* 1(1):6-8, 1982.
34. Rosskopf WJ, Woerpel RW, Pitts BJ: Paraphimosis in a California desert tortoise. *California Vet* 36(1):29-30, 1982.
35. Robinson PT, Sedgwick CJ, Meier JE, et al: Internal fixation of a humeral fracture in a Komodo dragon lizard. *VM SAC* 73(5):645-649, 1978.
36. Redisch RI: Management of leg fractures in the iguana. *VM SAC* 72(9):1487, 1977.
37. Redisch RI: Repair of a fractured femur in an iguana. *VM SAC* 73(12):1547-1548, 1978.
38. Hartman RA: Use of an intramedullary pin in repair of a midshaft humeral fracture in a green iguana. *VM SAC* 71(11):1634-1635, 1976.
39. Zwart P, Dorrestein GM, Stades FC, Broer BH: Vasectomy in the garter snake. *J Zoo Anim Med* 10(1):17-18, 1979.

UPDATE

Op-site® is not available in the United States, but Tegaderm™ (3M Health Care, St. Paul, MN) is a similar product that has proven to be very useful for wound management in reptile patients. It is semi-occlusive and allows oxygen and other gases to pass through the membrane while preventing water from entering the wound. This product is especially useful in aquatic reptiles. The membrane is secured in place and the edge sealed using a thin bead of cyanoacrylate adhesive around the periphery of the wound. Following application of this type of dressing, the patient may be allowed access to water.

The author prefers a paramedian incision for celiotomy in lizards to avoid damage to the ventral abdominal vein; others prefer a ventral midline incision. The ventral abdominal vein is suspended by a short ligament and, with careful dissection, the ventral midline may be incised without causing damage to the vessel.[1] It is suggested that there may be more hemorrhage following incision of the muscle through a paramedian incision. Since the skin is the main holding layer for closure of the celiotomy incision, wound healing does not appear to be affected by whether the incision is ventral midline or paramedian.

For celiotomy in chelonians, a three-sided plastron osteotomy is preferred. The fourth (caudal) side of the osteotomy is only partially cut and scored enough to be cracked, allowing the segment of plastron to be reflected caudally. This may provide some preservation of blood flow to the osteotomized segment through the cracked dermal bone. Additionally, as the body wall is subperiosteally elevated from the inner surface of the plastron and reflected caudally, the attachments of the pelvic musculature to the plastron should be preserved to maintain the periosteal blood supply to the plastron that has been cut. The caudal border of the plastron is only cracked and not completely cut; the muscular attachments continue to provide blood supply to the segment of bone. Once the body wall is exposed, the incision for the celiotomy is made in the midline. A flap technique, which results in destruction of the paramedian venous sinuses, is not recommended. Following closure of the ventral midline incision, the flap of plastron is replaced and secured using the technique described.

Green iguanas have become the most popular reptile pet in the United States. Since this article was published, reproductive surgery in green iguanas has become common. Related to many factors such as lack of appropriate nesting material, inadequate dietary calcium, and improper husbandry,[2] dystocia frequently requires surgery. Ovariohysterectomy may be recommended to prevent future episodes of dystocia. The technique has been described and is best accomplished using hemostatic clips (Hemoclips™; Solvay Animal Health, Mendota Heights, MN). The entire reproductive tract is removed, including both ovaries and both oviducts. In cases of postovulatory egg binding, the vessels that supply the oviduct are enlarged and numerous. Hemostasis is maintained by applying two clips to each vessel and transecting the vessel between clips. One clip will leave with the reproductive tract and the other will remain with the patient.

Many adult male green iguanas develop aggressive behaviors following sexual maturity, making them unacceptable pets as they can cause serious injury to their owners. Aggressive behavior has been linked to high testosterone levels and decreases following castration in many lizard species. Castration, performed through a ventral midline celiotomy, appears to reduce aggression in approximately 50% of green iguanas. The testicles are located dorsally in the middle of the abdomen and are adhered to the renal vein on each side. The attachment is short but contains small blood vessels that supply the testis. The testis is gently lifted to expose this short attachment. A hemostatic clip is placed between the renal vein and the testis. The tissue distal to the clip is then transected and the testis removed. With large testicles, two or more clips may be required. The adrenal glands are also attached to the renal veins in the same area as the testicles and must be avoided. It is im-

(continues on page 91)

Boas and Pythons

Justin Corliss
Veterinary Assistant and Amateur Herpetologist
Stroudsburg, Pennsylvania

Boas (Figure 1) and pythons (Figures 2 and 3) have become very popular reptile pets (Table I) and are frequently offered for sale in the pet trade. Boas are the smallest of the large tropical snakes and normally range from two to eight feet in length. Some boas, however, may possibly reach 13 feet. Pythons are the largest snakes and range from 3 to 27 or more feet in length. Boas and pythons are heavy-bodied snakes and are easily recognized by their color and pattern variations.

Boas are ovoviviparous (i.e., live bearing, producing 15 to 45 young at a time), crepuscular to nocturnal, terrestrial to arboreal, and basically new-world tropical snakes. Pythons are oviparous (i.e., egg laying, producing 3 to 100 eggs at a time), crepuscular to nocturnal, terrestrial to semiaquatic, and are rarely arboreal. In general, most pythons are from the Asian subcontinent, Australia, and Africa.

The diet of boas and pythons primarily consists of small to large mammals. When in captivity, boas and pythons are fed a diet that progresses from mice to rats to larger food/prey items. These snakes grow very rapidly when young and often eat more than once a week. Boas and pythons can go for long periods without food. This, however, normally depends on such factors as activity, breeding cycles, and yearly seasonal changes.

Boas tend to have small scales on their head in comparison with the large platelike scales of pythons. In the pelvic region, boas and pythons have two clawlike vestigial limbs (also known as anal or pelvic spurs) (Figure 4), one on each side of the cloaca. Males use these claws to stimulate females during mating. Many species of boas and pythons also have heat pits on the upper and/or lower jaws, which are used for prey identification based on temperature.

Thermoregulation

Like all snakes, boas and pythons require an external heat source for thermoregulation. Without optimum body temperature, all metabolic functions are reduced. These snakes should be provided with an ambient temperature between 82°F and 95°F with slight humidity depending on species. When handling reptiles in the veterinary practice, technicians should remember that drastic temperature fluctuations of any kind can severely affect the reptilian immune system. A warm treatment room as well as a warm treatment table must be provided. A cold, metal treatment table is not appropriate for snakes or any other reptile. A heated blanket or warm water pad should be used on countertops and treatment tables when reptiles are handled.

In relation to diet, if proper temperatures are not provided, ingested food will rot in the stomach when the metabolic rate of the snake drops with decreasing temperatures. Regurgitated food is a common problem associated with boas and pythons and is usually attributed to an inadequate heat supply. Heat can be provided in a number of ways. The most common method is an under-the-cage heating pad. Such pads warm the surface of the cage and provide warm, rising air directly above the pad and in the general vicinity. Ceramic heat lamps can also be used; however, direct access to these lamps by the snake must be avoided to prevent thermal burns. Open or screen-topped cages are problematic in terms of controlling cold air flow, which can be detrimental. Upper or lower respiratory infection by *Pseudomonas* is commonly caused by improper heating and drastic and/or prolonged temperature reductions.

Diet

Boas and pythons eat small to large mammals. Constrictors grab prey with an open mouth and quickly wrap their coils around the prey to suffocate it by constriction. Prey are then swallowed whole. Owners of boas should feed their snakes humanely prekilled food; this prevents the possibility of injury to the snake by live prey. Punctures, lacerations, trauma, and death to a snake can occur if offered live prey. While a snake is undergoing ecdysis (shedding), it should not be offered any food. Ecdysis causes the ocular scales to cloud and become opaque, reducing everything in the snake's field of vision to shadows. The offering of a food item during this time can cause considerable stress to a snake. It should be noted that the primary sensory perception of the snake is based on olfactory senses, not visual, as their eyesight is generally poor.

Prey selection in captivity is relatively basic for boas and pythons; rodents comprise most of the common diet. As boas and pythons grow, their diet should graduate from mice to small rats, large rats, and other large prey. Other rodents may be used if accepted by the snake. Prey identification, however, may be an important factor for accep-

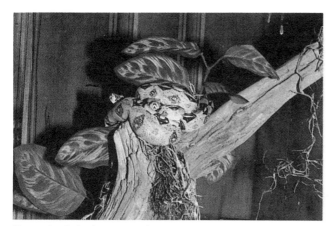
Figure 1—Baby boa constrictors.

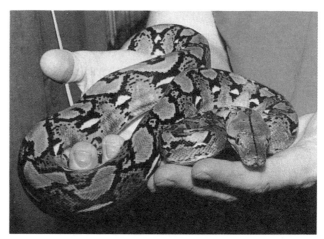
Figure 2—Baby reticulated python.

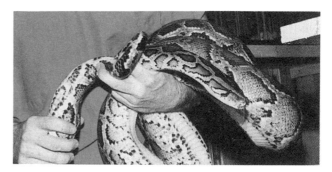
Figure 3—Burmese python.

tance. If the snake is not commonly fed alternate prey, it may not eat. The "prekilled prey offering rule" should always be in effect when snakes are fed vertebrate prey. Some snakes will eat chicks and other small fowl. There is no need for any dietary supplements or vitamin additives to the diet of large snakes as long as they receive quality food or prey. If the quality of prey is lacking, the diet of the prey should be improved to best accommodate the snake.

The size of a snake prescribes the basic requirements of food or prey selection. The first aspect of prey selection is based on the relative girth of a snake. A snake can ingest prey that is equal to its largest point of girth. The size of a snake's head is irrelevant due to its ability to separate its lower jaws in the front, and the skin of its chin and neck easily stretch to accommodate prey items. The stomach of a snake comprises approximately one fifth to one quarter of its overall length. If a snake is four feet in length, two or more small rats (based on equal girth) laid end-to-end that do not exceed one foot would be a sufficient amount of food.

Feeding regimens for large snakes vary in relation to age and size. Boas and pythons grow very rapidly during the first two years. As snakes reach sexual maturity during the third year, growth rate slows down. A juvenile snake may be fed one or more times per week. In adult snakes, the frequency of feeding may change to as little as once or twice a year. In general, small snakes are fed aproximately once a week whereas extremely large snakes are fed once or twice a year. Pet boas and pythons are usually fed once a week to once a month depending on size. A good guide in terms of when snakes should be fed is to wait for the snake to pass fecal matter (not urates) from a previous meal. Once fecal matter has been passed, the snake can be offered prekilled prey items one or two days later. As mentioned, snakes should never be fed during ecdysis.

Most snakes recognize their food/prey items by smell or heat radiation. This can be a very important factor when handling snakes and reptiles in the veterinary practice. It is important for technicians to wash their hands before and immediately after handling any pet. This is also true when handling reptiles. If a technician handles any animal (e.g., a rabbit) that smells like a food/prey item before handling a boa or python, he or she may be treated like a food item by the snake. A quick bite and then an attempt at constriction of the hand or arm may occur. Common sense should be used at all times when handling these snakes.

Basic Husbandry

Because boas and pythons have been kept and bred in captivity for many years, there are numerous books in the retail pet trade that provide extensive information on captive husbandry and propagation of these snakes. In general, a sturdy and large cage should be provided for large snakes. A hiding place, a water bowl for drinking only, and a climbing feature should also be provided. Heat is, of course, a primary concern and should be amply addressed.

Cage cleanliness is very important and easy to address because boas and pythons defecate infrequently compared with mammals. Bedding/substrate materials are commercially available; however, not all are sufficient. Pine or cedar shavings are not a good substrate due to phenol con-

TABLE I
Common Pet Boas and Pythons

Common Name	Genus and Species	Length (Feet)	Habitat	Origin
Boa constrictor	*Boa constrictor* species	5–13	T/A	South America
Dumerli's boa	*Acrantophis dumerili*	4–5	T/A	Madagascar
Emerald-green tree boa	*Corallus canius*	4–6	A	South America
Pacific tree boa	*Candoia* species	3–5	A	Pacific Islands
Rainbow boa	*Epicrates cenchria*	4–5	T/A	South America
Rosy boa	*Lichanura* species	2–4	T	Southwestern United States
Rubber boa	*Charnia* species	2–4	T	Southwestern United States
Sand boa	*Eryx* species	1–2	S/T	Middle East
African rock python	*Python sebae*	8–18	T	East Africa
Ball python	*Python regius*	2–4	T	West Africa
Blood python	*Python curtis*	2–4	T	Pacific and Malaysian Islands
Burmese python	*Python molurus bivittatus*	8–16	T	Burma
Green tree python	*Morelia viridis*	4–7	A	Thailand, South Asia, and North Australia
Reticulated python	*Python reticulatus*	12–28	AQ/T	Philippine Islands and Pacific Archipelago

Key: A = arboreal, AQ = aquatic, S = subterrestrial, T = terrestrial.

tent. Long-term aspiration has been linked to crystallization of phenols in the lungs. Corncob bedding tends to harbor bacteria and produces excessive fungal growth when wet. In addition, if corncob is ingested during feeding, it can swell and cause a blockage or impaction in the digestive tract of the snake. The best substrate is shredded newspaper. Newspaper is not aesthetically pleasing to most people; therefore, the alternative and safe wood product is aspen shavings. These shavings have been used successfully for many years without problems. Sand is acceptable to be used for the genera *Eryx*, *Charnia*, and *Lichanura* but should otherwise be avoided.

As previously mentioned, many boas and pythons are crepuscular to nocturnal reptiles, which means they are most active during the early evening, night, and morning. A hiding place is required for security during periods of inactivity. An overhead light that simply regulates the proper photo (daylight) period would be sufficient. There is no need for any type of specialized light for boas and pythons; however, a black light may be used during the evening for viewing.

Continuous ambient temperatures must be provided at all times. There are many ways to provide this requirement because of the availability of many commercial products. Reptiles in captivity need a continuous ambient temperature in their *entire* environment. There is, however, a need for a warm and a cool place. The cool place may simply be 8°F to 12°F lower in temperature and is normally out of the way of any direct heating source. This modification in environment is required for proper thermoregulation. A pool of water should not be part of the caging environment. Heat rocks are very inadequate heat sources

and should be avoided. This type of heat source is very local and insufficient for providing enough heat to warm an environment.

Common Maladies

Most ailments of large snakes are often related to improper husbandry practices. Often, when a boa or python is handled, common maladies can be observed. The general appearance of a healthy snake is that of an alert and strong animal. When presented to a veterinary practice, a healthy snake should flick its tongue repeatedly to sense its new environment. It should also grasp the handler very tightly. A soft or rubbery feel to boas, pythons, or any snake is not normal and could be related to obesity and general immunosuppression.

Upper and lower respiratory disorders have been previously mentioned. These conditions are normally caused by a reduction in the immune system. This reduction is associated with a drop in temperature as metabolic processes are unable to eliminate infectious agents. A snake with an upper or lower respiratory disorder commonly has bubbles or a mucous buildup around the nostrils and/or mouth, which is normally accompanied by gasping or wheezing.

Necrotic stomatitis or mouth rot is a common malady that invades the oral cavity. Mouth rot occurs around the gums and throughout the oral cavity. It is usually caused by infection due to unsanitary conditions (e.g., dirty water), a broken tooth, abrasion or impaction to the oral cavity, or a piece of foreign matter that gets stuck in the mouth. Mouth rot is easily identified by its yellowish "cheeselike" appearance in and around the base of the jaws. Stomatitis can become so caked in the upper oral

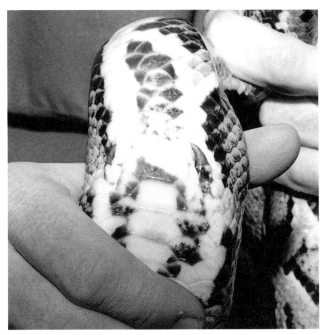

Figure 4—Male Burmese python showing vestigial limbs.

cavity that it may prevent normal breathing and therefore be confused with *Pseudomonas* infection. Necrotic stomatitis can normally be treated if diagnosed early.

Mites and ticks are common ectoparasitic problems, but the prevalence of these parasites has dwindled due to more snakes being bred in captivity. Ticks with blood-swollen abdomens can be found protruding from under the scales of snakes. Ticks should be soaked with alcohol and removed with tweezers. Mites (particularly *Ophionyssus* species) are smaller blood-sucking parasites. The presence of mites can be detected by spreading the scales, particularly the inframaxillary and gular scales (which are normally white with pink skin below) on a snake's bottom jaw, with the thumbs. Mites also tend to invade the ventral chutes. If small flecks of black are under the scales, this may indicate the presence of mites. Treatment of snakes with mite infestation varies; however, most methods include drowning the ectoparasites in such solutions as water or vegetable oil or by using a dichlorovinyl dimethyl phosphate-based pest strip. This strip should only be handled by an experienced veterinarian or herpetologist. Severe infections of ectoparasites can cause blood-borne parasitic infections, such as *Aeromonas* septicemia, and eventually lead to the death of the pet snake. Mites and ticks can be highly mobile; therefore, careful handling and quarantine of all reptiles in the veterinary practice is required.

Incomplete shedding and retained ocular scales (eye caps) are also common problems. Ecdysis is required for growth and is a sign of good health. Improper or incomplete sheds can lead to severe dermal infections and localized trauma. Most incomplete sheds are caused by a dry environment or poor diet. Boas and pythons should be soaked in water before shedding; this aids in moisturizing the skin prior to ecdysis. If a boa or python has a retained ocular scale or partial shed, the snake should be soaked in warm water. The skin is then rubbed off gently as it absorbs the water. Eye caps should be removed by an experienced veterinarian. The lack of humidity or a soaking regimen often leads to shedding problems.

Burns and dermal abrasions are problems associated with poor caging and/or heating systems. Some snakes have been known to escape their cage and seek heat by way of a furnace or electric water heater. These sources of heat may cause severe trauma to affected areas. Heat rock elements have been known to malfunction, thus producing an excessive hot spot that, in turn, produces thermal burns. Heat lamps, if used, should always be placed out of range of the snake.

Nose rubbing is a very common problem with wild-caught boas and pythons that are trying to escape or are seeking security. The rostral, nasal, and supraocular scales at the tip of the snout can become severely damaged, and nostrils can be rubbed down to the bone. Most often, these abrasions are exacerbated when the snake rubs its nose on wire or mesh screening used in the cage. Prevention of this problem is difficult; however, in time, the abrasions will heal. A radical change in the caging environment may be considered if the problem is severe. Boas and pythons require a hiding place to promote security and reduce stress in the animal; a hiding place may reduce the incidence of nose rubbing.

Blisters occur in snakes that are allowed to soak for prolonged periods of time or whose environments are excessively damp. In such instances, water seeps below the scales and is trapped, preventing air from getting in. Blisters can be identified during a visual inspection of the subcaudal chutes. These large, wide scales are normally opaque or white in appearance. Blistering causes the scales to appear enlarged and filled with fluid. In extreme cases, septicemia has been known to occur. Sometimes blood will be evident if it has progressed to septicemic conditions. A change in husbandry conditions to provide for a drier environment is often curative.

Endoparasites, commonly the roundworm and tapeworm, occur very frequently in wild-caught snakes and some captive raised snakes. Although normally not a serious problem in boas and pythons, stress and a general immune deficiency caused by other factors can lead to anemia and a general illness that results in death. Most endoparasites can be detected via a fecal examination. Protozoan infections are rare; however, dysentery has been caused by the protozoan *Entamoeba invadens* in some captive snakes.

Bacterial infections caused by *Salmonella* have been isolated in boas. The Centers for Disease Control have identified many new and rarely seen species of *Salmonella* recently associated with salmonellosis that was triggered by direct and indirect contact with reptiles. The need for proper hygiene when handling all types of reptiles cannot be understated; this holds true for veterinary technicians as well as pet owners. Proper hygiene is especially important when cleaning cages and handling feces. Pet owners who are immunosuppressed or have small children should be informed of the possible risk of zoonosis.

Stress

Stress has been associated primarily with the suppression of the immune system, thus causing other maladies to arise and take control of boas and pythons. The cause of stress is related to many factors, many of which must be weighed and considered when evaluating a pet snake. Improper caging, the lack of hiding spaces, live feeding, irregular feeding schedules, extended or prolonged photo periods, other cage mates, and many other factors can contribute to and cause stress. A general evaluation of husbandry practices of snake owners should be done to isolate any possible causes of stress on the animal. Reducing stress leads to the well-being of the snake in its captive environment.

Restraint

In general, boas and most pythons are very docile animals and are easy to control. Snakes should be grasped firmly behind the head with one hand while the other hand supports the rest of the animal. Large boas and pythons may require the assistance of other technicians. Shoulders are commonly used to provide a support surface for a large snake; however, in the veterinary practice, this should be avoided. Many large snakes have the ability to hold on very tightly during an examination and may slightly strangle an unsavvy technician. When drugs are administered, additional help may be needed to restrain a snake as it will instinctively coil during what may be perceived as an act of aggression.

Quarantine

It is necessary for veterinary practices that keep reptiles for extended periods to have a quarantine area. All reptiles should be housed separately from each other and in sterile conditions. When boas and pythons are kept overnight or for extended periods, all aspects of normal reptile husbandry should be provided. Heat, water, hiding places, and proper caging are imperative. Reptiles should also be isolated from other areas (e.g., the kennel) that house small animals or any rodents. The odor of food/prey may cause boas and pythons to search and seek aggressively for what

it believes may be prey; this may cause stress and other related problems.

Conclusion

In general, boas and pythons make excellent pets. They do not shed hair or make noise. In terms of feeding, they are very undemanding and far less expensive to feed than mammals. Boas and pythons do not scratch furniture or mark their territory. Snakes, like all reptiles, do not have hair, thus making them excellent pets for people with hair-related allergies. Due to these reasons and some inexplicable attraction to reptiles and large snakes, an enormous pet culture based around reptiles has arisen in the United States. Many veterinary practices do not currently handle reptiles and may have to do so to meet the demand. Technicians should be well informed and read as much as possible on reptiles and amphibians because they have become popular pets.

Acknowledgment

The author would like to thank photographer Steven Hauser for his assistance in taking photographs for this column.

Bibliography

Advanced Vivarium Systems, *General Care and Maintenance Series*. Lakeside, CA.
Bauchot R: *Snakes, A Natural History*. New York, NY, Sterling Publishing Co, 1994.
Coborn J: *The Atlas of Snakes of the World*. Neptune City, NJ, TFH Publications, 1991.
Frye F: *Reptile Care: An Atlas of Diseases and Treatments*. Neptune City, NJ, TFH Publications, 1990.
Mader D: *Reptile Medicine and Surgery*. Philadelphia, WB Saunders Co, 1996.
Obst J, et al: *The Completely Illustrated Atlas of Reptiles and Amphibians*. Neptune City, TFH Publications, 1988.
Ross R, Marzec G: *The Reproductive Husbandry of Pythons & Boas*. Stanford, CA, Institute of Herpetological Research, 1990.
Zug G: *Herpetology*. San Diego, CA, Academic Press, 1993. □

UPDATE

As the incidence of large boids held in captivity has increased, so too has scientific review of the myriad viral, bacterial, pathogenic, and genetic disorders and maladies experienced by these snakes. Proper and practicable husbandry of boas and pythons should be first and foremost in their care and medical management. The practitioners and clinicians who may encounter reptiles in practice will benefit from specific resources to supplement their experience. A number of texts have become available in the past few years and are listed in the bibliography. Certain professional organizations, such as the Association of Reptilian and Amphibian Veterinarians and the Society for the Study of Amphibians and Reptiles, are dedicated to the promotion of reptilian medicine practices. Boas and pythons will continue to remain in our presence, as they have for eons. The relevance of the information and scientific study we maintain will help dictate the future of these specialized animals.

Clinical Management of Tortoises

KEY FACTS

- Correction of poor husbandry techniques is the first step in medical management of tortoises.
- Maintaining tortoises in the preferred optimum temperature range of 26° to 32 °C (79° to 90 °F) is essential for normal physiologic function.
- Succinylcholine chloride at a dose of 0.25 to 1.5 mg/kg is safe and effective for immobilizing tortoises to facilitate diagnostic or therapeutic manipulations.
- An aggressive diagnostic approach and concomitant supportive treatment of moribund tortoises must take precedence over broad-spectrum therapy.
- The diagnostic procedures and therapeutic agents applicable to tortoises parallel those used in other species.

Jacksonville Zoological Park
Jacksonville, Florida
C. Douglas Page, DVM

University of Florida
Michele Mautino, MS, DVM

ORTOISES are an unusual and fascinating group of animals. Their unique anatomy and behavioral responses complicate clinical assessment and the performance of routine diagnostic and therapeutic procedures. Despite their unique characteristics, however, the diagnostic procedures and therapeutic agents applicable to tortoises parallel those used in other species. This article presents basic guidelines and techniques for proper husbandry, chemical restraint, and clinical management of tortoises.

TORTOISE HUSBANDRY

Correction of poor husbandry is often the first step in proper medical management of tortoises.[1,2] In addition to providing veterinary care, the clinician can be a valuable source of husbandry information for experienced as well as novice herpetologists.

Housing and Substrate

Small tortoises can be housed in glass aquariums with newspaper, pea-sized gravel, or alfalfa pellets as substrate. Newspaper is readily available; however, it does not absorb the large volumes of urine voided and must be changed frequently. Pea-sized gravel allows maintenance of a dry surface; but tortoises may accidentally ingest the gravel, and gravel may allow nitrogenous waste to accumulate and to irritate oral and nasal mucous membranes. Alfalfa pellets, such as rabbit ration, are absorbent and easily digested if consumed but must be changed regularly.

Sand, ground corncob, or resinous wood chips should not be used as substrate for housing tortoises. Sand is easily ingested and can cause intestinal obstruction. Ground corncob is hygroscopic and can dehydrate juvenile tortoises as well as cause obstruction if ingested. Resinous wood chips can cause localized or systemic toxicity.[3]

Large tortoises or groups of smaller tortoises are readily housed in galvanized troughs used to water livestock. Wooden boxes with open tops also make excellent cages. The wood should be sealed or painted to prevent absorption of excrement and to facilitate cleaning and disinfection. Dilute (3%) sodium hypochlorite solution is an effective and safe disinfectant for use on cages, water bowls, and other inanimate objects in the tortoise's environment. Any of the previously discussed substrates are suitable for these larger cages.

Whenever possible, outdoor pens that provide natural forage should be used; however, juvenile tortoises left unattended in outdoor pens are subject to predation. Regardless of the type of housing used, a shelter or hide box should be provided as a refuge for the tortoise.

Nutrition

Tortoises are predominantly herbivorous but accept certain other food items in their diet. Feed preparation techniques and presentation are crucial to consumption of a balanced diet. The ingredients must be chopped to a suitable size and then thoroughly mixed together. It is not unusual for a tortoise to select and ingest only favorite food items, thus consuming an unbalanced diet.

The composition of the standard tortoise diet used at the Jacksonville Zoo is presented in the box on page 83[4]; additional information on diets is available in the literature.[3] The prepared diet should be offered two times per week; greens, bean sprouts, or natural vegetation should be made available on alternate days. Vitamin and mineral supplements may be added but should not substitute for a properly balanced diet; oversupplementation must be avoided.

Water may be provided at all times, or the tortoise can be soaked in a shallow stand of water 1 to 2 cm deep for 15 to 30 minutes every other day.

Temperature, Humidity, and Lighting

Like all ectotherms, tortoises require a warm environment in order to maintain a functional and comfortable body temperature. The preferred optimum temperature range (POTR) for most tortoises is 26° to 32°C (79° to 90°F). Maintaining the animal in this range or preferably providing a temperature gradient in the cage is essential for normal physiologic function.[5] Infrared heat lamps suspended above the cage are an excellent heat source for tortoises of all sizes. Heat lamps provide a thermal gradient without lowering the humidity of the surrounding air.

A RELATIVE HUMIDITY of 55% to 65% is adequate for most tortoise species. If supplemental heat is provided by radiant or forced-air heaters to maintain the preferred optimum temperature range during winter months, low humidity and high temperature are likely to occur. These conditions can result in dehydration, which leads to constipation and damage to the oculonasal mucosa and predisposes the tortoise to secondary bacterial infections.

Vaporizers can be used to increase humidity, or the surface area of the water source in the enclosure can be increased. As mentioned, infrared lights provide excellent focal heat sources without decreasing environmental humidity. Excessive moisture in the environment can also be detrimental and result in fungal infections of the integument and lower respiratory tract.[3]

A balanced light–dark cycle (12 hours of light:12 hours of darkness) provides a suitable photoperiod for tortoises. Extremes in either phase constitute a stressor and are to be avoided. The type of lighting is not critical as long as it is within the range of visible wavelengths.[5] The exclusive use of indoor ultraviolet lighting as a source of photobiogenesis for cholecalciferol (vitamin D₃) is controversial. Exposure to natural sunlight is important to the well-being of tortoises.

CLINICAL ASSESSMENT
Anamnesis

The anamnesis must include a review of the conditions under which the patient has been kept, including cage de-

sign, environmental temperature, humidity, and photoperiod. The patient's diet should also be assessed with emphasis on the type of diet offered, frequency of feeding, amount normally consumed, and source and storage of the diet as well as frequency of watering or soaking. Poor husbandry techniques should be addressed in the treatment strategy. The condition of other animals in the collection as well as the performance of proper quarantine procedures should be considered.

SPECIFIC INFORMATION on the patient should include a history of previous disease problems, growth or weight changes, current attitude and behavior, appetite, food consumption, frequency of defecation, and consistency of feces. The origin of the tortoise, when it was acquired, and a description of its condition on acquisition are as important as the reason for presentation.

Recently acquired tortoises from pet shops or other dealers have often been subjected to stressful overcrowding and poor husbandry, which predispose the animals to parasites and infectious diseases. In contrast, captive-born animals acquired from knowledgeable herpetologists may be in excellent condition. Determining the initial condition of the animal and the time of acquisition are valuable in assessing the chronicity of the problem and the source of mismanagement.

Physical Examination

The physical examination should begin with assessment of body weight and the length of the dorsal shell (carapace). These measurements should be compared with reported data.[6] After examining several tortoises of a given size, the clinician will develop an ability to judge what body weight is normal.

The carapace, plastron (ventral shell), and integument should be evaluated for evidence of trauma, brightness of color, and presence of ectoparasites. If the tortoise presents its head, skin turgor over the dorsal aspect of the neck and the brightness and position of the globe in the orbit are useful in assessing the state of hydration. Structures of the eye, including the palpebrae and membrana nictitans, should be examined. Ocular, nasal, or oral discharge should be recorded. The tympanic membrane, which is located caudal to the orbit, should be inspected for swelling.

Although auscultation of the heart and lungs is not possible, the respiratory pattern can be assessed by observing the subtle forelimb movement, which creates a respiratory bellow effect in the absence of a diaphragm. Such abnormalities as open-mouthed breathing, wheezing, and a palpable rattle associated with respiration indicate respiratory tract disease.

The patient's motor function should be assessed. If the patient is willing to walk, its ambulation should be evaluated. A healthy tortoise elevates its plastron and keeps it parallel to the ground when walking. Abnormal locomotion may indicate a neuropathy, a musculoskeletal problem, or generalized weakness. All limbs should be assessed by palpation, and an attempt should be made to extend the limbs for further evaluation of muscle tone and strength. Chemical restraint of the tortoise may be necessary to facilitate clinical examination and diagnostic or therapeutic manipulations.

Restraint

Commonly recommended sedatives and anesthetics have variable effects on tortoises. Induction of anesthesia with volatile agents may be ineffective because tortoises may demonstrate apnea for extended periods. The most commonly used injectable anesthetic agent is ketamine hydrochloride at a dose of 20 to 80 mg/kg administered intramuscularly. Induction time may be more than one hour, and recovery time can be as long as 48 hours. Ketamine hydrochloride is a potentially dangerous drug, however, especially when administered to dehydrated and debilitated tortoises.[3]

Succinylcholine chloride is a depolarizing skeletal muscle relaxant that induces flaccid paralysis in tortoises. In our experience, succinylcholine chloride is the safest currently available drug to immobilize tortoises and facilitate clinical examination and manipulation. Immobilization also aids in positioning of the tortoise for radiographs of the extremities, obtaining diagnostic samples, and performing endotracheal intubation. An intramuscular dose of 0.25 to 1.5 mg/kg is effective for most tortoise species. The appropriate dose depends on the species, size, and health status of the patient.[7-9]

The use of reversible, nondepolarizing neuromuscular blocking agents in tortoises is being investigated and may be an alternative for chemical restraint of the tortoise.

Succinylcholine chloride should be administered intramuscularly in the thoracic limbs rather than the pelvic limbs to avoid possible drug transport through the renal portal system, which receives venous drainage from the pelvic limbs. If the drug is administered to the pelvic limbs, the patient's response to the drug may be unpredictable because of altered drug clearance from the vascular system.

Onset of action of intramuscular succinylcholine chloride varies from 20 to 45 minutes depending on the dose and on the condition of the individual tortoise. If the desired effect is not achieved with the initial dose, subsequent doses should not be given for at least 24 hours to avoid lethal overdose.

Succinylcholine chloride paralyzes the animal without providing analgesia; it should therefore be used in conjunction with an anesthetic agent for painful procedures. Depending on the extent of paralysis, the animal may require respiratory assistance by endotracheal intubation with positive-pressure ventilation or by pumping of the forelimbs to simulate the normal respiratory motion. Most tortoises recover from the drug sufficiently by one hour from the onset of action so that ventilatory assistance is no longer required.

One of the authors (CDP) has experienced problems with succinyl choline chloride at a dosage greater than 1.0 mg/kg. Two apparently healthy tortoises died following immobilization with this drug. Tiletamine plus zolazepam (Telazol) at a dose of 4 to 5 mg/kg IM may be used to facilitate diagnostic procedures or intubation.[9a]

Diagnostic Procedures

The reason for presentation and additional problems revealed by examination offer the clinician direction regarding applicable diagnostic procedures. Hypophagia, a common presenting sign, should be considered a serious problem because it is often associated with poor husbandry or systemic disease. The solution may involve correction of management practices, or it may require a barrage of diagnostic tests. More specific signs, such as oculonasal discharge or diarrhea, enable the clinician to be more selective in the diagnostic approach.

An aggressive diagnostic approach and concomitant supportive treatment of moribund patients must take precedence over broad-spectrum therapy. It must be emphasized that delaying diagnostic assessment and therapy until the tortoise is debilitated and easily manipulable worsens the prognosis considerably.

Parasitologic Examination

Tortoises should be examined for ectoparasites, particularly ticks, which may be found attached to the shell or integument covering the head, neck, and limbs. Mites are seldom a problem in tortoises. In tortoises, hemoparasites are rare and their clinical significance is unclear; in most cases, clinical signs (e.g., anemia) attributable to these parasites are absent even in severe infestations.[3]

Conventional diagnostic techniques can be used to investigate the presence of intestinal parasites. A direct fecal smear is useful for detecting such protozoa as amebae or flagellates. Flagellates are part of the normal intestinal flora; however, an increase in their number may signal primary or secondary gastrointestinal disease. Fecal flotation should be used to detect helminthiasis. If clinical signs indicate a gastrointestinal problem and a fresh fecal sample is not available, a cloacal lavage with normal saline should be performed to screen for parasites.

The helminth parasite ova found most commonly in the feces of tortoises are nematodes; cestode and trematode ova are found only rarely. Typically, helminthiasis is found in newly imported, wild-caught animals. Amebiasis is also common in recently imported tortoises[10] but may be associated with captive animals maintained on a high-carbohydrate diet, which allows amebae to proliferate rapidly.

Obtaining a blood sample from the tortoise patient can be an intimidating procedure for the clinician. Several peripheral sites for blood collection have been described in the literature[3,9]; but in our experience, the jugular vein provides the best source for blood samples that are of adequate volume and not diluted with lymph.

Blood smears should be made immediately after sample collection, preferably with blood collected without

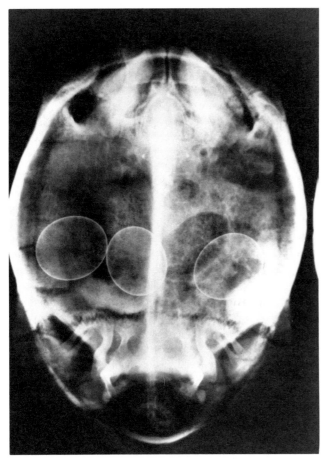

Figure 1—Radiograph of a female radiated tortoise (dorsoventral view). Note the skeletal structure, ceolomic cavity, and calcified eggs.

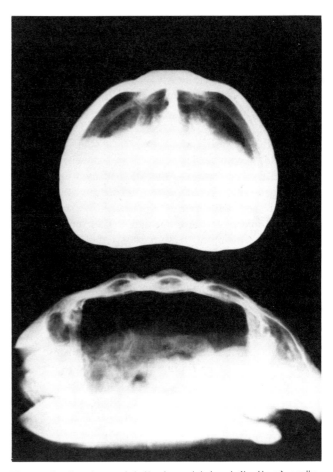

Figure 2—Craniocaudal (*top*) and lateral (*bottom*) radiographic views of a star tortoise. Note the skeletal structure and lung fields.

anticoagulant. The anticoagulant ethylenediaminetetraacetic acid (EDTA) lyses tortoise erythrocytes; heparinized blood yields a sample that is suitable for hematology. The sample can be centrifuged and the plasma analyzed for clinical chemistries.

Chemical restraint may be required for blood sampling except in weak or moribund patients. The reason for presentation and the physical findings help the clinician decide whether the diagnostic benefits outweigh the risk associated with chemical restraint. Also, the clinician must be willing to investigate the results and compare them with the scant published data on normal hematologic and serum chemistry values of tortoises.[3,9,11] In general, reptiles do not demonstrate the mechanisms for precise regulation of plasma constituents as do mammals and birds; individual variation may thus further complicate interpretation of laboratory results.

Microbiology

The clinician should not hesitate to perform bacterial and fungal cultures of skin or shell lesions, oculonasal discharge, feces, or cloacal swabs. Acquiring samples from deeper within the coelomic cavity, such as a tracheal aspirate or gastric lavage, requires chemical restraint. All bacterial isolates should be tested for antibiotic sensitivity. Cytologic evaluation and Gram staining of exudates and feces are quick screening methods for detecting infectious bacterial or fungal agents.

Radiology

Radiography is a valuable diagnostic aid for use in tortoises because it permits assessment of organ systems that are easily palpable in mammals. In most cases, whole-body views of unrestrained patients can be obtained. Dorsoventral, lateral, and craniocaudal projections are useful in investigating intracoelomic problems (Figures 1 and 2). The craniocaudal view is most useful for evaluating lung fields. The size of the tortoise and the equipment available dictate the radiographic technique.[12,13]

THERAPY
Fluid Therapy

Sick tortoises invariably have some degree of dehydration. The type of fluids used and the route of administration depend on the patient's condition and the accessibility of the jugular vein. The volume of fluid administered at any given time should not exceed 5% of the tortoise's body weight. Intravenous fluid administration should not exceed

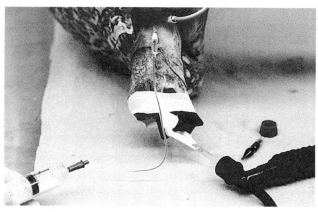

Figure 3—Leopard tortoise maintained under anesthesia via endotracheal intubation. The patient has a jugular catheter and an esophagostomy tube.

PREPARED TORTOISE DIET USED AT THE JACKSONVILLE ZOOLOGICAL PARK

8 cups alfalfa-based herbivore pellets, 15% to 16% protein.
8 cups sweet potatoes (finely chopped)
8 cups green beans (finely chopped)
8 cups carrots (finely chopped)
8 cups apples (finely chopped)
8 cups bananas (finely chopped)
6 tbsp. dicalcium phosphate powder

Ingredients are mixed and then divided to feed 35 tortoises. Approximately 250 g/kg should be offered. Exposure time should be four to eight hours per feeding.

1 ml/min; this rate of administration should be reserved for severely dehydrated and moribund patients.

Mildly dehydrated tortoises may respond favorably to being soaked in water as described. Subcutaneous fluids can be administered in the flexed forelimb on the dorsal surface or in the area overlying the ischium.

OTHER ROUTES include epicoelomic (which is approached by directing the needle caudally just ventral to the shoulder joint and dorsal to the plastron[5]) and intracoelomic (which is safest to approach just cranial to the hindlimb). Caution must be exercised when administering large amounts of fluids intracoelomically because direct infusion of the bladder or compression of the lungs may occur. Other than by the intravenous route, it is difficult to administer more than 2% to 3% of the body weight in a single dose.

In most instances, isotonic electrolyte solutions are suitable for restoring hydration in tortoises. For hypertonic dehydration, Jarchow prefers a mildly hypotonic solution consisting of two parts 2.5% glucose in 0.45% sodium chloride and one part Ringer's solution or its equivalent.[5]

Nutritional Support

Hypophagia or complete anorexia is common in tortoises that are presented to veterinarians. The chronicity of the problem and the animal's body weight should be considered in assessing the need for nutritional support. Other more urgent problems, such as dehydration and gross mismanagement, should be addressed first.

Basic nutritional support includes injectable vitamin preparations and the use of glucose in the rehydration fluids. Water-soluble vitamins (e.g., B-complex vitamins) should be given intramuscularly daily or every other day; the injection sites should vary to avoid painful swelling. Vitamins may instead be added to the rehydration fluids. The dose depends on the preparation and on the size of the animal.

Some authors believe that vitamin C is helpful if the tortoise has a bacterial infection; the recommended dose is 10 to 20 mg/kg given intramuscularly once daily.[3] A single intramuscular dose of vitamin A and cholecalciferol may be administered at a dose of 11,000 IU/kg and 1650 IU/kg, respectively. Repeat doses of these fat-soluble vitamins or higher initial doses may result in toxicity.

In cases of inanition, gastric intubation may be used to administer nutritional support. Physical or chemical restraint can be used depending on the size and strength of the tortoise. Placement of an esophagostomy tube is an alternative to reduce the stress associated with repeated restraint or immobilization and to permit frequent feeding (Figure 3).[8]

The use of the equine enteral diet, Equiprime®, is more calorically dense than other blended diets, and may be useful for tube feeding moribund tortoises.

THE TECHNIQUE FOR placement of an esophagostomy tube in a tortoise is analogous to placement of a pharyngostomy tube in other animals. General anesthesia or immobilization with succinylcholine chloride in conjunction with deep and superficial local anesthesia is required. The tube is placed to exit the cervical skin caudal to the rami of the mandible; the tube should be sutured to the skin to maintain placement. Soft, flexible polyvinyl

TABLE I
Therapeutic Agents Used in Tortoises[10,14-16]

Drug	Dose Regimen	Comments
Antibacterial		
Amikacin	5 mg/kg intramuscularly every 48 hours for 7 to 14 days	Aminoglycoside; maintain hydration orally or parenterally
Ampicillin	20 mg/kg intramuscularly once daily for 7 to 14 days	May be used concomitantly with aminoglycosides
Carbenicillin	200–400 mg/kg intramuscularly every 48 hours for 7 to 14 days	May be used concomitantly with aminoglycosides; may cause skin sloughing in desert tortoises
Cefotaxime	20–40 mg/kg intramuscularly once daily for 7 to 14 days	May be used concomitantly with aminoglycosides
Chloramphenicol	20 mg/kg intramuscularly or orally twice daily for 7 to 14 days	
Gentamicin	5 mg/kg intramuscularly every 72 hours for 7 to 14 days	Aminoglycoside; maintain hydration orally or parenterally
Trimethoprim–sulfonamide combinations	30 mg/kg intramuscularly or orally every 48 hours for 7 to 14 days	
Antifungal		
Ketoconazole	30 mg/kg orally once daily for two to four weeks	Use of this drug concomitantly with antibiotic therapy may prevent fungal superinfections
Parasiticide		
Metronidazole	Single oral dose of 250 mg/kg; repeat in two weeks	Effective against flagellated protozoans and amebae
Fenbendazole	Single oral dose of 50–100 mg/kg; repeat in two weeks	Effective against nematodes

chloride feeding tubes are well suited for this purpose and cause minimal trauma and discomfort.

A gruel made from commercial monkey biscuit blended in water or strained-vegetable baby foods may be fed via esophagostomy tube or stomach tube. A volume of 10 to 15 ml/kg may be administered once daily in an effort to provide nutritional support to an anorectic tortoise.[5] If an esophagostomy tube is used, it should be flushed with water after each feeding. The tortoise's body temperature should be maintained in the preferred optimum temperature range to encourage normal gastrointestinal function.

Anthelmintics and Antimicrobial Drugs

The pharmacokinetics of these therapeutic agents in tortoises have not been thoroughly researched. The drugs and doses used are often based on extrapolations from doses for mammals and other reptiles. Table I presents drugs and dose regimens commonly used to treat parasitic, bacterial, and mycotic infections in tortoises.[12]

The use of fluoroquinolone, enrofloxacin, at a dose of 5 mg/kg IM q 24 to 48 hr has been reported in treating upper respiratory tract disease in tortoises. It is also effective against gram-negative pathogens, including *Pseudomonas* spp.[17]

CONCLUSION

The clinician can be a source of husbandry information for tortoise owners in addition to providing medical management. Simple diagnostic and therapeutic techniques can be applied to tortoises in a manner analogous to their application in mammals. Therapeutic agents used in tortoises are commonly available drugs administered in dose regimens adapted to the unique physiology of this group of animals. A knowledge of basic techniques and therapeutics enables clinicians to address common problems associated with medical management of tortoises.

About the Authors
Dr. Page is Staff Veterinarian at the Jacksonville Zoological Park in Jacksonville, Florida. Dr. Mautino is affiliated with the Department of Toxicology of the College of Veterinary Medicine, University of Florida, Gainesville, Florida.

(continues on page 237)

Amphibian Husbandry and Medical Care

Terry W. Campbell, DVM, PhD
Colorado State University
Fort Collins, Colorado

The term *amphibian* is derived from the Greek word *amphibios*, which means double life—a reference to the two-stage life cycle of this class of animals. Familiar amphibians include frogs, toads, salamanders, and newts. Most adult amphibians are terrestrial; however, the eggs are laid in water and the larvae are aquatic. The larvae undergo metamorphosis, a process that involves the transformation of the body structure and most organs. During the metamorphosis, the mouth changes to adapt to different food, the gills are replaced by lungs for breathing air, and the eyes and other organs change to adapt to terrestrial life.

Terrestrial amphibians breathe in part through their skin, which is moist and contains a protective slime produced by mucous glands. In some instances, the slime may be poisonous to predators, as with the poison arrow frog of South America. Toads and frogs have special parotid glands behind the eyes that produce a milky, noxious or poisonous secretion. Secretions from the parotid gland of the marine toad (*Bufo marinus*) and the Colorado River toad (*Bufo alvarius*) contain a cardioactive glycoside (bufotoxin) that can be lethal to dogs. Amphibians periodically shed a thin layer of skin, which usually comes off in one piece and is eaten by the animal.

The collection and maintenance of amphibians are regulated by state laws; special permits may be required to possess native amphibians. Importation of amphibians into the United States is restricted by state and federal laws. Species commonly kept as pets are listed in the box.

Orders of Amphibia

The class Amphibia consists of three orders. Order Salientia (the anurans) includes frogs and toads; order Urodela (the caudates) includes salamanders, newts, and sirens; and order Gymnophiona (the apodans) includes rare legless, burrowing amphibians of the tropics. Approximately 2700 species of frogs and toads and 350 species of salamanders are known to exist worldwide.

The anurans have special skeletal adaptations that allow them to jump and hop. They have a short spine, short forelimbs, long hindlimbs, and a specialized pelvis. All adult frogs can swim. True frogs (ranids) have webbing between the toes of the hind feet; tree frogs have pads on the tips of the toes for clinging to leaves.

Most adult frogs and toads have no teeth in the lower jaw. They do, however, have large mouths and modified tongues for capturing prey. The feeding response is triggered by the prey's movement. Larval anurans (tadpoles) have mouth parts adapted for scraping algae off surfaces or for filtering water. The intestinal tract of a tadpole is long to allow digestion of vegetation.

Adult anurans have a Jacobson organ, a specialized smell–taste organ located in the nasal passages, which provides a keen sense of smell. Tadpoles, like fish, have chemoreceptors in the lateral line that are receptive to chemicals in the water. Also like fish, tadpoles have eyes that are adapted to aquatic life. Adult frogs and toads have eyes that are adapted for terrestrial life. The

Originally published in *Veterinary Technician*, Volume 14, Number 10, October 1993

Amphibian Species Commonly Kept as Pets

Bullfrog (*Rana catesbeiana*)
Clawed frogs (*Xenopus* species)
European green tree frog (*Hyla arborea*)
Green toad (*Bufo viridis*)
Green tree frog (*Hyla cinerea*)
Grey tree frog (*Hyla versicolor*)
Japanese fire-bellied newt (*Cynops pyrrhogaster*)
Northern leopard frog (*Rana pipiens*)
Red-bellied newt (*Taricha rivularis*)
Oriental fire-bellied toad (*Bombina orientalis*)
Red-spotted newt (*Notopthalmus viridescens*)
Southern toad (*Bufo terrestris*)
Tiger salamander (*Ambystoma tigrinum*)
Woodhouse's toad (*Bufo woodhousei*)

eyes are large, with slit pupils that are sensitive to light and to movement and that are effective at low light and for night vision. Adult frogs and toads also have a keen sense of hearing. The outer ear is a large, circular membrane (called a tympanum) that is located just behind the eye.

The caudates, unlike the anurans, have long bodies with numerous vertebrae. Salamanders do not have rib cages; their ribs are short and fused to the vertebrae. Specialized bones, called girdles, support the legs. The legs, which are short and extend away from the body, are too weak to lift the body during locomotion.

Salamander larvae have feather-like external gills and four legs. At several weeks of age, the larvae metamorphose into adults that have lungs rather than gills.

The senses of sight, smell, and touch are apparently well developed in salamanders. Aquatic salamanders have small eyes that do not protrude far above the skull; the small bulging eyes of terrestrial salamanders do protrude.

Adult and larval aquatic salamanders catch their prey by sucking it into the mouth. Adult salamanders usually are motionless until the prey approaches; then, stimulated by the prey's movement, the salamander grabs the food.

Care Requirements

Successfully maintaining amphibians in captivity depends on proper attention to temperature, humidity, diet, photoperiod, and housing. To ensure the best care for the pet, the owner of an amphibian should read as much as possible about the natural history of the animal before obtaining it. An attempt should be made to create a captive environment that closely resembles the animal's natural environment.

All amphibians rely on their environment and movements to regulate body temperature. Many species are active at or can tolerate temperatures of 4°C to 28°C (39.2°F to 82.4°F). The body temperature of an active amphibian tends to be lower than that of an active reptile because amphibians, which are active at night or live in microenvironments that are protected from sunlight, do not use the sun for thermoregulation. When temperatures are too low or too high, amphibians become inactive. Although some amphibians are able to change color in response to background color change, such transformation tends to occur in response to temperature: the animal becomes darker if the temperature drops or if the period of exposure to light shortens; it becomes lighter if the temperature or the period of exposure to light increases. A dull appearance to the skin may indicate an unhealthy amphibian.

Aquarium heaters can be used to maintain proper water temperature for aquatic cages; heating the terrestrial cage can be difficult unless it is kept in a room where the temperature is constant. Common methods of warming terrestrial cages include the use of heating pads, cables, or lamps. Horticultural soil-warming cables and heating pads can be used to heat the vivarium. For even heat distribution, soil warmers require sand, soil, or gravel on the cage floor; each product has a recommended depth of material to cover the heater. A barrier is suggested to prevent burrowing (fossorial) species from reaching the heat source.

High humidity is essential for the proper maintenance of amphibians. They should be housed in vivaria that provide aquatic and terrestrial environments. Clean water should be always available. With water constantly present, the humidity level is directly related to temperature and the amount of ventilation. If the temperature is held constant by a thermostat, humidity can then be regulated by the amount of ventilation provided.

The nutritional requirements of amphibians are unknown; most are fed diets based on knowledge of the animal's natural diet. Larval amphibians are herbivorous and feed primarily on algae; adult amphibians are carnivorous. Most captive adult amphibians should be fed twice weekly. Live food is usually necessary because feeding is stimu-

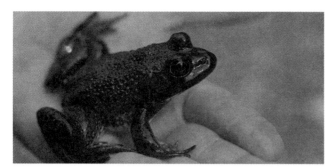

Figure 1—Bullfrog (*Rana catesbeiana*).

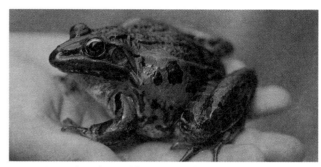

Figure 2—Southern leopard frog (*Rana sphenocephala*).

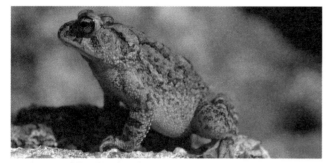

Figure 3—Southern toad (*Bufo terristris*).

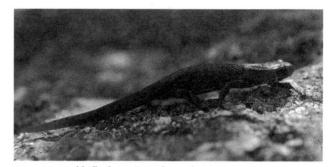

Figure 4—Red-bellied newt (*Taricha rivularis*).

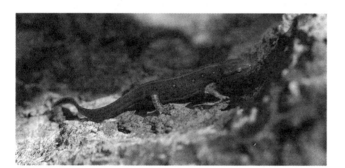

Figure 5—Eastern or red-spotted newt (*Notophthalmus viridescens*).

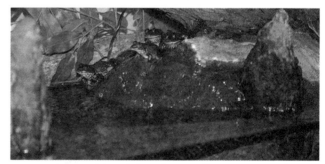

Figure 6—An amphibian habitat that provides an aquatic and terrestrial environment.

lated by the movement of the prey. Some species eventually learn to eat dead prey or prepared foods.

All frogs and toads are predators as adults and feed on invertebrates, primarily insects. Captive frogs and toads eat fruit flies, crickets, mealworms, and other live insects. Large toads eat mice. Aquatic species eat aquatic insects, earthworms, fish, and commercially prepared fish diets. Raw meat can be fed to amphibians, but it requires calcium supplementation—powdered calcium carbonate added at a ratio of 10 milligrams per gram of meat is recommended.

Adult terrestrial salamanders eat earthworms, slugs, insects, and commercially prepared fish diets. Aquatic salamanders can be fed tubifex worms, water fleas, freshwater shrimp, insect larvae, and earthworms. One species of earthworm commonly sold as fish bait is apparently toxic to salamanders. This earthworm, often referred to as a manure worm, is dark red with thin yellow bands near the caudal end.

In regard to the lighting requirements of amphibians, full-spectrum light bulbs are recommended if artificial light is used. The distance from the light source to the animals is an important consideration; for example, artificial light originating 60 centimeters from the cage floor provides only one quarter of the amount of light as the same source positioned 30 centimeters from the cage floor.

A natural photoperiod is best. Amphibians from temperate zones are accustomed to light cycles that vary from 16 hours in the summer to 8 hours in the winter.

Overcrowding should be avoided. Providing a hiding place is important; most amphibians are more likely to thrive if they can hide in or under objects in the cage or have access to soil or sand for burrowing. Aquatic amphibians should be kept in aquaria under conditions suitable for freshwater fish.

Diseases

Amphibians are subjected to a variety of diseases, the most common of which are bacterial and fungal infections, parasitic diseases, toxicities, and neoplasia. Clinical signs include dull color, lethargy, unresponsiveness to tactile stimulation, anorexia, weight loss, edematous limbs, neurologic disorders, and erosions on the head and limbs. Most of the health problems seen in pet amphibians (as with most exotic pets) result from environmental problems associated with poor husbandry practices; therefore, an assessment of the environmental conditions should always be a part of an examination.

A variety of bacteria can cause infection; *Aeromonas* species are most often isolated. Local bacterial infections can spread rapidly and result in fatal septicemia within 24 to 48 hours. Hyperemia, cutaneous hemorrhage (hemorrhage in the skin of the abdomen and appendages of frogs is known as red-leg disease), anorexia, depression, and dulling of the body color are common clinical signs.

Treatment of local and systemic bacterial infections in amphibians involves the use of a variety of antibiotics. Oral tetracycline given at a dosage of 0.16 mg/g twice a day has been recommended. One-hour dips using 50 milligrams of gentamicin per gallon of water or 250 milligrams of nifurpirinol per 10 gallons of water have also been suggested. Increasing the salinity of the water to a maximum of 0.6% may be helpful in aquatic species. Parenteral antibiotics, such as Amikacin given intramuscularly at a dose of 2.5 mg/kg every 72 hours have also been used in amphibians. The use of any medication in amphibians is dependent upon the environmental conditions. Therefore, an amphibian undergoing treatment should be housed under optimal environmental conditions to maximize the effect of the therapy.

Fungal infections often occur on wound sites and abrasions; such infections may appear as white, fluffy patches on the skin. Treatment may include a 2% malachite green bath for 30 to 60 minutes or a five-minute potassium permanganate (1:5000) bath. Systemic antifungal agents may be used on amphibians with systemic mycoses.

Aquatic amphibians are susceptible to the same cutaneous protozoa as are fish. Treatment regimens are the same as for fish. Although they may harbor a variety of internal parasites, amphibians rarely exhibit clinical signs of illness associated with such parasites. Ivermectin given orally or subcutaneously at a dose of 0.2 to 0.4 mg/kg has proven safe and effective in the treatment of nematode infestations in some amphibians. Fenbendazole used at an oral dose of 30 to 50 mg/kg is effective against intestinal nematodes in some species. Substances poisonous to amphibians include pesticides and excessive chlorine and copper in the water. Commercially available aquarium water test kits can be used to monitor the water quality of the amphibian habitat.

Conclusion

The goal of this article has been to provide the veterinarian and the veterinary technician with a general understanding of amphibians. Amphibians are kept by hobbyists, educational institutions, research facilities, and zoological parks. Although they are not a large part of the exotic animal practice, amphibians are occasionally presented for veterinary care. Veterinarians or technicians participating in wildlife rehabilitation efforts may also encounter amphibian patients. Amphibians can be cherished pets and can live for several years (adult anurans usually reach sexual maturity at one or two years of age) if proper attention is given to their environmental and nutritional needs.

BIBLIOGRAPHY

Ashton RE, Ashton PS: *Handbook of Reptiles and Amphibians of Florida. Part 3. The Amphibians.* Miami, FL, Windward Publishing, 1988.

Crawshaw GJ: Amphibian medicine, in Fowler ME (ed): *Zoo and Wild Animal Medicine, Current Therapy 3.* Philadelphia, WB Saunders Co, 1993, pp 131–139.

Fowler ME: Amphibians, in Fowler ME (ed): *Zoo and Wild Animal Medicine.* Philadelphia, WB Saunders Co, 1986, pp 100–105.

Mattison C: *The Care of Reptiles and Amphibians in Captivity.* London, Blandford Press, 1987.

Diagnostic Guide to Some of the Helminth Parasites of Aquatic Turtles

University of Prince Edward Island
G. A. Conboy, DVM, PhD

University of Minnesota
J. R. Laursen, PhD
G. A. Averbeck, MS
B. E. Stromberg, PhD

KEY FACTS

❏ Although aquatic turtles are known to be subject to infection with a wide variety of endoparasites, precise information on the clinical significance of most parasites is lacking.

❏ Parasites with direct life cycles can be numerous in turtles kept in captivity, especially in situations of poor sanitation, crowding, and nutritional stress.

❏ Spirorchid blood flukes are significant pathogens in aquatic turtles; the widespread deposition of fluke eggs affects many tissues.

❏ Other helminth parasites that are common in aquatic turtles include the nematodes *Serpinema trispinosus*, *Spiroxys* species, and *Falcaustra* species as well as acanthocephalans of the genus *Neoechinorhynchus*.

Freshwater turtles are popular pets. Species that are commonly kept as pets in the United States include the subaquatic (Family Emydidae) eastern diamondback terrapin (*Malaclemys terrapin*), red-eared slider (*Trachemys scripta elegans*), and painted turtle (*Chrysemys picta*) as well as the aquatic (Family Kinosternidae) musk turtle (*Sternotherus odoratus*) and soft-shelled (Family Trionychidae) turtles (*Trionyx* species).[1,2] With the inclusion of exotic-species medicine in many practices, turtles are presented with increasing frequency for veterinary care.

Turtles are subject to infection with a wide variety of arthropod, protozoan, and helminth endoparasites.[3,4] Although the prevalence of parasitic infection in turtles originating from the wild is known to be high,[5,6] the significance of parasitic infection in captive turtles is unclear. Most of the research literature that deals with the parasites of turtles is taxonomic in nature. Precise information on the clinical significance of most of the parasites is lacking. The clinical signs of parasitic infection in turtles are nonspecific and include progressive weight loss, decreased levels of activity, and anorexia.[7]

In turtles, the direct role of parasitism in overall health and the secondary role parasites may play in other disease conditions are mostly unknown. Accurate and specific antemortem and postmortem identification of parasites is a prerequisite for gaining an understanding of the relative importance of parasitism in turtles.

This article is intended to be a practical guide to the identification of some of the helminth parasites found in aquatic freshwater turtles. Parasite fauna differs between the terrestrial and aquatic species[5]; this discussion is limited to the freshwater aquatic species of turtles.

PLATYHELMINTHES

Numerous monogenetic (one host) and digenetic (two or more hosts)

Originally published in Volume 15, Number 9, September 1993

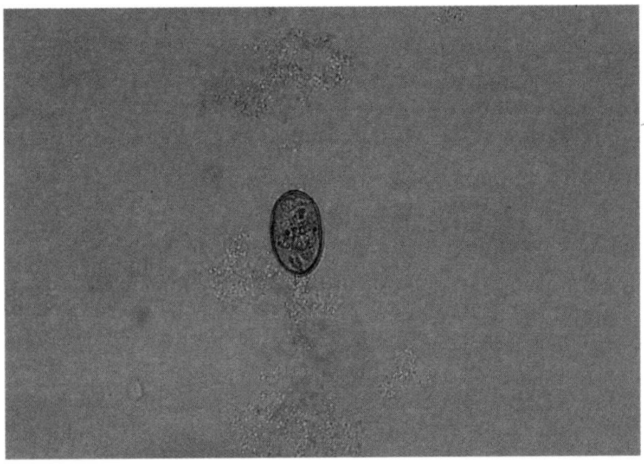

Figure 1—Egg of a *Telorchis* species, a nonpathogenic intestinal fluke recovered from a *Trachemys scripta elegans*. The egg is 30 × 16 μm in size, and the shell is operculate. (×140)

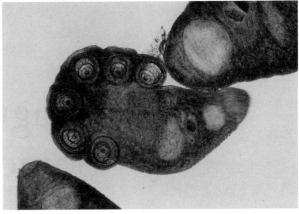

Figure 3—*Polystomoides* species recovered from the mouth of a *Trachemys scripta elegans*. The caudal end of the fluke is characterized by the hold-fast organ. (×14)

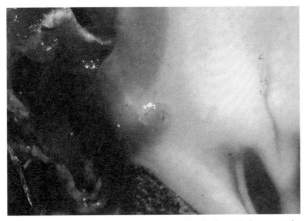

Figure 2—An immature monogenetic fluke, *Polystomoides* species, in the mouth of a *Trachemys scripta elegans*. (×1.2)

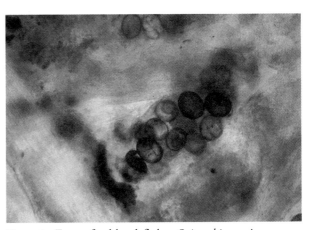

Figure 4—Eggs of a blood fluke, *Spirorchis* species, recovered from a *Trachemys scripta elegans*. (×35)

flukes can infect turtles. Monogenetic flukes inhabit the mouth, nasal cavity, and urinary bladder. Digenetic flukes that infect turtles mainly inhabit the stomach and intestine (Figure 1); the lungs, circulatory system, eyes, and urinary bladder are also infected. Currently, most species of monogenetic and digenetic flukes are considered to be nonpathogenic in turtles[1,8]; however, this phenomenon has not been thoroughly studied.

Various genera of monogenetic flukes infect turtles (*Polystomoides, Neopolystoma, Polystoma,* and *Polystomoidella*)[4] (Figure 2). The caudal end of the flukes is characterized by the hold-fast organ (opisthaptor), which consists of six suckers and a variable number of hooks (Figure 3). The life cycles are direct—eggs develop, hatch, and release the ciliated oncomiracidium. The oncomiracidia seek and infect the next host, developing from juvenile to adult flukes. The life cycle for *Polystomoides oris* in painted turtles takes one year to complete.[9] Large, operculate eggs (185 to 290 μm in diameter) can be detected in the feces of infected turtles via a simple sedimentation fecal exami-

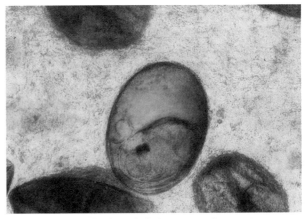

Figure 5—Eggs of a blood fluke, *Spirorchis* species, recovered from a *Trachemys scripta elegans*. The eggs measured 115 × 72 μm. (×140)

nation technique. Because egg production does not tend to be prolific,[9] monogenetic fluke eggs may not be commonly observed in fecal samples.

Although most of the flukes that infect turtles are

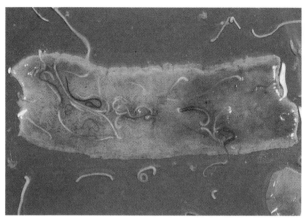

Figure 6—Segment of small intestine from a *Trachemys scripta elegans*. *Serpinema* (Camallanus) *trispinosus* (dark red worms 5 to 10 mm in length) and *Neoechinorhynchus* (stout, tan worms 14 to 40 mm in length) species are visible.

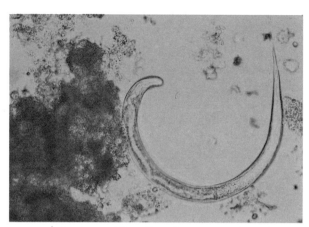

Figure 8—*Serpinema* (Camallanus) *trispinosus* larva (335 × 15 μm) recovered using a simple sedimentation fecal examination technique. (×140)

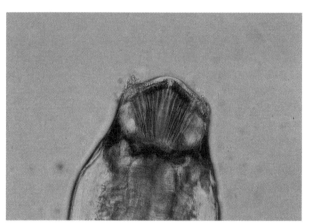

Figure 7—Cranial end of a *Serpinema* (Camallanus) *trispinosus* recovered from the intestine of a *Trachemys scripta elegans*. The sclerotized lateral valves resemble scallop shells. (×140)

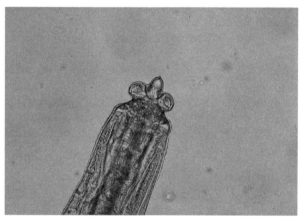

Figure 9—Cranial end of an adult *Spiroxys* species recovered from the stomach of a *Trachemys scripta elegans*. (×140)

considered to be nonpathogenic, the spirorchid blood flukes (*Spirorchis, Henotosoma, Unicaecum, Vasotrema,* and *Hapalorhynchus* species) are exceptions. Adult spirorchids are small (one to three millimeters in length) and inhabit the heart and lumina of blood vessels. Pathogenicity is apparently related to the widespread deposition of fluke eggs, which can be found in virtually any tissue (heart, lung, intestine, urogenital tract, brain, kidney, pancreas, spleen, spinal cord, liver, adipose, or skeletal muscle).[10–12] Spirorchid eggs may induce intense granulomatous tissue reactions, which can occlude blood vessels.

Heavily infected turtles exhibit listlessness and anorexia progressing to stupor and death.[11] Ulcerative lesions on the plastron and carapace occur in some infected turtles as a result of the occlusion of blood vessels. Flotation abnormalities can occur in turtles with extensive lung granulomas.[13] Adult *Spirorchis*

parvus infection of painted turtles is not restricted to the circulatory system and can be found in various tissues, most notably in the central nervous system. Severe neurologic disease has been reported in painted turtles experimentally infected with *S. parvus*; free adult flukes are present in the brain and spinal cord.[12]

At necropsy, adult spirorchids can be difficult to find. Diagnosis is usually made by examining tissue for the fluke eggs. The eggs, which may contain miracidia, can be demonstrated in the lungs by compressing a small piece of pulmonary tissue between a glass slide and coverslip and examining the tissue by microscope (Figures 4 and 5). Antemortem diagnosis is limited to observing fluke eggs (70 to 118 × 56 to 78 μm) on fecal examination. The eggs are not reliably detected by simple or centrifugal flotation techniques. A direct smear or preferably a simple sedimentation technique is recommended for fecal

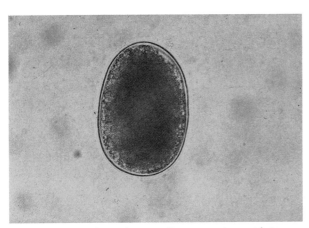
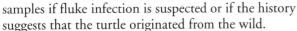

Figure 10—Egg of a *Falcaustra* (Spironoura) species from a fecal sample of a *Trachemys scripta elegans* (110 × 75 μm). (×140)

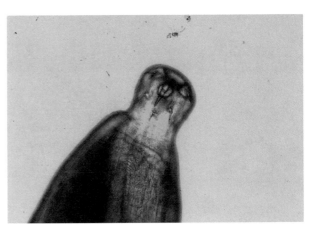

Figure 11—Cranial end of a *Neoechinorhynchus* species recovered from the intestine of a *Trachemys scripta elegans*. Prominent spines are visible on the proboscis. (×140)

samples if fluke infection is suspected or if the history suggests that the turtle originated from the wild.

Infections in captive turtles are usually believed to be self-limiting because of the complex parasite life cycle, which requires a snail intermediate host. Infection depends on the management system, however. Snails may be present as contaminants or as a food source provided to artificial ponds. Such contamination was observed in mariculture-reared green turtles in which spirorchid infection was reported.[14]

NEMATODES

Serpinema (Camallanus) *trispinosus* is a common nematode parasite that inhabits the stomach and small intestine of turtles.[4,15] Adults are 5 to 10 millimeters in length and are evident on necropsy because of their bright red color (Figure 6). Microscopically, camallanids are distinguished by the sclerotized lateral valves of the buccal cavity, which resemble scallop shells (Figure 7). Females are ovoviviparous.

The life cycle has not been determined but may be similar to that of the closely related *Camallanus oxycephalus*, in which copepods (*Cyclops* species) serve as intermediate hosts and fish serve as transport hosts.[16] There is some evidence that snails serve as transport hosts of *S. trispinosus*.[17] Because copepods may be present in artificial ponds and in tank or aquarium water, infections might occur in captive turtles. Signs of infection include weight loss; anorexia; and blood-stained, mucoid feces.[18] Antemortem diagnosis is made by finding the larvae, free or in eggs, on fecal examination (Figure 8). Larvae and eggs can be detected via simple flotation, centrifugal flotation, or simple sedimentation fecal examination techniques.

Spiroxys species (*S. contortus, S. constrictus*, and *S. amydae*) inhabit the stomach and small intestine of turtles (Figure 9). Adults are whitish in color and 15

to 40 millimeters in length. Small nodular thickenings of the gastric mucosa, visible to the naked eye, occur in response to the penetration of developing larvae in infected turtles. Adults inhabit the lumina of the stomach and small intestine. Clinical signs are the same as in *S. trispinosus*. Copepods serve as intermediate hosts; snails, fish, tadpoles, and dragonfly nymphs serve as transport hosts.[17,19] Antemortem diagnosis is made by demonstrating eggs (55 to 73 × 39 to 50 μm) on fecal examination. A simple or centrifugal flotation technique is recommended.

Some of the most common nematode parasites of turtles are members of the genus *Falcaustra* (Spironoura).[20] They are small (3 to 15 millimeters in length) pinworms that inhabit the intestine, cecum, and rectum. The worms have a direct life cycle and can be numerous in captive turtles. This is especially true in cases of poor management (i.e., substandard sanitation, overcrowding, or nutritional stress). Antemortem diagnosis is made by demonstrating eggs (79 to 119 × 62 to 83 μm) in the feces via simple or centrifugal flotation fecal examination techniques (Figure 10).

ACANTHOCEPHALANS

Aquatic turtles (*Trachemys scripta elegans, Chrysemys picta*, and *Trionyx* species) that originate in the wild are often infected with acanthocephalans of the genus *Neoechinorhynchus*.[4,21] These medium-sized worms (14 to 40 millimeters in length) (Figure 6) have a proboscis armed with teeth used to attach firmly to the mucosa of the stomach and intestine (Figure 11). The parasite life cycle includes an ostracod (crustacean) intermediate host and snail transport hosts. Turtles acquire infections after ingesting the infected snails.[22] Infection is believed to cause enteritis of varying severity.[7] Depending on the management system, infections in captive turtles may be self-limiting.

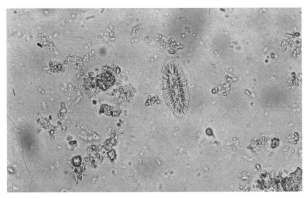

Figure 12—Egg of *Neoechinorhynchus pseudoemys* (42 × 18 µm) from a fecal sample of a *Trachemys scripta elegans*. Centrifugal flotation or sedimentation technique is required to detect such eggs. (×140)

Antemortem diagnosis is made by finding eggs (23 to 60 × 15 to 28 µm) on fecal examination (Figure 12). The eggs are not detected reliably unless a centrifugal flotation or sedimentation technique is used.[18]

TREATMENT

In many cases, turtles with fluke infections can be treated with oral or intramuscular praziquantel (8 mg/kg). Turtles with nematode infections should be treated with oral fenbendazole or thiabendazole (50 to 100 mg/kg).[23] Treatment with any of these anthelmintics should be repeated in two weeks. Because of reported toxicity, ivermectin is not recommended for use in chelonians.[24] Anthelmintic therapy should always be followed by fecal examination to monitor drug efficacy. Accurate diagnosis of the parasites that infect turtles presented for veterinary care is the first step toward a better understanding of the role parasites play in the overall health of these pets.

ACKNOWLEDGMENTS

The authors thank Robin Nelson, Nan Roberts, and Lauren Scheu for their assistance in the preparation of this article and Jerome A. Vanek, DVM, Department of Veterinary Pathobiology, College of Veterinary Medicine, University of Minnesota, for his editorial suggestions.

About the Authors
Dr. Conboy is affiliated with the Department of Pathology and Microbiology, Atlantic Veterinary College, University of Prince Edward Island, Charlottetown, Prince Edward Island, Canada. Drs. Averbeck and Stromberg are affiliated with the Department of Veterinary Pathobiology, College of Veterinary Medicine, University of Minnesota, St. Paul, Minnesota. Dr. Laursen is currently with the Department of Pathobiological Sciences, School of Veterinary Medicine, University of Wisconsin, Madison, Wisconsin.

REFERENCES

1. Rosskopf WJ: Medical care of aquatic turtles, in Kirk RW (ed): *Current Veterinary Therapy. VII.* Philadelphia, WB Saunders Co, 1980, pp 637–647.
2. Smith HM, Brodie ED: *A Guide to Field Identification—Reptiles of North America.* Racine, WI, Golden Press, 1982, pp 22–63.
3. Reichenbach-Klinke H, Elkan E: *Principal Diseases of Lower Vertebrates. Book III. Diseases of Reptiles.* London, Academic Press, 1965, pp 394–509.
4. Ernst EM, Ernst CA: Synopsis of helminths endoparasitic in native turtles of the United States. *Bull Maryland Herpetol Soc* 13:1–75, 1977.
5. Martin DR: Distribution of helminth parasites in turtles native to southern Illinois. *Trans Illinois Acad Sci* 65:61–67, 1972.
6. Frank W: Endoparasites, in Cooper JE, Jackson OF (eds): *Diseases of Reptilia,* vol 1. London, Academic Press, 1981, pp 291–358.
7. Marcus LC: Parasitic diseases of captive reptiles, in Kirk RW (ed): *Current Veterinary Therapy. VI.* Philadelphia, WB Saunders Co, 1977, pp 801–806.
8. Jacobson ER: Biology and diseases of reptiles—Parasitic, in Fox JG, Cohen BJ, Loew FM (eds): *Laboratory Animal Medicine.* Orlando, FL, Academic Press, 1984, pp 467–470.
9. Paul AA: Life history studies of North American freshwater polystomes. *J Parasitol* 24:489–510, 1938.
10. Goodchild CG, Dennis ES: Comparative egg counts and histopathology in turtles infected with *Spirorchis* (Trematoda:Spirorchiidae). *J Parasitol* 53:38–45, 1967.
11. Holliman RB, Fischer JE: Life cycle and pathology of *Spirorchis scripta* Stunkard, 1923 (Digenea:Spirorchiidae) in *Chrysemys picta picta. J Parasitol* 54:310–318, 1968.
12. Holliman RB, Fischer JE, Parker JC: Studies on *Spirorchis parvus* (Stunkard, 1923) and its pathological effects on *Chrysemys picta picta. J Parasitol* 57:71–77, 1971.
13. Jacobson E: Parasitic diseases of reptiles, in Fowler ME (ed): *Zoo and Wild Animal Medicine.* Philadelphia, WB Saunders Co, 1986, pp 162–180.
14. Greiner EC, Forrester DJ, Jacobson ER: Helminths of mariculture-reared green turtles (*Chelonia mydas mydas*) from the Grand Cayman, British West Indies. *Proc Helm Soc Washington* 47:142–144, 1980.
15. Reiber RJ: Nematodes of amphibia and reptilia. 1. Reelfoot Lake, Tennessee Report. *Biol Stat Tennessee Acad Sci* 5:92–99, 1941.
16. Stromberg PC, Crites JL: The life cycle and development of *Camallanus oxycephalus* Ward and Magath, 1916 (Nematoda:Camallanidae). *J Parasitol* 60:117–124, 1974.
17. Bartlett CM, Anderson RC: Larval nematodes (Ascaridida and Spirurida) in the aquatic snail, *Lymnaea stagnalis. J Invert Pathol* 46:153–159, 1985.
18. Wallach JD, Boever WJ: *Diseases of Exotic Animals—Medical and Surgical Management.* Philadelphia, WB Saunders Co, 1983, pp 1014–1026.
19. Hedrick LR: The life history and morphology of *Spiroxys contortus* (Rudolphi); Nematoda:Spiruridae. *Trans Am Microscop Soc* 54:307–335, 1935.
20. Kaplan HM: Parasites of laboratory reptiles and amphibians, in Flynn RJ (ed): *Parasites of Laboratory Animals.* Ames, IA, Iowa State University Press, 1973, pp 548–644.
21. Cable RM, Hopp WB: Acanthocephalan parasites of the genus *Neoechinorhynchus* in North American turtles, with the description of two new species. *J Parasitol* 40:674–680, 1954.
22. Hopp WB: Studies on the morphology and life cycle of

Neoechinorhynchus emydis (Leidy), an acanthocephalan parasite of the map turtle, *Graptemys geographica* (Le Suer). *J Parasitol* 40:284–299, 1954.

23. Jacobson ER: Reptiles. *Vet Clin North Am Small Anim Pract* 17(5):1203–1225, 1987.

24. Teare JA, Bush M: Toxicity and efficacy of ivermectins in chelonians. *JAVMA* 183:1195–1197, 1983.

Color Atlas of Reptilian Parasites
Part I. Protozoans

Susan M. Barnard, BS
Senior Keeper
Department of Herpetology
Atlanta Zoological Park
Atlanta, Georgia

It is impossible to duplicate a reptile's natural environment in captivity. Captivity therefore is stressful, predisposing reptiles to parasitic diseases.[1] Once an infected reptile is captive, those parasites having direct life cycles predominate over parasites requiring intermediate hosts. The consequence of this parasitism is competition with the host animal for food,[2] removal of tissue and fluid, blocking of lymph and blood vessels, edema, ulcerations, necrosis, and anemia.[2-4] Ultimately, death can occur.

The captive reptile's diet includes fruits, vegetables, invertebrates, birds and mammals, and a variety of amphibians and other reptiles. As a result, the feces of a captive reptile contain plant and animal artifacts that too often are mistaken for normal parasitic fauna, leading to unnecessary treatment.

Presented in this four-part series is a pictorial diagnosis of prevalent species of parasites affecting captive reptiles. Also presented are plant and animal artifacts that are commonly mistaken for parasites of reptilian hosts.

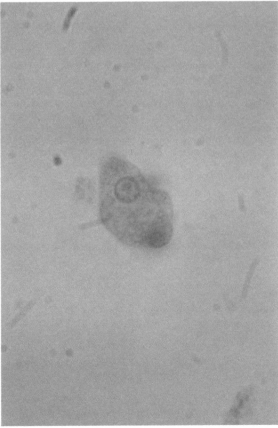 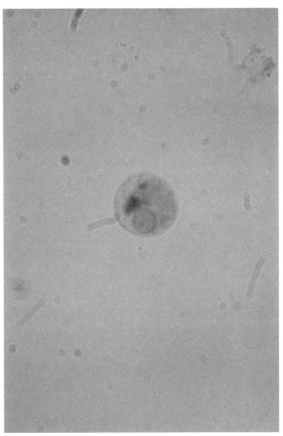

Figure 1A **Figure 1B**

Figure 1—(**A**) *Entamoeba* sp. trophozoite (×1000) and (**B**) *Entamoeba* sp. cyst (×1000). *Entamoeba invadens* is a highly pathogenic protozoan in lizards and snakes; the most severe damage occurs in the colon and liver. Clinical signs are usually limited to the terminal phase of infection and include anorexia, weight loss, blood and/or mucus in stools, and vomiting. *Entamoeba invadens* is transmitted by ingestion of infective cysts passed in feces. When chemically fixed, trophozoites average 16μ in diameter.[5,6] Cysts measure from 11 to 20μ in diameter and contain from one nucleus to four nuclei.[5,7]

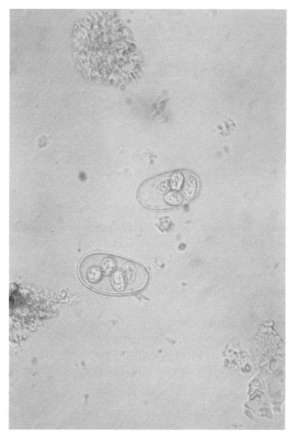

Figure 2A

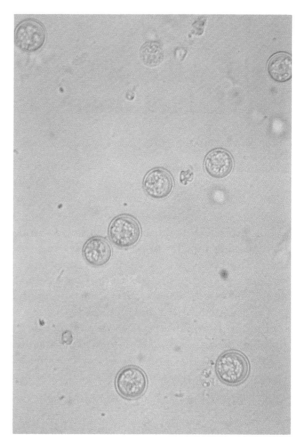

Figure 2B

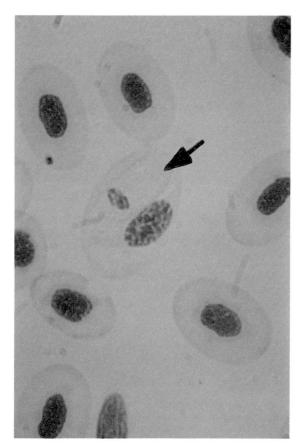

Figure 3

Figure 2—(**A**) *Eimeria* sp. measuring 10 to 15μ by 25 to 37μ (×400) and (**B**) unsporulated oocysts of *Caryospora simplex* measuring 13.5 to 16.2μ in diameter (×400). *Eimeria* is the primary coccidian found in reptiles[4,8-10]; but several others, such as *Caryospora, Isospora,* and *Sarcocystis,* are also common.[5,11] The intestinal tract and gallbladder are primarily affected, causing such clinical signs as restlessness, anorexia, and regurgitation. Transmission occurs by ingestion of sporulated oocysts from contaminated feces or soil. Oocysts vary in size according to species.

Figure 3—*Haemogregarina* sp. (*arrow*) (×1000). The major genera of blood sporozoans affecting reptiles include *Haemogregarina, Haemoproteus, Hepatozoon, Karyolysus, Plasmodium, Schellackia,* and *Simondia.*[7,12,13] Transmission occurs through the bites of leeches, ticks, and other blood-sucking invertebrates and by ingestion of mites.[4,7,14-16] A heavy infection of blood sporozoans has been known to cause anemia and inanition in snakes.[17,18]

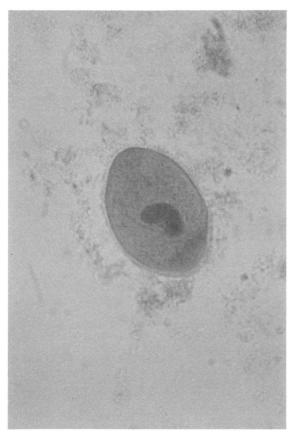

Figure 4A

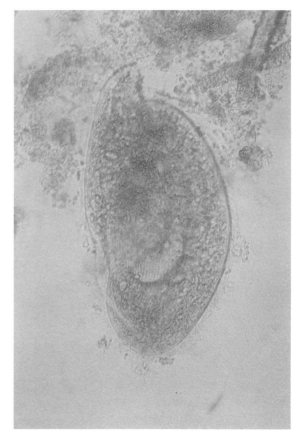

Figure 4B

Figure 4—(**A**) *Balantidium* sp. trophozoite (×400), (**B**) *Nyctotherus* sp. trophozoite (×200), and (**C**) *Nyctotherus* sp. cyst (×400). Although ciliates commonly affect tortoises, they have also been known to affect lizards and snakes. *Balantidium* and *Nyctotherus* are the two primary genera of ciliates affecting reptiles,[4] and they inhabit the host's intestines. *Balantidium* trophozoites vary in length from 70 to 300μ,[5] and *Nyctotherus* trophozoites vary in length from 60 to 190μ.[5] *Nyctotherus* is not known to be pathogenic[5,6]; however, *Balantidium* may be pathogenic in large numbers or in association with other parasites or pathogenic bacteria.[5,10] Transmission is by ingestion of the parasites passed in affected feces.

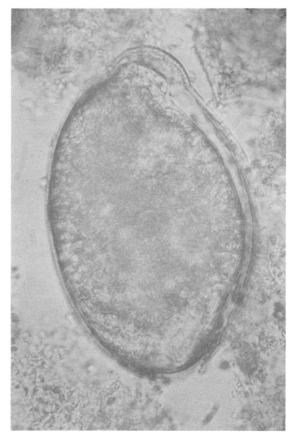

Figure 4C

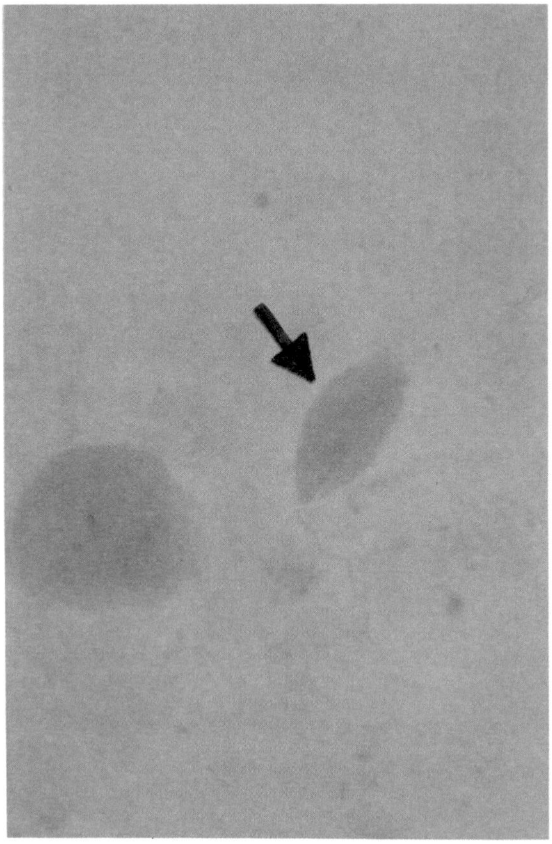

Figure 5—Trichomonad (*arrow*) (×1000). Pathogenicity caused by flagellates may vary according to a reptile's species, age, and general health. Young animals and those with other disorders are more likely to suffer deleterious effects. *Trypanosoma* and *Leishmania* commonly occur in reptiles and inhabit the circulatory system and intestines.[5,6] Flagellates affecting primarily the host's intestines include trichomonads, *Hexamastix*, *Hexamita*, *Monocercomonas*, and *Proteromonas*.[4-7] *Hexamita* also affects the urinary bladder of chelonians.[5,9] Trypanosomes are transmitted to reptiles by leeches and arthropod vectors. *Leishmania* can be contracted by either a bite or ingestion of an invertebrate intermediate host,[5,6] and the intestinal flagellates are contracted by ingestion of the organism passed in affected feces. Diagnosis is best made by direct smear because the movement of flagellates is easily observed.

REFERENCES

1. Telford SR Jr: Parasite diseases of reptiles. *JAVMA* (11)159:1644-1652, 1971.
2. Soulsby EJL: *Helminths, Arthropods, and Protozoa of Domestic Animals (Monnig)*. Philadelphia, Lea & Febiger, 1968.
3. Frank W: Endoparasites, in Cooper JE, Jackson OF (eds): *Diseases of the Reptilia*, vol 1. New York, Academic Press, 1981.
4. Reichenback-Klinke H, Elkan E: *The Principal Diseases of Lower Vetebrates*. New York, Academic Press, 1965.
5. Flynn RJ: *Parasites of Laboratory Animals*. Ames, IA, Iowa State University Press, 1973.
6. Frye FL: *Biomedical and Surgical Aspects of Captive Reptile Husbandry*. Edwardsville, KS, Veterinary Medicine Publishing Co, 1981.
7. Marcus LC: *Veterinary Biology and Medicine of Captive Amphibians and Reptiles*. Philadelphia, Lea & Febiger, 1981.
8. Bovee EC, Telford SR Jr: *Eimeria sceloporis* and *Eimeria molochis* ssp. n. from lizards. *J Parasitol* 51:85-94, 1965.
9. Keymer IF: Protozoa, in Cooper JE, Jackson OF (eds): *Diseases of the Reptilia*, vol 1. New York, Academic Press, 1981.
10. Kiel JL: A review of parasites in snakes. *Southwestern Vet* (3)28:209-220, 1975.
11. Pellerdy LP: *Coccidia and Coccidiosis*. Budapest, Akademiae Kiado, 1965.
12. MacKerras MJ: Hematozoa of Australian reptiles. *Aust J Zool* 9:61-122, 1961.
13. McGhee RB: Diseases caused by *Protista*, in Weinman D, Ristic M (eds): *Infectious Blood Diseases of Man and Animals*. New York, Academic Press, 1968.
14. Booden T, et al: Transfer of *Hepatozoon* sp. from boa constrictor to a lizard, *Anolis carolinensis* by mosquito vectors. *J Parasitol* 56:832-833, 1970.
15. Chao J, Ball GH: Transfer of *Hepatozoon rarefaciens* (Sanbon and Seligman, 1907) from the indigo snake to a gopher snake by a mosquito vector. *J Parasitol* 55:681-682, 1969.
16. Hazen TA, et al: The parasite fauna of the American alligator (*Alligator mississippiensis*) in South Carolina. *J Wildl Dis* 14:435-439, 1978.
17. Fantham HB, Porter A: The endoparasites of some North American snakes and their effects on the Ophidia. *Proc Zool Soc Lond* 123:867-898, 1953.
18. Fiennes RN T-W: Report of the society's pathologist for the year 1957. *Proc Zool Soc Lond* 132:129-146, 1959.

Acknowledgments

This study was supported, in part, by the Society for the Study of Amphibians and Reptiles, the American Association of Zoo Keepers, and the Atlanta Zoological Society. My deepest appreciation and thanks to Dr. Daniel R. Brooks, Dr. Steve J. Upton, and Dr. Nixon Wilson for their diagnostic expertise; to Mr. Rick Etzel, Ms. Tamara Romaine, and Mr. Fred Alvey for their assistance with the literature search; and to Ms. Susanne Wahlquist, Dr. Susan Wade, and the many individuals and institutions submitting fecal material, parasites, and prepared slides.

Color Atlas of Reptilian Parasites
Part II. Flatworms and Roundworms

Susan M. Barnard, BS
Senior Keeper
Department of Herpetology
Atlanta Zoological Park
Atlanta, Georgia

Flukes (class Trematoda) and tapeworms (class Cestoidea) are dorsoventrally flattened parasites that belong to the phylum Platyhelminthes. All flukes are parasitic, either as external parasites or as endoparasites. Two types of trematodes affecting reptiles are those requiring a single host (the monogenic flukes) and the more numerous digenic flukes. Digenic trematodes must parasitize two or more hosts before completing their life cycle.

The eggs of tapeworms vary considerably in form and size. Some eggs pass from the reptilian host intact within the proglottids; others escape from the tapeworm's uterine pore into the host's intestinal tract, where they can be observed in feces microscopically.

Parasitic nematodes (class Nematoda) of reptiles range in length from a few millimeters to over 30 centimeters. Their eggs may be observed microscopically in reptilian feces, uric acid, or sputum, depending on the species.

Some commonly occurring flatworm and roundworm eggs observed in reptiles after captivity are presented in this article. The other nematode genera will be reviewed in Part III of this series.

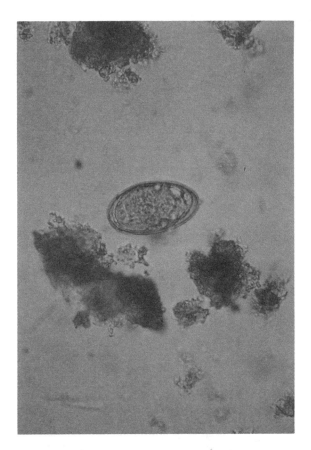

Figure 1—*Ochetosoma* sp. (×400). Flukes of the genus *Ochetosoma* are digenic trematodes that primarily inhabit a reptile's intestinal tract. Other commonly parasitized areas are the lungs, liver and gallbladder, circulatory system, and genital tract; trematodes also may be found free within the coelomic cavity.[5-10] Larval forms locate in the host's muscle, bile duct, skin, and various other tissues.[7,8] Transmission occurs when the reptile ingests such intermediate hosts as amphibians and crayfish. Severe infections can cause listlessness, anorexia, weight loss, dyspnea, uremia, pressure necrosis, and ultimately death. Digenic fluke eggs are gold to dark brown in color and measure 20 to 40μ long.[10]

Figure 2—(**A, B, C,** and **D**) Eggs from various cestodes observed in the feces of reptiles (×400). Cestodes affecting reptiles are hermaphroditic[9] and non-host specific.[8] Humans can become infected with some species by introducing contaminated material from their hands into their eyes.[8] Transmission to the reptile occurs by ingestion of intermediate hosts, such as ticks, copepods, fish, frogs, tadpoles, or other reptiles. Cockroaches can mechanically transfer cestode infections and are also a potential intermediate host.[8] Adult worms compete for nutrients and can cause chronic enteritis; large species may be pathogenic because of their size. Larval forms cause sparganosis in reptiles, and tissue damage can occur as larvae migrate throughout the body. Sparganosis should be suspected when subcutaneous or intramuscular lumps are detected on palpation.

Originally published in Volume 8, Number 4, April 1986

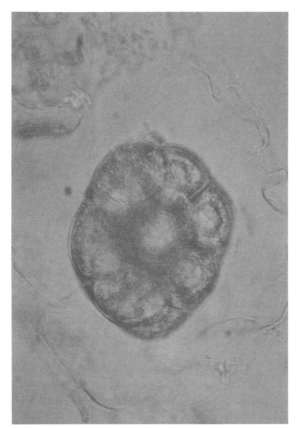

Figure 2A

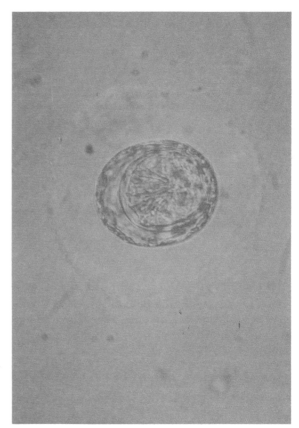

Figure 2B

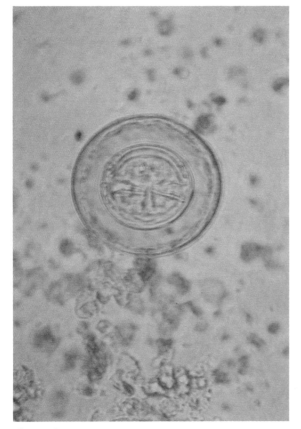

Figure 2C

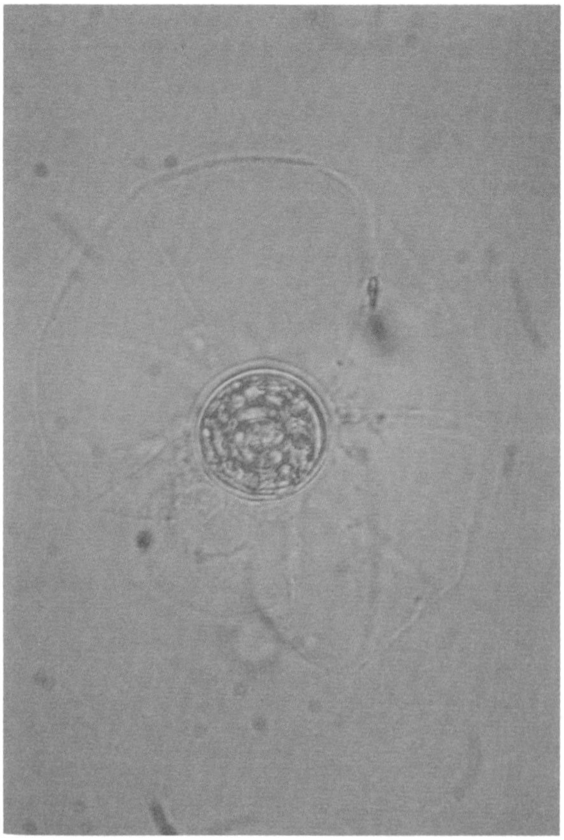

Figure 2D

Figure 3—(**A**) *Strongyloides* sp. egg (×400) and (**B**) *Strongyloides* sp. larva (×400). Based on egg size and description, the parasites in the genera *Strongyloides* and *Rhabdias* are impossible to differentiate solely on microscopic examination. If *Rhabdias* is suspected, diagnosis is possible if eggs can be demonstrated in wet mounts from tracheal washings. *Strongyloides* inhabits the small intestine or esophagus, while *Rhabdias* inhabits the host's lungs. Transmission occurs (1) by ingestion of embryonated eggs or infective third-stage larvae or (2) possibly by penetration of infective larvae through the skin. In both genera, the parasite can survive in a free-living form for several generations. Clinical signs of *Strongyloides* may be diarrhea, while *Rhabdias* may cause respiratory distress. Both parasites cause anorexia resulting in weight loss or death.

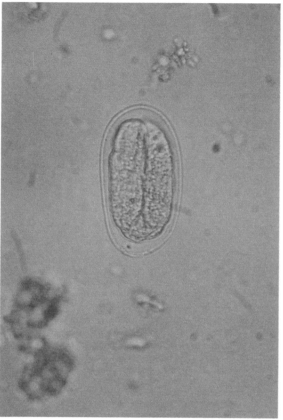

Figure 3A

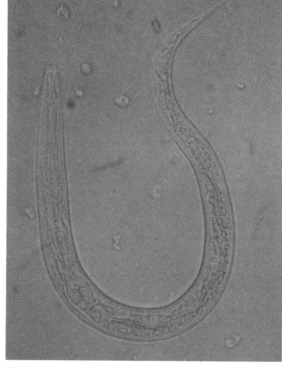

Figure 3B

Acknowledgments

This study was supported, in part, by the Society for the Study of Amphibians and Reptiles, the American Association of Zoo Keepers, and the Atlanta Zoological Society. My deepest appreciation and thanks to Dr. Daniel R. Brooks, Dr. Steve J. Upton, and Dr. Nixon Wilson for their diagnostic expertise; to Mr. Rick Etzel, Ms. Tamara Romaine, and Mr. Fred Alvey for their assistance with the literature search; and to Ms. Susanne Wahlquist, Dr. Susan Wade, and the many individuals and institutions submitting fecal material, parasites, and prepared slides.

REFERENCES

1. Cheng TC: *The Biology of Animal Parasites.* Philadelphia, WB Saunders Co, 1964.
2. Yorke W, Maplestone PA: *The Nematode Parasites of Vertebrates.* Philadelphia, Blakiston, 1926.
3. Ortlepp RJ: Observations on the nematode genera *Kalicephalus, Diaphanocephalus,* and *Occipitodontus* g.n., and on the larval development of *Kalicephalus philodryadus* sp. n. *J Heminthol* 1:165-189, 1923.
4. Harwood PD: The helminths parasitic in the amphibia and reptilia of Houston, Texas and vicinity. *Proc US Natl Mus* 81:1-71, 1932.
5. Frank W: Endoparasites, in Cooper JE, Jackson OF (eds): *Diseases of the Reptilia,* vol I. New York, Academic Press, 1981.
6. Reichenback-Klinke H, Elkan E: *The Principal Diseases of Lower Vertebrates.* New York, Academic Press, 1965.
7. Flynn RJ: *Parasites of Laboratory Animals.* Ames, IA, Iowa State University Press, 1973.
8. Frye FL: *Biomedical and Surgical Aspects of Captive Reptile Husbandry.* Edwardsville, KS, Veterinary Medicine Publishing Co, 1981.
9. Marcus LC: *Veterinary Biology and Medicine of Captive Amphibians and Reptiles.* Philadelphia, Lea & Febiger, 1980.
10. Kiel JL: A review of parasites in snakes. *Southwestern Vet* 28(3):209-220, 1975.

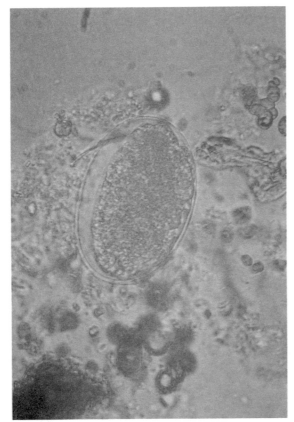 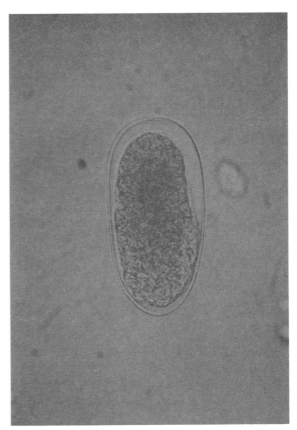

Figure 4A   **Figure 4B**

Figure 4—(**A**) *Oswaldocruzia* sp. (×400) and (**B**) *Kalicephalus* sp. (×400). *Oswaldocruzia* and *Kalicephalus* are hookworms that occur in reptiles worldwide and that inhabit the host's digestive tract. The two genera are similar in appearance. Transmission of *Oswaldocruzia* is probably direct, but little is known about its life cycle.[1,2] Transmission of *Kalicephalus* is (1) by ingestion of ova or infective third-stage larvae or (2) possibly by penetration of infective larvae through the skin. Severe infections of *Oswaldocruzia* may cause intestinal obstruction and peritonitis. *Kalicephalus* may cause anemia, hemorrhagic ulcers, and intestinal obstruction. A *Kalicephalus* organism measures 55 to 100μ long and 27 to 50μ wide[3]; *Oswaldocruzia* measures 75 to 80μ long by 42 to 50μ wide.[4]

Color Atlas of Reptilian Parasites. Part III. Miscellaneous Endoparasites and Ectoparasites

Susan M. Barnard, BS
Senior Keeper
Department of Herpetology
Atlanta Zoological Park
Atlanta, Georgia

Part III of this four-part series features diagnostic photomicrographs of nematode eggs (class Nematoda) commonly observed in reptilian feces as well as photomicrographs of a pentastomid egg (class Pentastomida) and the snake mite, *Ophionyssus natricis*.

Some pentastomid infections may infect reptiles for only about a year if the reptile is maintained under optimum hygienic conditions; however, those species of pentastomids that are capable of autoinfection may survive within the captive reptilian host for many years.

Ectoparasites often transmit other parasites and may be vectors for such diseases as Q fever, tularemia, and Russian spring and summer encephalitis. Common places where ectoparasites may be found are under a reptile's scales in the areas of the chin, eyes, cloaca, body folds, and buccal cavity.

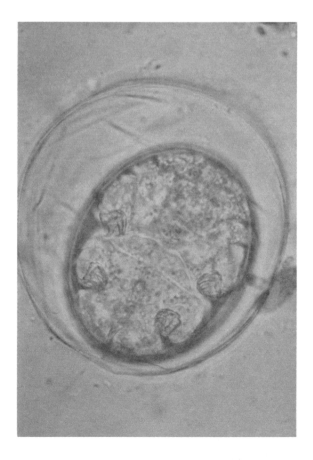

Figure 1—Pentastomid egg (×400). Pentastomids, also called *tongue-worms,* possess the qualities of both annelids and arachnids. The most common are *Porocephalus, Armillifer, Kiricephalus,* and *Raillietiella.* The lung is the primary host location for *Porocephalus* and *Armillifer.*[1,2] Adult *Raillietiella* and *Kiricephalus* also inhabit the lung,[1] while larvae and nymphs are found in subcutaneous tissue and the stomach wall.[3,4] All stages of *Raillietiella* have been reported in the lungs of a fer-de-lance snake (*Bothrops atrox*).[5] Transmission occurs from ingestion of an intermediate mammalian host. Therefore, feeding captured wild rodents to captive reptiles should be avoided. Because humans are an accidental host,[3] care should be exercised when handling infected animals. Clinical signs include lethargy, anorexia, dyspnea, and blood-tinged sputum. Some reptiles do not suffer deleterious effects from a pentastomid infection. Others, however, may suffer from hemorrhagic, acute inflammatory, or chronic granulomatous reaction in the colon, liver, or lungs from migrating larvae, nymphs, and adults.[3,6] Eggs measure approximately 130 to 140 μ.[7]

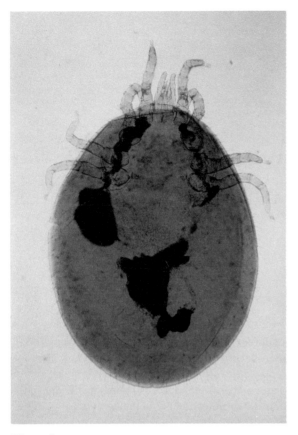

Figure 2

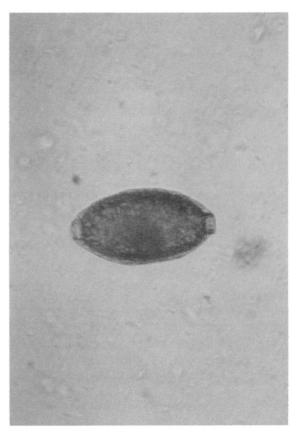

Figure 3

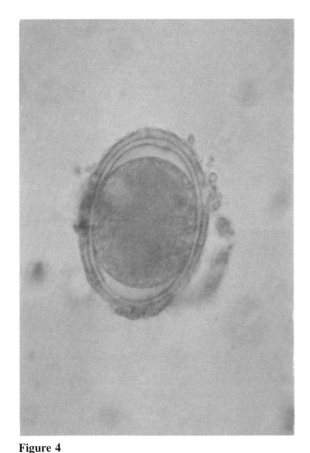

Figure 4

Figure 2—The snake mite, *Ophionyssus natricis* (×40). Of the 250 species of mites that affect reptiles, *O. natricis* is the most common to occur in captive reptiles. It is a mechanical vector for *Aeromonas hydrophila*,[8] the major causative organism of pneumonia. This ectoparasite is transmitted easily from one animal to another and causes irritation to the affected reptile. Infested animals may be observed soaking themselves excessively in their water-bowls or continually rubbing and twisting. Severe infestations can cause anemia and death.

Figure 3—*Capillaria* sp. (×400). *Capillaria* is the only known genus of trichurids to infect lizards and snakes.[3,5] These organisms primarily inhabit the host's intestines but have been observed in other organs.

Figure 4—*Ophidascaris* sp. (×400). *Ophidascaris* and *Hexametra* are the two most common genera of ascarids found in snakes.[3,4] They inhabit the host's stomach, esophagus, and/or small intestine. Severe infections of adult worms can occlude the stomach, causing the animal to regurgitate.[5] Diarrhea[3] and purulent pneumonia[9] are other frequent problems. The most probable source of infection in nature is by ingestion of such intermediate hosts as frogs and rodents.[10,11] Both genera measure 83 μ in diameter.[12]

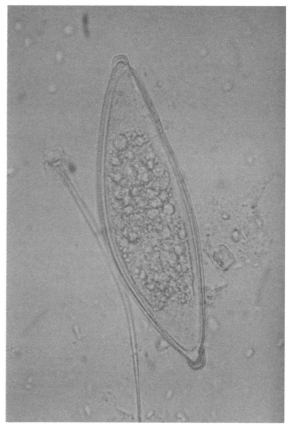

Figure 5A

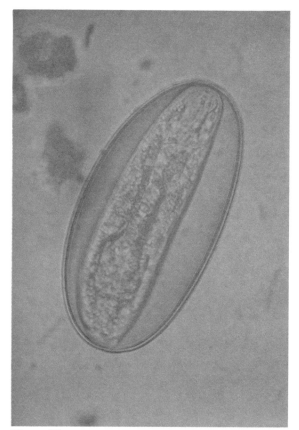

Figure 5B

Figure 5—(**A, B,** and **C**) Oxyurids commonly observed in the feces of reptiles (×400). *Falcaustra* and *Parapharyngodon* have been reported to be the most common oxyurids of reptiles in the United States.[13-16] Also common are (**A**) *Pharyngodon* in lizards and (**B**) *Tachygonetria* in chelonians of the family Testudinidae and lizards in the genus *Uromastix*.[1,5] Generally, oxyurids are nonpathogenic. They have a direct life cycle and inhabit the host's colon. (**C**) Oxyurid eggs are one of the most common helminths observed in lizards.

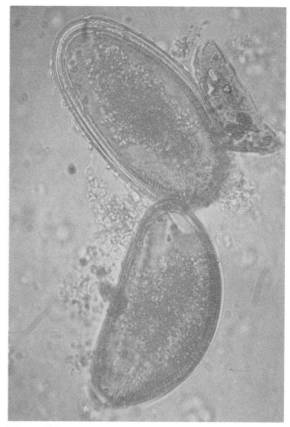

Figure 5C

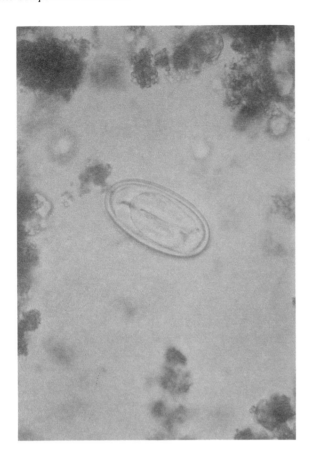

Figure 6—Spirurid ovum measuring 32.5 μ by 52.5 μ ($\times$400). The life cycles of spirurids include two or more hosts.[1] Reptiles may either act as the intermediate hosts for birds and mammals or serve as the final hosts.[1,4,5] Aquatic reptiles become infected by ingesting the larval stages when feeding on copepods. Insects and other arthropods serve as a source of infection for terrestrial reptiles. Ants are a common source of infection, and captive reptiles may become infected if ants gain access to caging. Some commonly occurring spirurids are *Abbreviata*, which infect lizards, and *Gnathostoma*, which parasitize crocodilians and other reptiles.[1] *Physaloptera, Skrjabinoptera*, and *Thubunaea* commonly infect snakes and other reptiles.[1,3] *Proleptus* is known to infect chelonians.[1] Spirurids are parasites of the mouth and gastrointestinal tract.

Acknowledgments

This study was supported, in part, by the Society for the Study of Amphibians and Reptiles, the American Association of Zoo Keepers, and the Atlanta Zoological Society. My deepest appreciation and thanks to Dr. Daniel R. Brooks, Dr. Steve J. Upton, and Dr. Nixon Wilson for their diagnostic expertise; to Mr. Rick Etzel, Ms. Tamara Romaine, and Mr. Fred Alvey for their assistance with the literature search; and to Ms. Susanne Wahlquist, Dr. Susan Wade, and the many individuals and institutions submitting fecal material, parasites, and prepared slides.

REFERENCES

1. Reichenback-Klinke H, Elkan E: *The Principal Diseases of Lower Vertebrates*. New York, Academic Press, 1965.
2. Frye FL: *Biomedical and Surgical Aspects of Captive Reptile Husbandry*. Edwardsville, KS, Veterinary Medicine Publishing Co, 1981.
3. Kiel JL: A review of parasites in snakes. *Southwestern Vet* 28(3):209-220, 1975.
4. Marcus LC: *Veterinary Biology and Medicine of Captive Amphibians and Reptiles*. Philadelphia, Lea & Febiger, 1981.
5. Frank W: Endoparasites, in Cooper JE, Jackson OF (eds): *Diseases of the Reptilia*, vol I. New York, Academic Press, 1981.
6. Deakins DE: Diagnosis and treatment of parasites of amphibians and reptiles. *Am Assoc Zoo Vet Ann Proc*:37-46, 1972-1973.
7. Slocombe JO, Budd J: *Armillifer brumpti* (Pentastomida) in a boa in Canada. *J Wildl Dis* 9:352-355, 1973.
8. Camin JH: Mite transmission of a hemorrhagic septicemia in snakes. *J Parasitol* 34:345-354, 1948.
9. Wallach JD: Medical care of reptiles. *JAVMA* 155:1017-1034, 1969.
10. Sprent JF: Studies on ascaridoid nematodes in pythons: The life history and development of *Ophidascaris moreliae* in Australian pythons. *Parasitology* 60:97-122, 1970.
11. Sprent JF: Studies on ascaridoid nematodes in pythons: The life history and development of *Polydelphis anoura* in Australian pythons. *Parasitology* 60:375-397, 1970.
12. Harwood PD: The helminths parasitic in the Amphibia and Reptilia of Houston, Texas and vicinity. *Proc US Natl Mus* 81:1-71, 1932.
13. Rausch R: Observations on some helminths parasitic in Ohio turtles. *Am Midl Nat* 38:434-442, 1947.
14. Walton AC: The parasites of amphibia. *J Wildl Dis* 40:(microcard), 1964.
15. Williams RW: Helminths of the snapping turtle, *Chelydra serpentina*, from Oklahoma, including the first report and description of the male of *Capillaria serpentina* (Harwood, 1932). *Trans Am Microsc Soc* 72:175-178, 1953.
16. Yamaguti S: The nematodes of vertebrates, in Yamaguti S (ed): *Systema helminthum*, vol 3. New York, Interscience Publications, 1961.

Color Atlas of Reptilian Parasites
Part IV. Pseudoparasites

Susan M. Barnard, BS
Senior Keeper
Department of Herpetology
Atlanta Zoological Park
Atlanta, Georgia

The diet of a captive reptile comprises various plant material and animals, including fruits, vegetables, invertebrates, birds, mammals, amphibians, and other reptiles. Consequently, the feces of reptiles contain remnants and/or spurious parasitic eggs from the food they eat; these artifacts can be mistaken for normal reptilian parasites, leading to unnecessary treatment.

The final part of this four-part series presents some common parasitic eggs of animals fed to reptiles in captivity. Also featured are the plant and animal artifacts frequently observed in reptilian feces. For additional information, the reader may wish to review the article by Habermann and Williams[1] and the book by Flynn.[2]

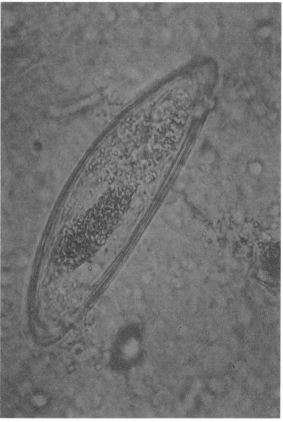

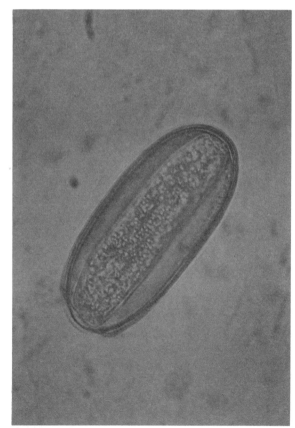

Figure 1A

Figure 1B

Figure 1—(**A**) *Syphacia obvelata* (×400) and (**B**) *Aspiculuris tetraptera* (×400). *Syphacia obvelata* and *Aspiculuris tetraptera* are pinworms of mice. Their eggs are the most commonly found in the feces of captive carnivorous reptiles. If observed, sequential fecal examinations should be performed. A series of negative findings may indicate that an infection was spurious, since these parasites would be expected to appear intermittently.[3] Ova of *S. obvelata* measure 118 to 153 μ by 33 to 55 μ and those of *A. tetraptera* measure 89 to 93 μ by 36 to 42 μ.

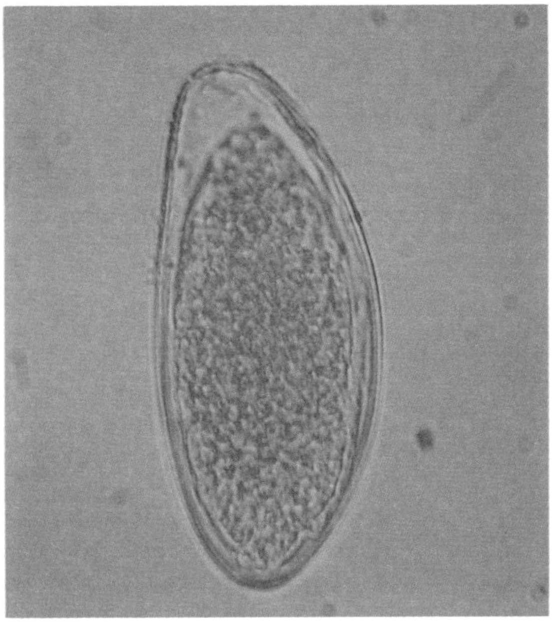

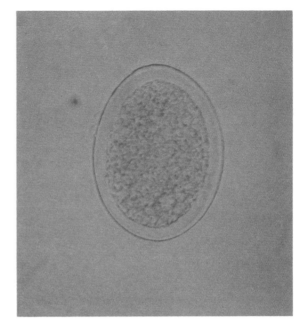

Figure 2A

Figure 2B

Figure 2—(**A**) *Passalurus ambiguus* (×400) and (**B**) *Ascaridia galli* (×400). Giant snakes, such as boas and pythons, are frequently fed rabbits and chickens and may exhibit parasites of these prey animals in their stools. Microscopic examination of the stools of prey animals before they are fed to a reptile may be beneficial in detecting spurious parasites. The eggs of *P. ambiguus*, a common pinworm of rabbits and hares, measure 95 to 103 *μ* by 43 *μ*. The eggs of *A. galli*, the common roundworm of domestic and wild birds, measure 70 to 80 *μ* by 45 to 50 *μ*.

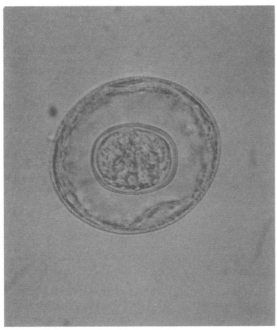

Figure 3A

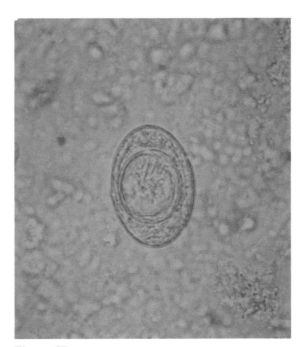

Figure 3B

Figure 3—(**A**) *Hymenolepsis diminuta* (×400) and (**B**) *Hymenolepsis nana* (×400). Although the tapeworm, *H. diminuta*, has an indirect life cycle, institutions breeding their own rodents may observe *H. diminuta* in the feces of captive reptiles when rodent colonies are exposed inadvertently to invertebrate intermediate hosts.[3] The dwarf tapeworm, *H. nana*, is the only known cestode with both direct and indirect life cycles.[4,5] *Hymenolepsis nana* ova are especially prevalent in the feces of carnivorous captive reptiles. Eggs of *H. nana* measure 44 to 62 *μ* by 30 to 55 *μ*, possess polar filaments, and contain an embryo measuring 24 to 30 *μ* by 16 to 25 *μ*. Ova of *H. diminuta* measure 62 to 88 *μ* by 52 to 81 *μ*, lack polar filaments, and contain an embryo measuring 24 to 30 *μ* by 16 to 25 *μ*.

Figure 4—(**A**) Partially digested mite (×100) and (**B**) invertebrate egg (×400). Mites commonly infest laboratory rodents. Invertebrate parts or eggs frequently appear in stools of reptiles. Although the mites parasitizing prey animals pose no threat to reptiles, the possibility of lethal consequences from the snake mite, *Ophionyssus natricis*, demands a thorough external examination of the reptile in question.[3]

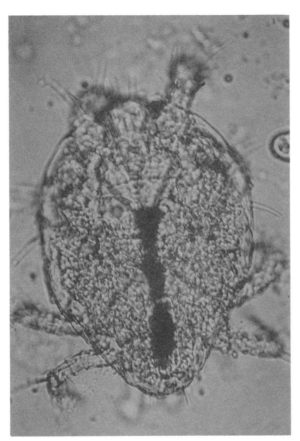

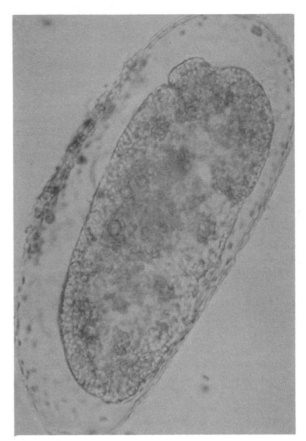

Figure 4A

Figure 4B

Figure 5—(**A**) Banana seeds (×100), (**B**) plant hair (×400), (**C**) animal hairs (×100), and (**D**) pine pollen (×400). Common artifacts observed in the feces of herbivorous reptiles include banana seeds and plant hairs. Animal hairs are routinely observed in the stools of carnivores, and pine pollen may be observed in the feces of all reptiles. Banana seeds can be mistaken for segmented tapeworms, while both plant and animal hairs have been confused with nematode larvae. The observer should note the obvious lack of internal structures in these artifacts, and their disparate sizes and shapes should minimize the possibility of mistaken identity.[3]

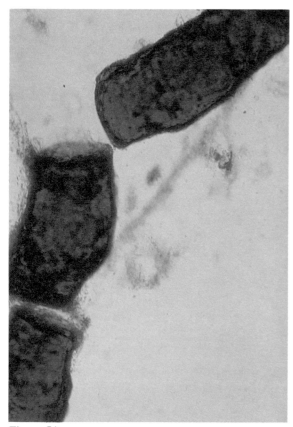

Figure 5A

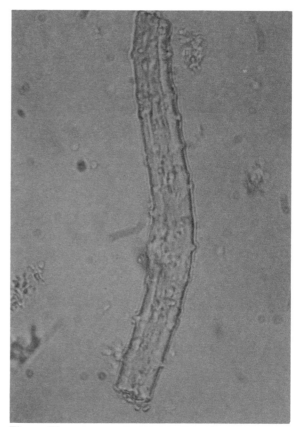

Figure 5B

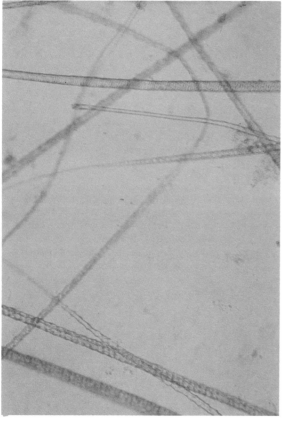

Figure 5C

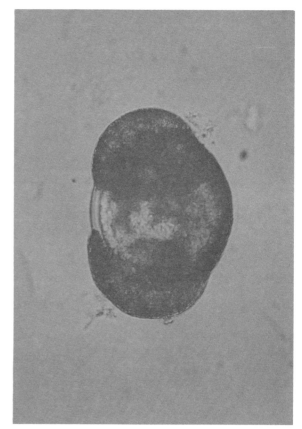

Figure 5D

Acknowledgments

This study was supported, in part, by the Society for the Study of Amphibians and Reptiles, the American Association of Zoo Keepers, and the Atlanta Zoological Society. My deepest appreciation and thanks to Dr. Daniel R. Brooks, Dr. Steve J. Upton, and Dr. Nixon Wilson for their diagnostic expertise; to Mr. Rick Etzel, Ms. Tamara Romaine, and Mr. Fred Alvey for their assistance with the literature search; and to Ms. Susanne Wahlquist, Dr. Susan Wade, and the many individuals and institutions submitting fecal material, parasites, and prepared slides.

REFERENCES

1. Habermann RT, Williams FP Jr: The identification and control of helminths in laboratory animals. *J Natl Cancer Institute* 20:979-1009, 1958.
2. Flynn RJ: *Parasites of Laboratory Animals.* Ames, IA, Iowa State University Press, 1973.
3. Barnard SM: A review of some fecal pseudoparasites of reptiles. *J Zoo Ann Med* 14:79-88, 1983.
4. Cheng TC: *The Biology of Animal Parasites.* Ames, IA, Iowa State University Press, 1973.
5. Wardle RA, McLeod JA: *The Zoology of Tapeworms.* Minneapolis, MN, University of Minnesota Press, 1952.

Reptilian Surgery, Part I. *(continued from page 42)*

REFERENCES

1. Allen DG, Pringle JC, Smith D: *Handbook of Veterinary Drugs.* Philadelphia, J.B. Lippincott, 1993, pp 534–567.
2. Young LA, Schumacher J, Jacobson ER, et al: Pharmacokinetics of enrofloxacin in juvenile Burmese pythons (*Python molurus bivattutus*). *Proc Assoc Rept Amph Vet/Am Assoc Zoo Vet*: 97, 1994.
3. Jenkins JR: Diagnostic and clinical techniques, in Mader DR (ed): *Reptile Management and Surgery.* Philadelphia, WB Saunders, 1996, pp 264–276.

Reptilian Surgery, Part II. *(continued from page 53)*

portant to advise clients that a decrease in aggression should not be anticipated until the following breeding season (usually in the fall). Prepubertal castration may prevent the development of aggressive behavior although research in this area is lacking.

Since publication of this article, new information has become available on the causes and treatment of nutritional secondary hyperparathyroidism and metabolic bone disease in green iguanas; however, much remains to be learned.[3]

The best recommendation for the prevention of this common disease of green iguanas is exposure to direct sunlight and a diet with a proper (2:1) calcium:phosphorus ratio.

REFERENCES

1. Bennett RA, Mader DR: Soft tissue surgery, in Mader DR (ed): *Reptile Medicine and Surgery.* Philadelphia, WB Saunders, 1996, pp 287–299.
2. DeNardo D: Dystocia, in Mader DR (ed): *Reptile Medicine and Surgery,* Philadelphia, WB Saunders, 1996, pp 370–374.
3. Boyer TH: Metabolic bone disease, in Mader DR (ed): *Reptile Medicine and Surgery.* Philadelphia, WB Saunders, 1996, pp 385–392.

Parasites of Domesticated Pet Ferrets

Judith A. Bell, DVM, PhD

KEY FACTS

❏ Intestinal worms are not a problem in ferrets; however, coccidiosis is common in kits and may cause diarrhea.

❏ Common ectoparasites of ferrets include ear mites and fleas.

❏ Ferrets that have ear mites are best treated locally with ivermectin; safe and effective remedies for cats can be used to treat ferrets that have fleas.

❏ Ferrets that are housed outdoors require heartworm prophylaxis during mosquito season.

❏ Potential zoonoses include cryptosporidiosis, giardiasis, and toxoplasmosis.

Ferrets (*Mustela putorius furo*) are mustelids that have been kept as domesticated pets for thousands of years. These animals are most likely descended from wild polecats that still exist in Europe and Asia; they were brought to America approximately 300 years ago to control vermin on ships and in homes and barns[1] and were later used to hunt groundhogs and rabbits. Ferrets have also been raised for their fur. *Fitch* is a term that denotes the fur made from the coat of a ferret, polecat, or hybrid as well as the ferret itself when domesticated for fur production.

NEMATODES AND CESTODES

Fitch are sometimes housed with ranch mink (their close biologic relatives) and fed raw meat and fish—the intermediate hosts for some endoparasites. Fitch and mink seem to be resistant to intestinal nematodes and cestodes that are commonly found in other carnivores. Although the literature suggests prophylactic treatment of fitch and mink for gastrointestinal helminths,[2] veterinarians who treat many pet ferrets or ranch mink[3] rarely find worms in the animals or nematode eggs in stool samples.

There are no reports of roundworms or hookworms naturally infecting ferrets or mink. *Baylisascaris devosi*, also known as *Ascaris mustelarum*, is an intestinal roundworm of two wild mustelids, marten and fisher.[4] The parasite has been transmitted to ferrets via mice (that are used for food) infected with L2 larvae; however, natural infection has not been reported. *Dipylidium caninum*, a tapeworm transmitted to dogs and wild canids by fleas, has not been reported in either pet or fitch ferrets.

The giant kidney worm (*Dioctophyma renale*) and lung fluke (*Paragonimus kellicotti*) are common in wild and ranch mink that feed on freshwater fish and crayfish. Other wild mustelids have also been naturally infected,[5] as have pet dogs and cats,[6] but there are no reports of these two parasites in ferrets.

Most pet ferrets are housed indoors or in cages off the ground and have no opportunity to eat intermediate hosts. The natural prey of escaped pets are small rodents, rabbits, and birds; ferrets rarely eat fish by choice. It is unlikely that endoparasites of wild mustelids will ever become a diagnostic problem for veterinarians who treat confined, domesticated ferrets.

Dirofilaria immitis is a nematode that occasionally causes a significant problem in pet ferrets.[1] A small number of adult worms can cause congestive heart failure. Clinical signs may be confused with signs indicative of hypertrophic cardiomyopathy (a disease of idiopathic origin in ferrets) or lymphosarcoma with thymic or hepatic involvement. Diagnosis is complicated by the possibility that all worms in the heart are of one sex; therefore, failure to find microfilariae in the blood of ferrets does not rule out heartworm disease. Heartworm antigen tests may be falsely negative because so few worms are present. The prognosis for ferrets with clinical signs of heartworm disease is poor. Thiacetarsamide sodium treatment may be attempted using the recommended dosage for dogs (0.2 ml/kg intravenously twice daily for two consecutive days). Because thiacetarsamide sodium is very irritating, placing a jugular catheter in an anesthetized patient may be considered for administration of the solution.

Ferrets that are housed outdoors in areas infested with heartworms should be treated prophylactically. Ivermectin should be given monthly either orally or subcutaneously during mosquito season. Even high doses (1 mg/kg) of ivermectin are safe to use in ferrets. The microfilaricidal dose is 6 µg/kg. For practical purposes, doses that vary from 0.5 milligrams injected subcutaneously to one quarter of the smallest dog tablet (17 µg) have been used safely in ferrets weighing more than 500 grams.

Administering a heartworm tablet to a ferret is difficult and can be avoided. Tablets should be ground to powder and mixed with something sweet and sticky (e.g., malt-based nutritional cat supplements or corn syrup) to accommodate both patient and owner.

PROTOZOANS

Protozoans are common gastrointestinal parasites of ferrets. Oocysts of *Isospora* species are frequently found in fecal flotation samples from young ferrets. *Cryptosporidium parvum* has been detected in histologic sections of the small intestine from clinically healthy kits. Other protozoans reported to infect ferrets are *Giardia* species[2] and *Toxoplasma gondii*.[7] Infections with all species (except *Isospora*) are usually subclinical.

Oocysts of *Isospora* species are most commonly shed by ferrets that are 6 to 16 weeks of age and are rarely shed by adults. The species of coccidia that infects ferrets most likely infects puppies and kittens.[5] Occasionally, young ferrets develop bloody diarrhea shortly after being purchased from pet stores and large numbers of oocysts are found in fecal flotation samples. Oocysts are more often found in fecal flotation samples of formed stools from apparently healthy ferrets. After infected kits are treated to reduce coccidial burden, their growth rate increases and they have healthier coats.

Several coccidiostats (that is, sulfadimethoxine, trimethoprim–sulfadiazine, amprolium, and decoquinate) are safe and effective for the treatment of ferrets but are not specifically labelled for this use. Ferrets should be treated for at least two weeks with any coccidiostat and should have a follow-up fecal flotation one week after the last treatment to verify elimination of the infection.

Cleanliness of the living area is vital to controlling parasites. Ferrets fastidiously keep one area of their enclosure for elimination, but litter training is not usually accomplished until a few weeks after kits are acquired. Oocysts become infectious in one to two days in a temperate environment[6] and are rapidly transmitted if feces accumulate for more than one day. Because ferrets are playful and clumsy, they may come in contact with contaminated feces and spread the infection when playing with each other or sleeping in heaps. Contamination of food may also occur. When ferrets are eating, they usually contact the feed container with their front paws and sometimes walk or stumble on the dish. Open water dishes invite play and are easily contaminated with infectious fecal material.

Selection of a coccidiostat depends on the number of animals involved as well as housing conditions. Sulfadimethoxine may be added to the drinking water if groups of kits are infected. Ferrets drink approximately three times more water than the volume of dry food consumed. Sulfadimethoxine is bitter and may therefore reduce water intake. An effective and safe dose of sulfadimethoxine for ferrets is 300 mg/kg daily, which is approximately 0.5 ml/kg of a 12.5% solution. The volume of consumed water should be recalculated one or two days after the drug has been added, and the concentration of sulfadimethoxine should be adjusted (if necessary) to ensure adequate dosing. No other source of water should be available for two weeks. If animals must be individually treated, sulfadimethoxine can be given to each animal via a medicine dropper; ferrets may resist treatment after the first dose.

Cherry-flavored trimethoprim–sulfadiazine oral suspension is effective and easy to administer. This drug is well accepted by ferrets of all ages and only requires once-daily treatment. The dose of the oral suspension (48 mg/ml) for ferrets is 30 mg/kg. A seven-week-old male kit that weighs approximately 400 grams requires 0.4 milliliters of the suspension daily. Kits, however, double their weight between 7 and 10 weeks of age; therefore, the dose must be adjusted for the second week of treatment. Underdosing may lead to drug resistance.

Amprolium is a thiamine inhibitor. Well-nourished young ferrets, however, have been treated with this drug for more than six consecutive weeks with no signs of toxicity. The daily dose of the 9.6% oral solution is 19 mg/kg (0.2 ml/kg) given by syringe or added to the drinking water. Amprolium is not as bitter as sulfadimethoxine but causes a noticeable reduction in water intake. The crumble form of amprolium used to treat cattle can be mixed with moist food without affecting palatability. Crumbles are packaged in large quantities that are impractical for most small animal practices to use within the shelf-life of the product. Amprolium solution is likewise available only in large volumes and must be kept away from heat and direct sunlight. After six months, the solution begins to lose its effectiveness, even if stored properly.

Decoquinate, a coccidiostat labelled for use in cattle and poultry, is safe for prolonged use in ferrets at a daily dose of 0.5 mg/kg. Because the drug is insoluble, it comes in crumble form, which is only practical for treating large groups of kits, and must be mixed with moist food.

In humans, *Cryptosporidium parvum* causes mild to severe self-limiting gastrointestinal disease; symptoms often include vomiting, watery diarrhea, fever, and malaise.[9] Immunologically normal animals and humans eliminate the parasite in two to three weeks. The parasite may persist in immunocompromised humans and cause severely debilitating chronic diarrhea. The life cycle of *C. parvum* includes autoinfectious oocysts that amplify the initial infection without fecal–oral contamination. There are no drugs to control this parasite in humans or animals, and oocysts are resistant to common disinfectants. Hot water and sodium hypochlorite, however, destroy oocysts in the environment.

Cryptosporidiosis is rarely found in kits older than 10 weeks and is not usually associated with diarrhea in ferrets. Heavy parasitism may reduce feed efficiency in growing animals, but zoonosis is the major concern when ferrets are infected with *C. parvum.* Uncooked beef by-products (e.g., tripe and liver) are palatable to ferrets and have been commonly fed to mink and fitch. Raw by-products, however, are a poor food choice for pet ferrets because of contamination with *Cryptosporidium* species and other parasites.

Cryptosporidiosis is not easily diagnosed in live animals. The oocysts are very small (approximately 5 microns) and may not be found in sodium nitrate flotation samples. Oocysts, however, will rise in concentrated sugar solutions with centrifuging. Highly refractive oocysts may be found in fresh fecal smears that are examined by phase-contrast microscopy *immediately* after acid-fast staining.[8] If the smears are left for more than a few minutes before examination, the oocysts will stain acid-fast and be difficult to find. Oocysts resemble bright, little lightbulbs against a red background immediately after staining (Figure 1).

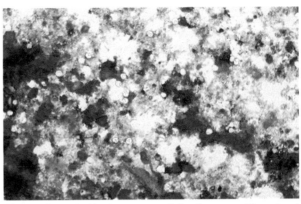

Figure 1 Carbolfuchsin-stained fecal smear. Unstained *Cryptosporidium* oocysts are distinct against the acid-fast stained background. (×100)

The literature indicates that ferrets are susceptible to toxoplasmosis[2]; however, clinical cases in pet ferrets have not been reported. Mink that were fed infected muskrats and rabbits developed toxoplasmosis; spontaneous abortion was the common clinical sign.[7] Ferrets that are permitted to hunt and eat prey are most likely to become infected. The possibility of zoonosis from a ferret with toxoplasmosis is remote. The serologic test for toxoplasmosis in dogs and cats is diagnostic in mink and probably is effective in ferrets.

Clinical giardiasis is not described in the literature pertaining to mustelids, but mink and ferrets are believed to be susceptible to infection.[2] Kits in pet stores may possibly be infected by contaminated food or water that has been handled by attendants coming in contact with infected puppies before caring for the ferrets. Ferrets have been treated with metronidazole (a common treatment for giardiasis) for weeks at a time without ill effects. The suggested dose is 35 mg/kg daily, but one quarter of a 200-mg tablet (the smallest available) given daily for at least five days is safe for a 400- to 500-gram ferret.

ECTOPARASITES

Most ferrets have ear mites (*Otodectes cynotis*) at some time in their lives but rarely show evidence of distress. Ferrets do not scratch their ears or shake their heads even when the ear canal is full of dark-red waxy discharge. Treatment at three- to six-week intervals controls and eventually eliminates mites and keeps the ear canal clean. Feline ear mite remedies[1] or diluted ivermectin solution can be instilled locally. Injectable ivermectin is mixed with propylene glycol at a ratio of approximately 1:20; 0.2 to 0.3 milliliters (10 to 15 milligrams) is dropped into each ear canal. If the ferret is on seasonal heartworm prophylaxis, ear mites will be affected by the systemic drug and no further treatment will be necessary.

Female ferrets (jills) can be safely treated with iver-mectin during the latter stages of pregnancy and again before the ear canals of kits open (at three to four weeks of age) to reduce the number of mites that may potentially infest the litter. Cats or other suscep-tible animals that are kept in the same household as ferrets should also be treated.

Ferrets acquire fleas (*Ctenocephalides* species) from either cats or dogs[1] and may be infested heavily enough to become anemic. Many ferrets are allergic to flea bites and develop areas of alopecia that regrow hair when fleas are controlled. Fleas are most easily found between the shoulder blades of heavily para-sitized or allergic ferrets. The skin may be excoriated and the hair may be sparse in this area.

Any flea treatment that is safe for use in cats is therapeutically safe for ferrets when used correctly, including dips, shampoos, sprays, and collars. Ferrets have oily coats and skin and must be shampooed and rinsed before being submerged in a dip to allow the solution to thoroughly wet the hair. Even very young kits can be sprayed with pyrethrins with impunity. If females nursing kits must be treated, it is better to treat the nest material daily rather than applying medication (that may be licked off by the kits) direct-ly on the jill. Flea collars may be hazardous to ferrets that are permitted to run loose in the house and climb inside furniture or appliances because they may get caught on projections.

The environment must be very thoroughly treated, particularly in small spaces where ferrets have been sleeping. Bedding should be changed or treated regu-larly. Cedar litterbox filler helps to control fleas in the cage and does not harm or irritate ferrets. Ferrets should be confined to a small area until the fleas are completely eliminated. Other animals in the house should also be treated for fleas at the same time or ferrets will quickly become reinfested.

Ferrets that have escaped and spend even a short time on the ground or wooded areas may be infested with ticks of several *Ixodes* species. Ticks may attach themselves to the head, neck, and abdomen of ferrets. Sprays and dips that are safe for use on cats may be used to remove ticks from ferrets. Lyme disease has not been reported in ferrets.

Pet ferrets that are well housed and well fed are probably not as susceptible to sarcoptic mange (*Sar-coptes scabiei*) as fitch that were previously kept for fur production. Ferrets with mange have itchy, swollen, red, and weeping paws and legs that progressively get worse. Untreated fitch may lose their claws because of the severe damage done to their feet.[2] A skin scraping should be performed by a veterinarian if a lesion that resembles mange is discovered on a ferret. The tradi-tional remedy for mange in fitch was a lime-sulfur dip that did not provide a complete cure. Ivermectin, however, most likely works well in ferrets because it is effective in other animals that have mange.[10]

CONCLUSION

Health problems in mature ferrets housed indoors are rarely caused by parasites; therefore, other causes should be investigated. Ferrets, like other animals, de-velop resistance to coccidia and *Cryptosporidium* species (their most common endoparasites) as they mature. Complications that result from ear mite and flea infestation are easy to diagnose and can be per-manently eliminated if ferrets are not reexposed.

About the Author

At the time of original publication, Dr. Bell was staff veteri-narian with Marshall Farms USA Inc, North Rose, New York.

REFERENCES

1. Fox JG: *Biology and Diseases of the Ferret.* Philadelphia, Lea & Febiger, 1988, pp 6, 242–245.
2. Ryland LM, Bernard SL, Gorham JR: A clinical guide to the pet ferret. *Compend Contin Educ Pract Vet* 5(1):25–32, 1983.
3. Allen JA, Kirk RJ: *The Principles of Mink Ranching: Mink Ranching in Manitoba.* Game and Fisheries Branch Depart-ment of Mines and Natural Resources, 1940, p 121.
4. Anderson RC: *Nematode Parasites of Vertebrates: Their De-velopment and Transmission.* Wallingford, CT, CAB Interna-tional, 1992, p 274.
5. Sloss MW, Kemp RL: *Veterinary Clinical Parasitology.* Ames, IA, Iowa State University Press, 1989, pp 65–69.
6. Georgi JR: *Parasitology for Veterinarians.* Philadelphia, WB Saunders Co, 1985, p 80.
7. Leonard A: *Modern Mink Management.* Ralston Purina Company, 1966, p 125.
8. Garcia LS, Bruckner DA, Brewer TC, et al: Techniques for the recovery and identification of *Cryptosporidium* oocysts from stool specimens. *J Clin Microbiol* 18:185–190, 1983.
9. Current WL, Bick PH: Immunobiology of *Cryptosporidium* spp. *Pathol Immunopathol Res* 8:141–160, 1989.
10. Roken BO: Parasitic diseases of carnivores, in Fowler ME (ed): *Zoo and Wild Animal Medicine, Current Therapy,* ed 3. Philadelphia, WB Saunders Co, 1993, pp 399–404.

Rabbit Anesthesia

University of Bern
Bern, Switzerland
Gina Neiger-Aeschbacher, DrMedVet

KEY FACTS

❏ Doses of anesthetic drugs for rabbits are relatively high when compared with other animals of similar size.

❏ Use of short-acting or reversible substances and inhalant anesthetics facilitates control over the depth of anesthesia.

❏ Oxygen supplementation and endotracheal intubation enhance anesthesia safety and recovery.

❏ The criteria for assessing the depth of anesthesia in rabbits vary from those used for cats and dogs.

The domesticated or European rabbit *(Oryctolagus cuniculus)* is a lagomorph of the family Leporidae,[1] which includes several breeds (e.g., Dutch, Polish, New Zealand white). An approved research animal for decades, the rabbit has gained a secure place as a family pet among other household animals. The indications for general anesthesia in the rabbit are numerous (e.g., dental work, wound cleaning, otitis treatment, ovariohysterectomy and castration). In a nervous animal, heavy sedation may also be required to assist diagnosis and treatment.[2] Rabbits are considered one of the most difficult and unpredictable species to anesthetize.[3–5] This perception is attributed to the apparent sensitivity of the rabbit's respiratory center to anesthetic agents, the narrow range between anesthetic and toxic doses, and the wide species variability to the depressant effects of anesthetics.[3,4] This article summarizes the perianesthetic management of rabbits.

PREANESTHETIC EVALUATION

A clinical evaluation of the rabbit's health status should be performed prior to anesthesia. Special attention should be given to signs of disease involving the respiratory system (respiratory noises, changed respiratory pattern, sneezing, coughing), the digestive tract (status of teeth and buccal mucosa, appetite, weight loss, consistency of feces), and fluid homeostasis (skin turgor, moistness of mucous membranes).[6] Any abnormalities or disease conditions should be corrected to minimize anesthetic risk.

ROUTES OF DRUG ADMINISTRATION

The marginal ear veins, because of their prominence and ease of access, are considered the veins of choice for intravenous injections.[4,7] A 22-gauge, 1.5-inch, over-the-needle catheter can be used for venous cannulation in most rabbits. It is not advisable to puncture the vein directly from above because the pressure applied to the ear will flatten the vein and hinder penetration.[4] Dilatation and visibility of the vein can be enhanced by rubbing the vein, applying heat (e.g., heat lamp), alcohol, and/or xylene.[1,3,8,10,11] A topical anesthetic can be used to reduce discomfort.[12] Intravenous injections should always be given slowly, titrated to effect, and preferably given as dilute solutions.

Intramuscular injection is the most common route of drug administration because of the ease of execution. Injections should be made into large muscle masses. Volumes up to one milliliter can be injected with a 22-gauge (or smaller) needle into the quadriceps, posterior thigh, or lumbar muscles.[1,9,13]

The administration of drugs into the subcutaneous tissue at the dorsal as-

TABLE I
Drugs Used for Premedicating Rabbits[5,7,11,13,27–29,a]

Substance (Dose and Route)	Effects	Comments
Atropine (0.8–1.0 IM, IV up to 3.0 IM, SC)	Reduces salivary and bronchial secretions; protects heart from vagal inhibition	Endogenous atropinase levels make repeated injections every 10–15 min necessary
Glycopyrrolate (0.011 IV)		Advantageous over atropine
Diazepam (2.0 IV, 4–10 IM)	Good sedation and muscle relaxation; no analgesia; broad therapeutic index	Broad therapeutic index, insoluble in water
Midazolam (2.0 IV, 4.0 IM)		Broad therapeutic index, water soluble
Acepromazine (0.5–2.0 IM)	Moderate sedation, tranquilization, no analgesia; hypotensive and hypothermic effects	
Chlorpromazine (20–25 IM)		
Morphine (2.0–5.0 IM, SC)	Sedation, analgesia, degree of respiratory depression drug dependent	
Meperidine (10 IM, SC)		
Butorphanol (0.1–0.5 IM, IV)		
Xylazine (1.0–3.0 IV, 4.0–5.0 IM)	Sedation, some analgesia, cardiac dysrhythmias, respiratory depression	
Medetomidine (0.3–0.5 SC)		
Ketamine (15: IV, 25 IM)	Sedation, muscle rigidity	Chemical restraint
Fentanyl/droperidol (0.2 ml/kg: IM)	Good analgesia, bradycardia possible, injection painful	Naloxone (0.1 mg/kg IV) to reverse effects of fentanyl

[a]If not stated otherwise, all doses are in mg/kg. IV = intravenously, IM = intramuscularly, SC = subcutaneously.

pect of the neck (scruff) or flank is straightforward.[1,13] A 20-gauge needle can be used and volumes up to 50 milliliters can be injected. The rate of absorption and onset of drug action is less predictable with this route of administration.

GENERAL CONSIDERATIONS

In general, the doses of anesthetic drugs are higher for the rabbit than for a cat or dog of similar size. In the rabbits, response to anesthetic agents is affected by many factors, including age, sex, breed and strain, body weight, and time of day.[1,5] Widely varied dose requirements within the species have been described.[5]

Rabbits should always be weighed before anesthesia because estimations of body weight are not reliable. It should be kept in mind, however, that the body weight of the rabbit may overestimate lean body mass due to the voluminous intestinal tract, particularly the large ingesta-filled cecum.[1,5]

It may be beneficial to calculate the drug dose based on metabolic body size ($W_{kg}^{0.75}$). This formula takes into account the fact that smaller animals require larger doses of anesthetic drugs than larger animals to achieve the same drug effect. Further, it is recommended that all intravenously administered drugs be given to effect for the individual rabbit and not given according to fixed, calculated dose rates. For intramuscularly administered drugs, it is recommended to start at the lower end of the recommended dose range when titrating for drug effect in an individual animal.

Fasting for more than one hour before anesthesia is not indicated due to a rabbit's high metabolic rate[14] and the low risk of vomiting[13] occurring during anesthesia induction. Fasting also can cause potentially

TABLE II
Injectable Drugs Used for Induction of Anesthesia in Rabbits[5,7,13,36,a]

Substance (Dose and Route)	Duration of Anesthesia	Effects	Comments
Thiopental (30–45 slowly IV) Thiamylal (30–40 slowly IV) Methohexital (10 slowly IV)	5–10 min (allows for endotracheal intubation)	Little analgesia, transient apnea possible, hypotensive, can cause abundant bronchial and salivary secretions	Incremental doses with little risk of accumulation
Ketamine (10–20 IV, 25–60 IM, SC)	20 min	Respiratory depression dose dependent, tachycardia and hypotension possible, can cause abundant bronchial and salivary secretions	
Propofol (8–12 slowly IV)	5 min (allows for endotracheal intubation)	Respiratory depression dependent on speed of injection and dose, no analgesic properties, hypotensive, induction and recovery free of excitement	Do not mix with other drugs, can be diluted with dextrose (5%) in water; little risk of accumulation with incremental injections; expensive
Fentanyl/droperidol (0.2–0.3 ml/kg IM)	30–60 min	Good analgesia, respiratory depression and bradycardia possible, injection painful	Incremental doses (0.1 ml/kg) every 30–40 min to prolong anesthesia; naloxone (0.1 mg/kg IV) to reverse fentanyl

[a]If not stated otherwise, all doses are in mg/kg. IV = intravenously, IM = intramuscularly, SC = subcutaneously.

detrimental side effects, such as hypoglycemia and acid–base imbalance.[10]

PREANESTHETIC MEDICATION

The primary indications for preanesthetic medication of rabbits are the same as in other species. Such indications include alleviation of apprehension and anxiety and reduction of excitement during the induction of and recovery from anesthesia. Whenever possible, rabbits should be sedated before being removed from the cage or accustomed surroundings to reduce possible stress and anxiety, to decrease the possibility of injuries, and to prevent additional catecholamine release.[13] Also, as part of preanesthetic preparation, bland, sterile ophthalmic ointment or drops should be used to prevent corneal drying and irritation.[1]

Anticholinergic agents may be indicated in rabbits, especially when salivation (e.g., ketamine and barbiturate use) and bradycardia (e.g., opioid and α_2-agonist use) are anticipated. The use of atropine as a standard premedication is controversial because the effectiveness varies among strains of rabbits. High levels of endogenous atropinase are present in 30% to 50% of all rabbits.[5,7] Glycopyrrolate is a better choice than atropine in rabbits because of the longer duration of action.[a]

[a]Webb AI: Personal communication, College of Veterinary Medicine, University of Florida, Gainesville, FL, 1992.

Table I summarizes the most frequently used substances for premedication in rabbits.

INDUCTION AND MAINTENANCE

Selection of an anesthetic agent is governed by the length of the anesthetic period needed and the health status of the animal. Rabbits are not considered good candidates for intravenous anesthetics[9] because even the small incremental doses that are needed to maintain anesthesia may cause respiratory arrest.[14] Slow, intravenous injections given to effect are important to avoid overdose and acute toxicity. Anesthesia depth is more easily controlled by intravenously administered short-acting and/or reversible drugs and inhalant anesthetics. Although desirable, oxygenation via a face mask frequently prohibits smooth induction of anesthesia.

When a rabbit has been anesthetized with ketamine, it is difficult to determine whether body movements made during the anesthetic period are due to central nervous system stimulation by the drug or inadequate anesthetic depth and pain sensation.[7] Ketamine has limited use as a sole anesthetic because of muscle rigidity, inadequate analgesia, and possible seizure activity; therefore, it is more frequently used in combination with other anesthetic agents. Tissue irritation and muscle necrosis are other possible adverse effects of intramuscular injection of ketamine.[1]

TABLE III

Inhalant Anesthetics for Induction and
Maintenance of Anesthesia in Rabbits[4,13,14,18]

Substance	Induction Dose	Maintenance Dose	Comments
Halothane	3.0% to 4.0%	1.0% to 2.0%	Narrower margin of safety than methoxyflurane; cardiovascular depression stronger than methoxyflurane
Isoflurane	3.5% to 4.5%	1.5% to 3.0%	Resembles halothane in its effects, but respiratory depression stronger and cardiovascular depression less than with halothane
Enflurane	3.0% to 5.0%	0.5% to 2.0%	Resembles halothane with regard to cardiovascular and respiratory depression
Methoxyflurane	3.0%	0.4% to 1.0%	Safe, effective, good muscle relaxation; analgesic properties that extend into recovery period; cardiovascular and respiratory depression occur but less than halothane at comparable anesthetic levels

If only a short (30-minute) to moderate (60-minute) period of anesthesia is required, an intramuscularly administered drug combination is adequate. Suitable anesthetic regimens include ketamine with an α_2-agonist or a benzodiazepine and neuroleptoanalgesic combination. The combination of tiletamine and zolazepam has been used in rabbits for sedation and induction of anesthesia. Nephrotoxic effects of this drug combination have been described.[15] Although these effects could not be demonstrated by other researchers,[16] this drug combination does not offer significant advantages over ketamine and diazepam to justify its continued use in rabbits.

The use of barbiturates for anesthesia induction has exhibited large variations in dose requirements and has a recovery period that can be accompanied by excitatory behavior unless appropriate premedication is given. Less concentrated barbiturate solutions (e.g., thiamylal and thiopental less than 2%, methohexital not more than 1%) should be used to reduce pain on injection, to facilitate titration to effect, and to decrease the risk of overdose. Pentobarbital has shown a marked variability in response, a low therapeutic index, and high mortality; as a result, it is best avoided in rabbits.[13] Long-term anesthesia (longer than 90 minutes) can be maintained with injectable anesthetics, but inhalant anesthetic agents or a combination of injectable and inhalant anesthetics in a balanced regimen are considered safer.[9,17] An oxygen source should always be available,[9] and endotracheal intubation should be performed if anesthesia is going to be prolonged.[5,7] Table II lists the most frequently used injectable induction agents for rabbit anesthesia. After premedication with a sedative or tranquilizer, the induction doses of most injectable anesthetic drugs can be reduced by 30% to 50%.

ADMINISTRATION OF INHALANT ANESTHETICS

Anesthesia can be induced by only using inhalant anesthetics via a mask or chamber, but these procedures can be very stressful for rabbits. Premedication with a sedative or tranquilizer followed by an injectable agent helps produce a smooth induction and transition to maintenance of anesthesia. Inhalant anesthetics administered via an endotracheal tube is the safest technique for rabbit anesthesia. Maintenance of anesthesia with inhalant anesthetics administered by mask is acceptable for 30 to 45 minutes,[9] but administration by endotracheal intubation is preferable. Respiratory depression with hypoxia is the most frequently encountered side effect in anesthetized rabbits.[4] During the anesthetic period, it is recommended to support respiration by intermittent, positive-pressure ventilations (sighs) every 15 to 25 spontaneous breaths[7] or about once per minute. Because of the rabbit's small respiratory tidal volumes,[1] a pediatric circle breathing system or nonrebreathing circuits (e.g., Ayre's T-tube, Bain coaxial system) are recommended for rabbits. These breathing systems offer the least resistance to breathing and minimal dead space.[13,14] All commercially available inhalant anesthetics have been used in rabbits,[4,13,14,18] and oxygen and nitrous oxide can be used simultaneously as carrier gases in a ratio of 1:1. Table III lists the common inhalant anesthetics used in rabbits.

ENDOTRACHEAL INTUBATION

Prolonged anesthesia with injectable or inhalant anesthetic agents is safer with an endotracheal tube in place.[5] The anatomic characteristics of the rabbit head and neck make visualization of the epiglottis and larynx difficult. I use the blind, oroendotracheal method exclusively: intubation is guided by respiratory sounds and tube insertion timed during an early inspiration. Laryngospasm has been described as a possible complication during rabbit intubation.[19] Application of a local anesthetic to the larynx or the endotracheal tube can be helpful.[6,9,13,19] Depending on the size of the animal, a 2.0-mm to 4.0-mm inner diameter (3.3-mm to 6.0-mm outer diameter; 10-French to 18-French) endotracheal tube will be adequate. The internal diameter of the adult rabbit trachea is approximately five millimeters. Although intubation is easier with uncuffed tubes, cuffed tubes can be used. The cuff should be inflated just enough to preclude leakage around the cuff and to allow a peak pressure of about 15 cm H_2O with positive-pressure ventilation.[20] This level of inflation allows sufficient blood supply to the underlying tracheal mucosa. The length of the endotracheal tube should be long enough to prevent inadvertent extubation. Accidental bronchial intubation is rare because the trachea bifurcates into the smaller right and left main-stem bronchi at equal obtuse angles.[21] After correct placement and patency has been confirmed, the tube should then be secured in place.

MONITORING AND CARE DURING THE ANESTHETIC PERIOD

Careful monitoring of the anesthetized rabbit is essential to assure appropriate anesthesia depth (i.e., unconsciousness, analgesia, muscle relaxation) for the procedure, to maintain an airway and correct ventilation, to support adequate circulation, to preserve renal function, and to maintain normothermia. Anesthesia depth is continuously assessed by monitoring different body systems. The use of monitoring devices depends on availability. The physiologic parameters should be monitored and recorded according to a standard written protocol.

Body temperature should be continuously monitored. The high ratio of body surface to body weight (despite the heavy fur) predisposes the rabbit to hypothermia. Hypothermia increases the susceptibility to complications (e.g., sudden death, prolonged recovery, distress, and exacerbation of clinically silent respiratory disease) both during and after surgery. To prevent or minimize heat loss, the following precautions can be taken: increase the temperature in the operating or procedure room; create a draft-free environment; wrap the animal in aluminum foil, plastic

Indicators of Planes of Anesthesia in the Rabbit

Light: Chewing and head lift[6]; nystagmus[26]

Safe: Rate and depth of respiration is regular but deeper and slower than in the awake animal[5,9] with more pronounced abdominal features[3]; respiratory frequency not less than 40 breaths per minute[26]

Deep: Respiration shallow and intermittent[3]

Dangerously deep: Exophthalmus and strong protrusion of third eyelid[6]; wide pupils, pale mauve "fish eye"[9]; loss of corneal[9] and anal[26] reflex

Signs of Surgical Anesthesia

Unreliable: Response to pin prick on abdomen and skin sensitivity of trunk[13]

Reliable: Negative pedal withdrawal[3,17,26]; negative ear pinch[9,17,23,26]

wrap, or a warm-water circulating heating pad; humidify and warm the inspired anesthetic gases; and warm the intravenous and surgical irrigation fluids.

The respiratory pattern and rate should be regular with deep, uniform breaths. An esophageal stethoscope and direct observation of the reservoir bag are methods for monitoring respiration rate. An electrocardiogram is helpful in monitoring heart rate and rhythm. An estimate of pulse quality can be made by palpating a peripheral artery—the central ear artery is the best choice.

Adequate peripheral perfusion is indicated by pale pink mucous membranes and a capillary refill time of less than two seconds. A fluid replacement rate of 10 ml/kg/hr[13] is necessary to maintain normovolemia in all but the shortest anesthetic periods. Continuous infusion of lactated Ringer's solution or a mixture of dextrose (5%) in water and normal saline are appropriate replacement fluids. The total blood volume of the rabbit is between 6% to 8% of the body weight.

The criteria for assessing anesthesia depth in rabbits vary from those used for other small animals and seem to be more complex. The rabbit pupil is slow to react and is not reliable in predicting anesthesia depth.[3] The palpebral reflex often persists after surgical anesthesia stage has been achieved[3] and becomes absent only at dangerously deep anesthesia stages[13] and low arterial oxygen tensions.[22] Eye reflexes, position, and movement are of limited use and should not be relied on because they vary with the drugs used.[13] At deep levels of anesthesia and with many anesthetic regimens, the pedal withdrawal reflex may remain strong even if the animal is very close to death, again demonstrating the strong reflex activity in the rabbit.[6,14] The reliability of accepted reflex tests as indicators of anesthesia level has been rated (most to least reliable) as follows: pinna, pedal, corneal, palpebral reflex.[23] Reaction to ear pinch (i.e., vocalizing, head shaking) is regarded as the most sensitive test for assessing analgesia and surgical depth of anesthesia[23] (see the box).

Bradycardia (i.e., an approximate 20% reduction in heart rate from preanesthetic values[7]) can be a sign of very deep anesthesia. Blood pressure, but not heart rate, is a good indicator of systemic response to a noxious stimulus.[24] Increased respiratory rate in response to surgical stimulation can be a sign of inadequate anesthesia depth or can be due to hypercarbia.[13] Respiratory rate is a reasonable indicator of respiratory depression, which is commonly associated with deep anesthesia levels, especially in rabbits with subclinical respiratory disease.[25]

CONCLUSION

Rabbit anesthesia has become safer with the increased knowledge about the physiologic characteristics of the species and with the availability of potent, short-acting, and reversible anesthetic agents. Neuroleptoanalgesic combinations with fentanyl, inhalant anesthetics (i.e., halothane, isoflurane), or balanced anesthetic combinations provide reliable and predictable anesthesia. Oxygen supplementation for all but the shortest anesthetic periods is recommended. Although successful endotracheal intubation requires patience and practice, the advantage of a patent airway is indisputable. Until complete recovery has been achieved, anesthesia monitoring and patient care are of utmost importance. Providing analgesia during and after the surgical intervention contributes to the patient's well-being and anesthesia outcome.

About the Author

Dr. Neiger-Aeschbacher, who is a Diplomate of the American College of Veterinary Anesthesia and the European College of Veterinary Anesthesia, is affiliated with the Department of Anesthesia, Small and Large Animal Clinics, School of Veterinary Medicine, University of Bern, Bern, Switzerland.

REFERENCES

1. Harkness JE, Wagner JE: *The Biology and Medicine of Rabbits and Rodents*, ed 3. Philadelphia, Lea & Febiger, 1989, pp 9–11, 61–65.
2. Wood C: The pet rabbit–Veterinary problems. *Vet Rec* 102: 304–308, 1978.
3. Murdock HR: Anesthesia in the rabbit. *Fed Proc* 28(4): 1510–1516, 1969.
4. Bivin WS, Timmons EH: Basic biomethodology, in Weisbroth SH, Flatt RE, Kraus AL (eds): *The Biology of the Rabbit*. New York, Academic Press, 1974, pp 76–83.
5. Harvey RC, Walberg J: Special considerations for anesthesia and analgesia in research animals, in Short CE (ed): *Principles and Practice of Veterinary Anesthesia*. Baltimore, Williams & Wilkins, 1987, pp 380–392.
6. Erhardt W: Anaesthesieverfahren beim kaninchen. *Tieraerztl Prax* 12:391–402, 1984.
7. Sedgwick CJ: Anesthesia for rabbits. *Vet Clin North Am Food Anim Pract* 2:731–736, 1986.
8. Clifford D: Restraint and anesthesia of small laboratory animals, in Soma LR (ed): *Textbook of Veterinary Anesthesia*. Baltimore, Williams & Wilkins, 1971, pp 377–379.
9. Green CJ: *Animal Anesthesia, Laboratory Animal Handbooks*, ed 8. London, Laboratory Animals LTD, 1979, pp 131–138.
10. Bonath K, Hirche H, Lange S: Einfluss der ketamin-hydrochlorid/halothan-sauerstoffnarkose auf atmung, blutgase und saeurebasenhaushalt des kaninchens. *Berl Munch Tierarztl Wochenschr* 93:462–468, 1980.
11. Portnoy LG, Hustead DR: Pharmacokinetics of butorphanol tartrate in rabbits. *Am J Vet Res* 53(4):5441–543, 1992.
12. Flecknell PA, Liles JH, Williamson HA: The use of lignocaine-prilocaine local anesthetic cream for pain-free venipuncture in laboratory animals. *Lab Anim* 24:142–146, 1990.
13. Flecknell PA: *Laboratory Animal Anaesthesia*. London, Academic Press Ltd, 1987, pp 2–100.
14. Hall LW, Clarke KW: Anaesthesia of birds, laboratory animals and wild animals, in *Veterinary Anaesthesia*, ed 9. London, Bailliere Tindall, 1991, pp 339–351.
15. Brammer DW, Doerning BJ, Chrisp CE, et al: Anesthetic and nephrotoxic effects of Telazol® in New Zealand White rabbits. *Lab Anim Sci* 41(5):432–435, 1991.
16. Popilskis SJ, Oz MC, Gorman P, et al: Comparison of xylazine with tiletamine-zolazepam (Telazol®) and xylazine-ketamine anesthesia in rabbits. *Lab Anim Sci* 41(1):51–53, 1991.
17. Peeters ME, Gil D, Teske E, et al: Four methods for general anesthesia in the rabbit: A comparative study. *Lab Anim* 22: 355–360, 1988.
18. Allan DJ, Blackshaw JK: The anaesthesia and euthanasia of small rodents and rabbits. *Aust Vet Prac* 16(2):81–86, 1986.
19. Wixson SK: Intubation of rabbits and rodents. *Proc North Am Vet Conf* 6:719–720, 1992.
20. Boothe HW, Hartsfield SM: Use of the laboratory rabbit in the small animal student surgery laboratory. *JVME* 17(1): 16–18, 1990.
21. Davis NL, Malinin TI: Rabbit intubation and halothane anesthesia. *Lab Anim Sci* 24(4):617–621, 1974.
22. Wyatt JD, Scott RAW, Richardson ME: The effects of pro-

longed ketamine-xylazine intravenous infusion on arterial blood pH, blood gases, mean arterial blood pressure, heart and respiratory rates, rectal temperature and reflexes in the rabbit. *Lab Anim Sci* 39(5):411–416, 1989.

23. Borkowski GL, Danneman PJ, Russel GB, et al: An evaluation of three intravenous anesthetic regimens in New Zealand rabbits. *Lab Anim Sci* 40(3):270–276, 1990.
24. Danneman PJ, White WJ, Marshall WK, et al: An evaluation of analgesia associated with the immobility response in laboratory rabbits. *Lab Anim Sci* 38(1):51–57, 1988.
25. Flecknell PA, Liles JH, Wooton R: Reversal of fentanyl/fluanisone neuroleptanalgesia in the rabbit using mixed agonist/antagonist opioids. *Lab Anim* 23:147–155, 1989.
26. Genevois JP, Autefage A, Fayoll P, et al: L'anesthesie des es-

peces insolites en pratique veterinaire courante. 3. L'anesthesie du lapin et des rongeurs. *Rev Med Vet* 135(5):273–279, 1984.
27. Marini RP, Avison DL, Corning BF, et al: Ketamine/xylazine/butorphanol: A new anesthetic combination for rabbits. *Lab Anim Sci* 42(1):57–62, 1992.
28. Mero M, Vainionpaeae S, Vasenius J, et al: Medetomidine-ketamine-diazepam anesthesia in the rabbit. *Acta Vet Scand* 85:135–137, 1989.
29. Zornow MH, Spooner ML, Bloom AE, et al: The sedative and ventilatory effects of dexmedetomidine in rabbits. *Anesth Analg* 70:S449 (abstract), 1990.
30. Aeschbacher G, Webb AI: Propofol in rabbits. Part I: Evaluation of an induction dose. *Lab Anim Sci* 43(4):324–327, 1993.

UPDATE

ROUTES OF DRUG ADMINISTRATION

Although the marginal ear veins are easily accessible in rabbits of all sizes, the vein on the cranial aspect of the front limb (*Vena cephalica*) offers an alternative for intravenous (IV) drug injection or venous cannulation in the conscious or sedated animal. In the anesthetized animal, the jugular or femoral veins are other choices.

DRUGS

The α_2–agonist medetomidine has become quite popular in small animal veterinary anesthesia in Europe. I use it frequently for the sedation of healthy rabbits. While more expensive than other sedative drugs (e.g., acepromazine), medetomidine offers the advantage of potent sedation with some analgetic action, reducing the anesthetic requirements dose dependently (up to 50% to 80%). Additionally, all its effects can be antagonized using the α_2–agonist atipamezole, which is specific but also costly. I use medetomidine in a dose of 0.1 to 0.25 mg/kg intramuscularly (IM). A noticeable decrease in heart and respiratory rate occurs, along with the effects already mentioned. Blind oroendotracheal intubation, which is guided by respiratory sounds, becomes more challenging: The reduction in respiratory frequency renders timing during early inspiration more difficult independent of the drug used for induction of anesthesia. The grade of sedation will also influence the coughing reflex. In my experience, this sometimes prohibits the early recognition of correct endotracheal placement of the tube.

It appears that the production of the combination fentanyl/droperidol (Innovar–Vet®) has been discontinued. In many countries, it is no longer available for the veterinary market although it is still offered for use in humans (Innovar®). It remains unclear whether or when it will become obtainable again. Although much more expensive and less concentrated (resulting in a larger volume), the ratio of the two drugs in the human preparation is equal to that in Innovar-Vet®.

The following drug combinations are suggested in substitution of fentanyl/droperidol:

- Fentanyl/fluanisone (Hypnorm®) 0.2 to 0.5 ml/kg IM: Some sedation and analgesia with the lower doses; with the higher doses, sufficient analgesia for smaller interventions (drainage of abscess). Hypnorm® 0.3 ml/kg IV in combination with a benzodiazepine (e.g. midazolam 2 mg/kg IM) provides 20 to 40 minutes of surgical anesthesia, which can be prolonged if necessary with Hypnorm® 0.1 ml/kg IV or IM every 30 to 40 minutes. Naloxone (0.01 to 0.1 mg/kg IV or IM) antagonizes respiratory depression, sedation, and analgesia and speeds recovery. Using an opioid antagonist/agonist (e.g. butorphanol, buprenorphine, nalbuphine) maintains analgesia.
- Ketamine alone is not very suitable for rabbit anesthesia but in conjunction with other drugs becomes a good alternative to fentanyl combinations: Xylazine 1 to 3 mg/kg slowly IV, 3 to 5 mg/kg IM; medetomidine 0.1 to 0.25 mg/kg slowly IV or IM; acepromazine 0.5 to 1.0 mg/kg IM; or diazepam or midazolam 2 to 4 mg/kg IM, each followed by ketamine 10 mg/kg IV or 30 to 50 mg/kg IM will provide surgical anesthesia for approximately 30 minutes.

ANALGESIA

Analgesia during recovery is an important requirement. Several analgetic agents have been used in the rabbit:

Substance	Dose (mg/kg) & Route	Interval (hours)
Buprenorphine	0.01–0.05 IM, SC, IV	8–12
Butorphanol	0.1–0.5 IM, SC, IV	2–4
Meperidine (Pethidine)	10 IM, SC	2–3
Morphine	2–5 IM, SC	2–4
Nalbuphine	1–2 IM, SC; IV	4–5
Pentazocine	5–20 IM, SC, IV	2–4

MASK OR CHAMBER INDUCTION WITH INHALANT ANESTHETICS

Without sedative premedication, induction of anesthesia using a mask or chamber for administration can lead to severe struggling and to breath-holding for up to two minutes, accompanied by significant bradycardia and moderate hypercapnia. Premedication does not prevent the breath-holding response, but does reduce the degree of heart rate decline.[1]

ENDOTRACHEAL INTUBATION

Although advantageous in some aspects, endotracheal intubation in the rabbit should not be persistently pursued. Several unsuccessful attempts at intubation can lead to trauma, hematoma and edema formation at and around the tracheal opening, followed by obstruction and respiratory distress.

REFERENCE

1. Flecknell PA: Influence of medetomidine, acepromazine or midazolam on the adverse effects of induction of anesthesia with halothane. Abstract. *Proceedings of the Spring Conference of the Association of Veterinary Anaesthetists*, p 69, 1995.

Nutrition and Pet Rabbits

Susan Donoghue, VMD
Nutrition Support Services, Inc.
Pembroke, Virginia

Domesticated rabbits can be great pets. Naturally quiet yet alert and inquisitive, they come in a variety of sizes, colors, and appearances. Short haired or long haired; large, medium, or small sized; erect eared or lop-eared—all make fine companions. Some pet rabbits are kept outdoors in hutches; others are kept indoors, trained to use a litter box, and given the run of the home.

Although owners are usually responsible and well-meaning, the nutritional needs of pet rabbits are sometimes not met. Owners that are familiar with the feeding of dogs and cats may lack understanding of the needs of nonruminant herbivores. A veterinary technician's counsel of rabbit owners about diet may prevent nutritional disease. In addition, the technician's experiences with rabbit nutrition are applicable to hospital care because sick rabbits that are presented to veterinary hospitals may require nutrition support.

Nutritional Problems
Supermarket Diets

Pet rabbits that are fed only foods from supermarkets are at risk for malnutrition. Individual foods for humans are not complete and balanced as are many commercial diets for animals. Most human foods lack one or more essential nutrients; humans achieve nutritional completeness by selecting a variety of foods and by taking supplements (e.g., multivitamin pills). Owners often fail to achieve such balance for their rabbits.

Most technicians know of house rabbits that are fed produce and cereals. Much of the produce commonly fed to rabbits is low in calories and deficient in several essential nutrients (Table I). Many cereals (e.g., granola) contain too much fat (for rabbits) and too few essential nutrients, such as calcium. Almost all supermarket foods, even those labeled "high fiber," contain an inadequate amount of fiber for rabbits.

Fiber

Gastrointestinal disease caused by low fiber intake may be the most prevalent feeding problem in house rabbits.

Rabbits have a simple stomach and a specialized lower bowel. They are hindgut fermenters, as are other companion animals (e.g., horses and iguanas), but have special adaptations. Large fiber particles quickly transit the ileum and colon; fine low-fiber particles travel backward (via reverse peristalsis) from the colon into the cecum for fermentation.[1] Cecal fermentation yields short-chain volatile fatty acids (propionate, butyrate, and acetate) that are absorbed and used for energy.

The fiber residue is excreted as hard fecal pellets. The nonfiber portions are excreted and consumed (coprophagy) and are referred to as soft feces or night feces. Compared with hard feces, soft feces contain less fiber and more water, protein, volatile fatty acids, vitamins, and minerals.[1] Coprophagy is normal in rabbits and, incidentally, in hares, lemmings, and koalas.

Rabbits that are fed low-fiber diets may be presented with signs of gastrointestinal disease, such as diarrhea or constipation. Some patients exhibit such behavioral signs as hair chewing. Many are very sick and anorectic.

Improving Supermarket Diets

Supplements can be added to supermarket foods to increase fiber and to improve levels of calories, calcium, and other essential nutrients. Such diets are difficult to balance without training in ration formulation, however. A diet change is usually safer, cheaper, and more convenient for owners.

Diets of hay, commercial rabbit food, and treats usually ensure nutritional completeness and adequate fiber intake. These diets are considered in more detail here.

Finding Fiber

High-fiber plant foods, referred to as roughages or forages, include fresh grasses and legumes, hay, pellets, and cubes. Forage in pellets and cubes has been chopped into small pieces and then compressed. Research in cattle suggests that grinding and pelleting forage increases food intake and utilization of digestible energy.

TABLE I
Calorie and Nutrient Contents of Supermarket Foods[a]

Food Item	Energy (kcal/g as fed)	Protein	Fat	Nonfiber Carbohydrate	Fiber	Calcium	Phosphorus
		----------------------		(% dry-matter basis[b])	----------------------		
Romaine lettuce	0.18	21	5	56	11	1.1	0.4
Spinach	0.26	36	3	48	7	1.0	0.6
Dandelion greens	0.44	18	5	61	11	1.2	0.4
Beet greens	0.24	24	3	51	14	1.3	0.4
Alfalfa sprouts	0.39	37	4	39	12	0.2	
Carrots	0.42	9	2	82	8	0.3	0.3
Granola	4.5	11	18	70	1	0.1	0.3
Puffed oats	4.0	16	7	74	2	0.1	0.5
Flaked bran	3.3	13	2	82	4	0.1	0.5
Bran and fruit cereal	3.1	10	1	84	4	0	0.6

[a]Pennington JAT, Church HN: *Bowe's and Church's Food Values of Portions Commonly Used.* Philadelphia, JB Lippincott Co, 1985.
[b]Water contents vary greatly.

In herbivores, fiber aids gut motility and water balance and yields calories via fermentation. Herbivores generally prefer and maintain better gut motility and function with long-stem fiber (found in hays, fresh forage, and coarsely chopped cubes) rather than short-stem fiber (found in meals, pellets, and, recently, some small cubes).

Hay can be purchased from feed stores and farms. Alfalfa cubes are readily available from pet shops but are relatively expensive. The cubes also can be purchased from feed stores in 50-pound (22.7-kg) bags and stored in metal trash cans in a cool, dry room. Such a purchase is suitable for a large rabbitry, but consumption is too slow if 50 pounds of cubes are fed to a few rabbits—vitamin A activity is diminished. This loss of activity is the primary nutritional change that is likely to cause a clinical problem.

For pet rabbits, product quality and owner convenience may be the primary determinants of the form of roughage selected. Suburban owners may find small bags of pellets or cubes easier to manage than hay bales. Forage need not be of the highest quality if the remaining diet of commercial pellets and treats is of superior quality.

Commercial Diets

Rabbit pellets are designed to be complete feeds (Table II). Such diets are formulated to provide all nutrients and fuel sources necessary to meet the particular requirements at a given stage of the animal's life cycle. Pellets are easy to store and feed, can be offered free choice, and minimize waste. They contain 12% to 28% crude fiber and 14% to 19% crude protein. Occasionally, commercial diets cause nutritional problems.

At the North American Veterinary Conference in Orlando, Florida, in January 1992, vitamin A deficiency was described in an unpublished report of a rabbitry that fed pellets composed of old alfalfa hay. Carotene, the precursor of vitamin A, is lost as hay ages; the pellets in question were made from two-year-old hay. The purchaser should look for pellets that are bright green; brown pellets may contain scant carotene. Rabbits that are deficient in vitamin A exhibit increased mortality, poor reproduction, birth deformities, and (in erect-eared rabbits) drooping ear tips.

In another rabbitry, vitamin A intoxication was diagnosed.[2] The problem was caused by errors in pellet preparation—10 times the recommended level of vitamin A was added inadvertently. Clinical signs of vitamin A intoxication are similar to those of vitamin A deficiency: poor reproduction and birth defects. Despite occasional problems with commercial feeds, rabbit pellets are the safest and most convenient way to provide balanced and complete nutrition to pet rabbits.

Snacks

Supermarket produce and cereals make fine treats and snacks for pet rabbits. Small amounts of greens, vegetables, cereals, and low-fat snacks (e.g., rice cakes) are well accepted by rabbits. Owners should be counseled to limit snack feeding and to ensure that most of the daily food consumed is pellets and forage.

Snacks offered should be fresh and washed. Produce must be free of foreign objects (e.g., plastic twist ties and rubber bands) and washed thoroughly before feeding.

TABLE II
Examples of Forages and Rabbit Feeds

Food Item	Energy (kcal/g as fed)	Protein	Fat	Nonfiber Carbohydrate	Fiber	Calcium	Phosphorus
				(% dry-matter basis[b])			
Alfalfa hay[a] (sun-cured early bloom)	1.50	18	3	46	23	1.4	0.2
Timothy hay[a] (sun-cured, midbloom)	1.64	9	3	51	31	0.5	0.2
Clover[a] (red, fresh)	0.46	21	3	42	26	1.7	0.4
Alfalfa meal[a] (dehydrated, 15% protein)	1.50	17	3	41	29	1.4	0.2
High-fiber pelleted diets[b]	1.80	16	2	44	28	—	—
Pelleted diets for growth and reproduction[b]	2.40	19	2	50	20	—	—
Pelleted diets for all life stages[b]	2.20	16	2	49	22	—	—

[a]Committee on Animal Nutrition: *United States–Canadian Tables of Feed Composition*, ed 3. Washington, DC, National Academy Press, 1982.
[b]Data are calculated from guaranteed analyses on labels.

Feeding Management

Rabbits adjust their food intake according to the energy content of the diet.[1] For example, when a diet is changed from low-energy supermarket produce to high-energy pellets, fewer pellets (than produce) are consumed. Pet rabbits may overeat, however, and obesity can be a problem. It is usually controlled by adding high-fiber, low-energy coarse hays to the usual diet.

Depending on their size, age, environmental temperature, reproductive status, and health, rabbits consume approximately 150 to 400 calories (kcal) of metabolizable energy (ME) daily.[3] Energy needs are determined by calculating basal metabolic rate (BMR = $70 \times$ body weight in $kg^{0.75}$) and then multiplying by a maintenance factor (1.5 for adults with limited activity; 2.0 for growth).

Dry feeds, such as pellets and hay, contain approximately 1.5 to 2.5 kcal of metabolizable energy per gram (43 to 71 kcal per ounce). A healthy, three-year-old, male house rabbit that weighs two kilograms (4.4 pounds) thus requires approximately 175 kcal daily, or approximately four ounces of pellets. If the pet is very active or the house is cold, more calories are needed.

Water is provided by sipper-tube bottles or bowls and must be clean and wholesome. Rabbits drink approximately 5 to 10 milliliters per 100 grams of body weight daily.[4]

Nutrition Support

Sick rabbits that are presented to veterinary hospitals may need nutrition support. Such common disorders as hairballs and respiratory disease lead to anorexia. In order to avoid catabolism of vital tissue protein as a result of low calorie intake, nutrition support is recommended.

Selecting Diets for Sick Rabbits

Enteral diets, or slurries made with enteral diets, may be fed to rabbits via syringe or nasogastric tube. In selecting ingredients for rabbits and other herbivores (unlike ingredients for carnivores), it is necessary to look for products with less fat and protein and more complex carbohydrates and fiber.

Although enteral diets fed to sick rabbits provide needed calories and nutrients, none is ideal for hindgut fermenters. The enteral diets are made for humans. Even less acceptable are products made specifically for dogs and cats; these products contain more fat and protein, relatively few carbohydrates, and no fiber.

Enteral diets are relatively isosmolar (300 mOsm/kg) or hyperosmolar (greater than 400 mOsm/kg). Feeding isosmolar enteral diets can begin with minimal dilution for the first few meals. Feeding hyperosmolar diets begins with a 50:50 dilution with water to avoid stomach upset.

Although ideal for humans, enteral diets contain relatively high fat and low fiber levels for rabbits. Most of the fiber-containing enteral diets use soy polysaccharide to provide approximately 2 to 10 milligrams of fiber per milliliter. Alfalfa hay, by comparison, has 200 milligrams of long-stem fiber per gram; the fiber in enteral diets is of insufficient quantity and less-than-ideal physical form. Nevertheless, enteral diets provide a useful adjunct to medical and surgical care and save the lives of anorectic patients.

Slurries

Enteral diets may be blended with other ingredients to increase fiber and palatability. Two successful ingredients are yogurt and alfalfa meal.

A recipe used successfully in sick rabbits by Julie Langenberg, VMD, at the School of Veterinary Medicine of the University of Wisconsin-Madison consisted of the following: a commercial enteral diet (8 ounces; 227 grams), low-fat fruit yogurt (8 ounces; 227 grams), and alfalfa meal (4 tablespoons; 54 grams). This mix provides approximately 8% crude fiber, 1.1 kcal/ml, 17% protein (on a dry-matter basis), 8% fat, and approximately 60% carbohydrate. The alfalfa meal increases fiber (although not long-stem fiber) in a form that is more appropriate for rabbits. The diet can be fed via syringe or tube and can be managed easily by owners.

The three-year-old, male house rabbit, when sick, requires approximately 160 ml/day of slurry to meet its need for 175 kcal daily. Nutrition support would entail 20 milliliters administered four times daily for the first day, followed by 30 milliliters four times daily for the next day and then 40 milliliters four times daily.

REFERENCES

1. Partridge GG: Nutrition of farmed rabbits. *Proc Nutr Soc* 48:93–101, 1989.
2. DiGiacomo RF, Deeb BJ, Anderson RJ: Hypervitaminosis A and reproductive disorders in rabbits. *Lab Anim Sci* 42:250–254, 1992.
3. National Research Council: *Nutrient Requirements of Rabbits.* Washington, DC, National Academy Press, 1977.
4. Harkness JE: Rabbit husbandry and medicine. *Vet Clin North Am Small Anim Pract* 17:1019–1044, 1987.

Bibliography

Harkness JE, Wagner JE: *The Biology and Medicine of Rabbits and Rodents*, ed 3. Philadelphia, Lea & Febiger, 1989.

UPDATE

FEEDING FOR LIFE STAGES

Although production rabbits may eat to meet their energy needs, pet rabbits may overeat, consume too much energy, and risk obesity. Alternatively, poor diets with low protein and extremely fibrous, stemmy ingredients may limit a rabbit's energy intake, resulting in weight loss or poor growth. Many diseases and conditions, including stress, also reduce food intake in rabbits. Energy intakes may be compared to recommended energy needs in order to diagnose energy excess and deficiency.

Most commercial rabbit diets and hays provide about 2.5 to 3 calories (kcal) of metabolizable energy (ME) per gram of dry matter (DM). These foods are about 90% DM; fresh grasses may contain about 30% to 70% DM.

For rabbits at maintenance (defined as healthy adults in comfortable surroundings), energy requirements (kcal/day) are estimated to be $100W^{0.75}$ (W = body weight in kg). Energy needs increase for growth, pregnancy, and lactation: Growth, 190 to $210W^{0.75}$; early gestation, $135W^{0.75}$; late gestation, $200W^{0.75}$; lactation $300W^{0.75}$.[1]

Growing rabbits should be expected, therefore, to eat up to twice the amount of food consumed by an adult rabbit at maintenance. Juvenile rabbits often lose weight at weaning, but compensatory growth following the stress of weaning permits a return to rapid growth.[2]

Pregnant rabbits eat amounts of food that gradually increase above maintenance. By the time of late gestation, the doe is consuming twice the maintenance level. Does in late pregnancy may reduce food intake briefly, presumably because of extreme abdominal fill from the conceptus. Lactating does may eat up to three times maintenance. For lactating does, energy needs often surpass the capacity for food intake; weight will be lost but regained following the cessation of lactation.

Requirements for essential nutrients change little for different life stages, and rabbits thrive when fed diets containing 12% to 18% protein, 2% to 5% fat, at least 14% crude fiber, and a balanced and complete complement of vitamins and minerals. Optimal intakes of B-vitamins are assured through coprophagy, but clinical deficiencies of vitamins A, E, and K have led to supplementation of commercial diets with these three essential nutrients. Most commercial rabbit diets provide all the micronutrients known to be essential.

NUTRITIONAL DISORDERS

Problems associated with diet and feeding management often reflect the rabbit's relatively unique gastrointestinal physiology. For example, obesity may occur even when high fiber diets are fed, because rabbits digest fiber with greater efficiency than observed for most companion animals.

Low fiber ($\leq$ 14%) diets may cause diarrhea, leading to debilitation, as well as excessive grooming leading to hairballs and anorexia. Provision of supplementary loose grass hay reduces hair chewing, even for rabbits fed high-fiber pelleted diets.[3]

Rabbits demonstrate little control of calcium absorption from the gastrointestinal tract, excreting excess dietary calcium in urine (a system similar to that observed in horses).

(continues on page 111)

Pseudomonas aeruginosa Pneumonia in Vietnamese Potbellied Pigs

Texas A&M University
P. R. Woods, DVM, PhD, MRCVS
D. B. Lawhorn, DVM, MS

Texas Veterinary Medical Diagnostic Laboratory
College Station, Texas
W. L. Schwartz, DVM, MS

Parker County Veterinary Clinic
Weatherford, Texas
P. D. Jarrett, DVM

Miniature pigs have been used extensively by the biomedical community and continue to play a valuable role in basic research. The recent appearance and popularity of Vietnamese potbellied pigs as pets has created an interesting challenge for veterinarians. As pets, these pigs apparently have considerable individual economic and emotional value but are often owned by a relatively poorly informed clientele. Clients present sick Vietnamese potbellied pigs to small and large animal veterinarians, providing a diagnostic challenge to both groups.

Relatively little has been published regarding management and diseases of Vietnamese potbellied pigs because of the assumption that they are identical to commercial pig breeds. Although many of the diseases of commercial pigs have been diagnosed in Vietnamese potbellied pigs, it is probable that there are some conditions (caused by management or genetics) peculiar to Vietnamese potbellied pigs of which veterinarians are just becoming aware. Regular vaccination against *Erysipelothrix rhusiopathiae*, *Pasteurella multocida*, *Mycoplasma hyopneumoniae*, *Bordetella bronchiseptica*, *Escherichia coli*, *Actinobacillus pleuropneumoniae*, parvovirus, coronavirus, rotavirus, and *Leptospira* serovars is currently recommended for breeding and neutered Vietnamese potbellied pigs in addition to regular deworming.

Nutrition of Vietnamese potbellied pigs may be woefully inadequate and may lead to a variety of mineral and vitamin deficiencies. A commercial balanced feed specifically marketed for Vietnamese potbellied pigs is available. A pig's environment also can contribute to disease; we recently identified pruritus in a Vietnamese potbellied pig associated with hypersensitivity to cedar shavings in the pillow that the pig slept on at night.

The three cases of *Pseudomonas* pneumonia in Vietnamese potbellied pigs reported in this article exemplify the peculiarities of the disease that may present a challenge to the diagnostician. This report publicizes what may be a newly identified susceptibility of these pigs.

CASE REPORTS

Case 1. A two-year-old Vietnamese potbellied sow was presented to the Texas Veterinary Medical Center at Texas A&M University for reproductive evaluation subsequent to abortion. The pregnant sow had been purchased and transported to the owner several weeks earlier. The sow was kept outside as part of a herd of potbellied pigs. No abortions occurred in the other pigs, but coughing and nasal discharge were noted in some. The pregnant sow went off feed 7 to 10 days before aborting eight late-gestation piglets, three weeks before presentation. No obvious vaginal discharge was seen subsequent to abortion. The patient was vaccinated against *B. bronchiseptica*, *E. rhusiopathiae*, *P. multocida*, parvovirus, and six serovars of *Leptospira* after it went off feed. The sow was noted by the owners to have had a low-grade respiratory problem for an unknown period; the problem was treated with oxytetracycline and vitamin B_{12} injections.

At presentation, the sow was in good flesh and well hydrated but in obvious respiratory distress. She had a respiratory rate of 200 breaths/min and cyanotic mucous membranes. The sow became extremely distressed with any form of handling. Auscultation of the thorax revealed very harsh lung sounds, tachypnea, and tachycardia. Because of the severity of dyspnea, the patient was immediately placed in a humidified oxygen cage with an oxygen level of 40% and an oxygen flow rate of 7 L/min.

The pig's condition stabilized to the point that a detailed physical examination could be performed. The examination was unremarkable except for tachycardia, dyspnea, tachypnea, and harsh lung sounds over left and right lung fields. Mucous membrane color had improved subsequent to placing the patient in the humidified oxygen cage. Only one blood sample (in EDTA) was obtained before the pig again became dyspneic. Results of the complete blood count indicated 21,300 white blood cells/μl with 18,531 segmented neutrophils/μl, 1491 lymphocytes/μl, and 1278 monocytes/μl, consistent with a stress leukogram. Plasma protein was 8.2 g/dl, and fibrinogen was marginally elevated at 500 mg/dl. Because of the extreme condition, it was decided not to stress the patient by further diagnostic procedures. A presumptive diagnosis of acute pneumonia was made.

The sow was medicated with ceftiofur (2.5 mg/kg intramuscularly every 12 hours), flunixin meglumine (1 mg/kg intramuscularly every 12 hours), and dex-amethasone (0.1 mg/kg intramuscularly, single dose). The pig was kept in the oxygen cage overnight with ad libitum water. The patient's condition remained stable throughout the night. Radiographs of the thorax taken the next morning demonstrated a diffuse interstitial and alveolar pattern, multiple circumscribed soft tissue densities, and increased density throughout the lungs (which obscured the cardiac silhouette). The radiographic diagnosis was diffuse bronchial pneumonia with multiple areas of abscess formation. Thoracic ultrasonography was attempted; during the procedure, the patient again became distressed and cyanotic, began coughing up bloody foam, and died.

Necropsy revealed severe chronic-active pneumonia with chronic lesions in the cranioventral lung tissue and acute lesions in the dorsal lung tissue. There was no evidence of pleural effusion. The reproductive tract was apparently normal. The nasal turbinates did not demonstrate lesions consistent with atrophic rhinitis. Tissue samples were submitted for microbiologic evaluation. A pure growth of *P. aeruginosa* isolated from all tissues submitted (lung, kidney, liver, spleen, and uterus) suggested septicemia. Lung tissue assayed for mycoplasma was found to be negative.

Case 2. A four-month-old Vietnamese potbellied boar with a two-day history of anorexia and respiratory distress was kept in an outdoor environment with approximately 50 other such pigs. The herd was in good health and under regular veterinary care. All of the pigs were immunized against *B. bronchiseptica*, *E. rhusiopathiae*, *P. multocida*, and *A. pleuropneumoniae*. The owner noted the patient to have progressively worsening respiratory distress, behavioral depression, and anorexia during a two- to three-day period. The referring veterinarian made a presumptive diagnosis of acute pneumonia and administered corticosteroids, nonsteroidal antiinflammatory drugs, and antibiotics. Moderate improvement occurred for 12 hours; the pig then died.

At necropsy the lungs were firm, fibrotic, and dark with some abscess formation. Fibrinous pleuritis and interlobular and proteinaceous alveolar edema were found. More than 90% of the lung parenchyma was affected. Lesions noted at necropsy were highly suggestive of *A. pleuropneumoniae*. *Pseudomonas aeruginosa* was isolated from lung tissue at necropsy; *A. pleuropneumoniae* was not isolated.

Case 3. A yearling Vietnamese potbellied neutered male was kept in an outside environment with other pigs. The herd was vaccinated regularly against *A. pleuropneumoniae*, *B. bronchiseptica*, *E. rhusiopathiae*, *P. multocida*, *E. coli* pilus antigens, six serovars of *Leptospira*, rotavirus, parvovirus, and coronavirus. The patient developed a cough on day 1 and had a rectal temperature of 104.5°F (40.3°C). Based on physical examination, a presumptive diagnosis of *Actinobacillus* pleuropneumonia was made. The pig was treated with a combination of dexamethasone, dipyrone, and ceftiofur for five days. By day 2, the cough had resolved. On day 5, the patient was found to be in acute respiratory distress with cyanosis and open-mouthed breathing. The pig died on day 5.

A full necropsy revealed lesions limited to the lungs. The lungs were edematous; more than 90% of the parenchyma was affected. Serosanguineous fluid and pus were found in the pleural space. No pulmonary abscesses were seen. A pure culture of *P. aeruginosa* was isolated from purulent material collected from pus in the pleural fluid. The referring veterinarian subsequently noted that only pigs kept outside developed clinical signs of respiratory disease; cohorts that were kept in an air-conditioned indoor environment had no respiratory problems.

DISCUSSION

Pseudomonas aeruginosa is a gram-negative aerobic microaerophilic bacillus with a wide environmental distribution (soil and standing water). The bacillus is often identified as a contaminant of animal feed and drinking water.[1] It has considerable resistance to a variety of antimicrobials and disinfectants and produces pathogenic factors that include endotoxins, exotoxins, protease, and phospholipase.[2] *Pseudomonas aeruginosa* is believed to be a major cause of secondary opportunistic infections in compromised or chronically diseased animals. Its involvement is best described as sporadic and late in the disease process.

Pseudomonas aeruginosa (although not recognized as a significant respiratory pathogen in pigs) has been well documented as a pathogen in abortion and infertility in pigs and horses; mastitis in cattle, pigs, goats, and horses; lower urinary tract infections in horses; bronchopneumonia in cattle, sheep, and goats; and corneal ulcers in horses.[3] *Pseudomonas aeruginosa* is the major pathogen in cystic fibrosis in humans.[4]

Porcine pneumonia is usually associated with a limited number of pathogens; *M. hyopneumoniae, A. pleuropneumoniae, P. multocida, Salmonella cholerasuis* and influenza type A are the most significant.[5] Although *P. aeruginosa* is not a primary pathogen in porcine atrophic rhinitis, the agent is easily isolated from the nasal conchae of chronic cases and from lung tissue of chronic porcine pneumonia cases.[1]

The identification of *P. aeruginosa* as the major isolate from pneumonic pigs is very unusual. A survey of porcine bacterial pneumonia cases reported to the Veterinary Medical Data Base at Purdue University

did not identify any associated with *P. aeruginosa*. A herd outbreak of *P. aeruginosa* pneumonia in pigs adjacent to cattle with *P. aeruginosa* septicemia and dyspnea was reported in 1962.[6] The affected pigs in the report had a constellation of clinical signs similar to that reported here; respiratory distress and death occurred in one to three days.

The finding of these cases of *P. aeruginosa* pneumonia in Vietnamese potbellied pigs is intriguing. All of the affected pigs were kept outside. Dr. Jarrett noted that the pigs kept in an air-conditioned environment apparently did not demonstrate clinical signs associated with respiratory disease (cough and runny nose), whereas pigs housed outside did.

The patients described were under good veterinary supervision and vaccinated against significant pathogens on a regular basis. Several stressors and predisposing factors can be identified in these cases. Case 1 was associated with recent transportation and abortion; in case 2, there may have been underlying primary pleuropneumonia; and in case 3, extremely hot and humid weather was associated with coughing and nasal discharge in the pigs kept outside compared with those kept in an air-conditioned environment.

The gross and microscopic pulmonary lesions from these and other cases of *Pseudomonas* pneumonia can easily be ascribed to many causative agents. It is possible that an initial insult by another respiratory pathogen predisposes Vietnamese potbellied pigs to *Pseudomonas aeruginosa* pneumonia, somewhat analogous to the shipping fever complex of cattle.

In the herd from which case 3 came, two other pigs subsequently developed the same clinical signs. There was no antemortem attempt to isolate a respiratory pathogen. Based on the antibiotic sensitivity pattern of *P. aeruginosa* isolated from case 3, the affected pigs were medicated with enrofloxacin (2.5 mg/kg intramuscularly every 12 hours) and recovered.

The number of cases reported here is small. Nevertheless, another parameter that should be considered is the possible genetic susceptibility of Vietnamese potbellied pigs to *P. aeruginosa*, given their presumably limited genetic pool within the United States.

The treatment of *Pseudomonas*-associated disease entails specific patient therapy and environmental control. Specific antibacterial treatment has traditionally involved the use of aminoglycosides, oxytetracycline, and chloramphenicol. If possible, treatment should be based on antibiotic sensitivity, as was used presumptively in the case 3 herd. Environmental control includes good hygiene, chlorination of drinking water, a warm and dry environment with minimal temperature fluctuation (low stress), and an appropriate vaccination and deworming program to limit opportunistic secondary infection.[7,8] Veterinarians should consider *P. aeruginosa* as a significant pathogen in cases of pneumonia in Vietnamese potbellied pigs.

About the Authors

Drs. Woods and Lawhorn are affiliated with the Department of Large Animal Medicine and Surgery, College of Veterinary Medicine, Texas A&M University, College Station, Texas. Dr. Lawhorn is also with the Veterinary Extension Education Department at Texas A&M University. Dr. Jarrett is affiliated with the Parker County Veterinary Clinic, Weatherford, Texas. Dr. Schwartz is with the Texas Veterinary Medical Diagnostic Laboratory, College Station, Texas.

REFERENCES

1. Taylor DJ: *Diseases of Swine*, ed 7. Ames, IA, Iowa State University Press, 1992, pp 627–629.
2. Doring G, Maier M, Muller E, et al: Virulence factors of *Pseudomonas aeruginosa. Antibiot Chemother* 39:136–148, 1987.
3. Smith BP: *Large Animal Internal Medicine.* Toronto, CV Mosby Co, 1990.
4. Dinwiddie R: Clinical aspects of mucoid *Pseudomonas aeruginosa* infections, in Gacesa P, Russell NJ (eds): *Pseudomonas Infection and Alginates. Biochemistry, Genetics and Pathology.* London, Chapman and Hall, 1990, pp 13–28.
5. Walton J: Differential diagnosis of lower respiratory disease in pigs. *In Pract* 12:126–129, 1990.
6. Baker WL: *Pseudomonas* pneumonia in swine. *VM SAC* 57:232–233, 1962.
7. Bradford JR: Caring for potbellied pigs. *Vet Med* 86:1173–1181, 1991.
8. Reeves DE: *Care and Management of Miniature Pet Pigs: Guidelines for the Veterinary Practitioner*, ed 1. Santa Barbara, CA, Veterinary Publishing Co, 1993.

Nutrition and Pet Rabbits *(continued from page 107)*

High dietary calcium levels and naturally alkaline rabbit urine may predispose to calcium-containing uroliths. Dietary calcium is recommended not to exceed 0.5% of dry matter for rabbits at maintenance, and 0.8% for growth and breeding.[1] Vitamin D is recommended not to exceed 1000 IU/kg diet.[1] Intake of alfalfa and other high-calcium foods (clover and supplements containing limestone, dicalcium phosphate, or calcium salts) may be restricted in rabbits with a history of calcium-containing uroliths. Access to high-calcium house plants, such as ficus, should be prevented in pet rabbits with urolithiasis

REFERENCES

1. Tobin G: Small pets—food type nutrient requirements and nutritional disorders, in Kelly NC, Wills JM (eds): *BSAVA Manual of Companion Animal Nutrition & Feeding.* Gloucestershire, UK, 1996.
2. Petersen J, Klausdeinken FJ: The importance of weaning age of young rabbits for the development of the kits and the food consumption. *Deutsche Tierartztliche Wochenschrist* 99:510–513, 1992.
3. Beynen AC, Mulder A, Nieuwenkamp AE, Vanderpalen JGP, Vanrooijen GH: Loose grass hay as a supplement to a pelleted diet reduces fur chewing in rabbits. *J Anim Physiol An Nutr* 68:226–234, 1992.

Anesthesia in Potbellied Pigs

Colorado State University
Etta M. Wertz, DVM, MS   Ann E. Wagner, DVM, MS

KEY FACTS

❏ Potbellied pigs can be anesthetized in a manner similar to that of farm pigs.

❏ Endotracheal intubation is easily performed after the unique pharyngeal and laryngeal anatomy is understood.

❏ Several techniques are available to practitioners to induce anesthesia in pigs, such as intravenous injection, deep muscular injection, and mask administration of inhalant anesthetics.

❏ Malignant hyperthermia, a possible anesthetic complication, is uncommon in potbellied pigs.

Potbellied pigs are becoming increasingly popular as house pets. Because of this, they are being presented to veterinarians for numerous procedures (e.g., ovariohysterectomy, castration,[1] laceration repair, and umbilical and inguinal hernia repair),[2] which require general anesthesia. They can be safely anesthetized using many of the same drugs and techniques used to anesthetize research or domesticated farm pigs. Inhalation equipment used for dogs and cats may be used to deliver inhalant anesthetics to pigs weighing up to 140 kg (300 lbs).

PRESURGICAL CONSIDERATIONS

A thorough physical examination should be performed, and the animal should be assessed before being anesthetized.[3] Such procedures help determine the patient's physiologic status and anesthetic risk (normal values are listed in Table I[4,5]). Presurgical laboratory assessment should be completed at this time, and all pertinent information should be reviewed to determine an appropriate anesthetic protocol.

Food is withheld for 12 hours, and water is withheld for four to six hours before general anesthesia is induced for elective procedures in pigs older than eight weeks of age. This decreases the incidence of vomiting and potential aspiration of foreign matter as well as the incidence of tympany produced after anticholinergic administration. In piglets younger than eight weeks, food and water withheld for one to two hours before anesthesia is induced. These guidelines are similar to recommendations for the young of other species.

Pigs should be handled gently to avoid injuries and problems caused by increased stress. The animals are difficult to restrain because of their size and shape, and they are often intolerant of even minimal restraint techniques. A pig restraint chute, Panepinto (pipe-framed) sling,[6] or transport cart with webbing is ideal for restraint; however, these methods are not available in many practices. A makeshift restraint chute can be made by squeezing the pig behind a cage door. Construction of a Panepinto sling or webbed table may be a better option if many potbellied pigs are seen by the practice. This is easily done using PVC pipe and seat belt webbing or canvas material with holes cut out and padded for limbs.

TABLE I
Ranges of Normal Heart Rate, Respiratory Rate, and Body Temperature of Piglets and Pigs[4,5]

Age	Heart Rate (BPM[a])	Respiratory Rate (BPM[b])	Temperature (°C)
6 to 15 weeks	80 to 100	25 to 40	39 to 40.5
15 to 26 weeks	75 to 85	25 to 35	38 to 40
Adult	63 to 92	13 to 18	38 to 40

[a]BPM = beats per minute.
[b]BPM = breaths per minute.

TABLE II
Hematologic and Serum Biochemical Values for Mature Yucatan Pigs[a] (n = 30)[7]

Component	Mean	Observed Range
RBC ($10^6/\mu l$)	7.0	5.6 to 8.8
Hematocrit (%)	44.6	36.3 to 53.7
Hemoglobin (g/dl)	14.9	13.1 to 17.0
Platelets ($10^3/\mu l$)	440.6	217 to 770
WBC ($10^3/\mu l$)	12.6	6.9 to 21.2
Total protein (g/dl)	7.5	6.3 to 9.4
Albumin (g/dl)	4.7	4.1 to 5.6
Globulin (g/dl)	2.8	1.4 to 3.6
Albumin:globulin ratio	1.8	1.11 to 3.49
Creatinine (mg/dl)	1.6	1.2 to 2.0
AST (IU/L)	28.2	15 to 53
ALT (IU/L)	33.6	20 to 48
Glucose (mg/dl)	79.8	56 to 153

[a]Yucatan and Vietnamese potbellied pigs are individual breeds of miniature pigs. The values for Yucatan pigs are consistent with other breeds of miniature pigs.
RBC = red blood cells, WBC = white blood cells, AST = aspartate transaminase, ALT = alanine transaminase.

Holding only the forelimbs or hindlimbs should be avoided as a method of restraint because joint dislocation may result. A hog snare, more commonly used with farm pigs, should also be avoided because pet pigs often fight this restraint technique. Lumbar and hindlimb injuries may result from the use of a snare,[3,6] and the pig may become quite excited—increased excitement should be avoided before general anesthesia.

Blood for presurgical laboratory evaluation (packed cell volume and total protein) can be collected by percutaneous puncture of the cranial vena cava or brachiocephalic vein (normal values are listed in Table II[7]). This technique has been previously described.[8,9] Using these routes (cranial vena cava or brachiocephalic vein) for administration of intravenous drugs is discouraged because most pigs will not remain immobile for the injection, and complications resulting from perivascular injection or laceration of the vessels may result.

PREANESTHETIC MEDICATIONS

Preanesthetic tranquilization or sedation, as is commonly done in dogs and cats, is difficult to achieve in pigs. Acepromazine is a phenothiazine tranquilizer with antagonistic effects at α_1 receptors. Published doses for acepromazine vary greatly (0.03 to 2.0 mg/kg).[10,11] Acepromazine reportedly does not produce reliable sedation in pigs. When a high dose is administered to a healthy pig, only minimal sedation is produced. Acepromazine can potentially cause hypotension through peripheral α_1 blockade; because of this, acepromazine is contraindicated for sick, debilitated, or hypovolemic animals as well as those in shock. Acepromazine may predispose the patient to hypothermia due to peripheral vasodilatation; however, incidence of halothane-triggered malignant hyperthermia syndrome in susceptible individuals is decreased after acepromazine administration.[12]

Because pigs are relatively resistant to the sedative effects of xylazine, which is an α_2 agonist, doses higher than those administered to dogs and cats are used. Although xylazine does not produce reliable sedation and some investigators report that it is ineffective in pigs,[13] the agent is useful for preanesthesia because it potentiates the sedation, muscle relaxation, and analgesia produced by other anesthetic agents. Administration of xylazine with tiletamine HCL–zolazepam enables endotracheal intubation, which is not possible with tiletamine HCL–zolazepam alone. In the latter situation, the pig must receive an inhalant anesthetic to reach an adequate depth of anesthesia for successful tracheal intubation.

Diazepam reportedly provides adequate tranquilization in pigs when administered at a dose of 5.5 to 8.5 mg/kg.[14] At this dose, diazepam causes moderate to severe hindlimb ataxia within five minutes and complete recumbency within 10 minutes. Lower doses (0.05 to 0.1 mg/kg) are administered intravenously during ketamine anesthesia to provide muscle relaxation and have a duration of one to four hours.[13]

A combination product containing fentanyl (a short-acting opioid) and droperidol (a butyrophenone tranquilizer) is available. This agent has been administered to pigs to facilitate face mask administration of inhalation agents,[15] although it can cause excitement and goose-stepping[14] when administered alone. It has been administered before ketamine with satisfactory results, although movements reportedly

TABLE III
Dose Information on Preanesthetic Agents for Potbellied Pigs[a]

Drug	Dose (mg/kg)	Comments
Acepromazine	0.03 to 0.1[10] 2.0	Slow onset of action, 20 to 30 minutes to peak effect Light, unreliable sedation No analgesia Maximum dose, 15 mg
Xylazine	2.2[10,18] 4.4	Minimal sedation May cause vomiting before surgery or during recovery Administer with atropine to block increased vagal tone Will potentiate other anesthetic drugs Will offset hyperanalgesic effect produced by thiobarbiturates Use with ketamine or tiletamine HCL–zolazepam anesthesia recommended High dose used by authors in combination with atropine (0.04 mg/kg, IM) and tiletamine HCL– zolazepam (6 mg/kg, IM) in healthy pigs
Diazepam	0.5 to 1.0[13,19] 5.5 to 8.5[14]	High therapeutic index Effective central muscle relaxant High doses produce ataxia and recumbency
Fentanyl citrate and droperidol	1.0 ml/10 kg[14] 1.0 ml/11 kg[13] 1.0 ml/14.6 kg[17,20] 1.0 ml/12–25 kg[10]	Administer with atropine Administer 20 to 30 minutes before catheterization and induction May cause excitement and goose-stepping
Azaperone	0.23 to 1.0[13]	Light sedation produced after IM sedation Decreases aggressiveness

[a]All agents are delivered via the intramuscular (IM) route.

occur continually throughout anesthesia.[16]

Lastly, azaperone, a butyrophenone tranquilizer, produces tranquilization after intramuscular administration. Excitement can occur initially, however. The primary use of azaperone has been to decrease stress and aggression in weanling pigs when they are initially grouped together.

The administration of an anticholinergic drug as a preanesthetic agent to potbellied pigs is a matter of practitioner discretion. Advantages for anticholinergic administration include a decrease in the production of respiratory and salivary secretions, which improves visualization of the larynx during intubation. Anticholinergic drugs prevent the increased vagal tone that occurs during tracheal intubation. Administration of anticholinergic drugs with anesthetic agents that cause bradyarrhythmia (e.g., xylazine and opioids) counteract and help prevent such effects. Increased salivary and respiratory secretions are prevented with anticholinergic administration either before or in conjunction with ketamine or tiletamine HCL–

zolazepam. When tachycardia is present, administration of anticholinergic agents is not recommended because of possible progression of dysrhythmia (e.g., ventricular tachycardia). Drugs used as preanesthetic medications in potbellied pigs are summarized in Table III.[10,13,14,17–20]

GENERAL ANESTHESIA
Induction
Several techniques are available to induce general anesthesia in pigs (Table IV[10,16,18,19,21–25]), including intravenous injection (e.g., thiobarbiturates, dissociative agents, or combinations of these drugs), deep intramuscular injection (e.g., xylazine or diazepam with dissociative agents), or mask administration of inhalant anesthetics (e.g., halothane or isoflurane).

Unless a venous catheter is placed to ensure access, intravenous administration of anesthetic drugs is not recommended because of such possible complications as lacerated veins during injection or perivascular drug injection. For intravenous injection in domesti-

TABLE IV
Dose Information on Induction Agents for Potbellied Pigs

Drug	*Dose (mg/kg)*	*Route*	*Comments*
Injectable Single Drugs			
Ketamine	20[10]	IM	Poor analgesia and muscle relaxation when used alone
Tiletamine HCL–zolazepam	4.4[18]	IM	Inadequate for endotracheal intubation
			Rough recovery, characterized by vocalization, excessive salivation, and paddling motions
Thiobarbiturates			
Thiopental	10 to 20[10]	IV	Concentration should be 5% or less
Thiamylal	6 to 18[10]	IV	Administer $^1/_3$ to $^1/_2$ as rapid bolus to unpremedicated pig; titrate to effect
			Supplemental doses to prolong anesthesia will prolong recovery
Injectable Drug Combinatios			
Atropine	0.044[19]	IM	Mix together in one syringe to administer
Xylazine	4.4		Satisfactory short-term anesthesia
Ketamine	2.2		Prolong anesthesia with xylazine-ketamine combination (100 mg ketamine added to 50 mg xylazine); titrate *slowly* to avoid apnea
Acepromazine	0.5[16]	IM	Onset of recumbency within 5 minutes after ketamine; unreliable
Ketamine	15 (given 30 minutes after induction of acepromazine)	IM	
Acepromazine, wait 30 minutes, ketamine	0.39[21]	IM	Recovery 65 to 80 minutes
	15 (given 30 minutes after induction of acepromazine)	IM	
Diazepam	1.0 to 2.0[19]	IM	Analgesia not as profound as xylazine–ketamine
Ketamine	10 to 18		Smooth recovery
Xylazine	2.2[18]	IM	Mix together in one syringe to administer
Tiletamine HCL–zolazepam	4.4		Good induction combination, recumbency within 5 minutes
			Endotracheal intubation easily performed
			Acceptable short-term anesthesia
			Initial inhalation vaporizer setting should be low to prevent over-anesthesia
			Smooth recovery, standing in approximately 70 minutes
Atropine	0.044	IM	Similar to the xylazine/tiletamine HCL–zolazepam combination
Xylazine	4.4		Smooth recovery; standing in approximately 120 to 150 minutes
Tiletamine HCL–zolazepam	6.0		Combination routinely used in laboratory setting by authors
Xylazine[a]	1 ml/75 kg[22]	IV	Anesthesia can be maintained with 0.5 ml/75 kg, IV; must be given slowly (over 60 seconds) to minimize respiratory depression
Ketamine			
Tiletamine HCL–zolazepam			
Xylazine[a]	2.2[18]	IM	Good induction combination
Ketamine	2.2		Endotracheal intubation possible
Tiletamine HCL–zolazepam	4.4		Recovery smoother than tiletamine HCL–zolazepam alone; rougher than when xylazine included in protocol
			Time to standing approximately 80 minutes

TABLE IV (continued)

Drug	Dose (mg/kg)	Route	Comments
Xylazine	2.20[23]	IV	Mix together in one syringe to administer
Ketamine	2.0		Suitable for short-term anesthesia and minor surgery
Oxymorphone	0.075		Breathing is rapid and shallow
			Duration of anesthesia and recumbency approximately 20 to 30 minutes
			Smooth, rapid recovery
			All doses may be doubled for IM administration
GKX[b] for swine (triple drip)	0.5 to 1.0 mg/kg[19,24] (to induce unpremedicated pig)	IV	Decrease induction dose 50% if tranquilizer or sedative administered before induction
			Administer atropine IM before beginning induction
	2.0 ml/kg/hr (constant infusion to maintain anesthesia)		Rapid recovery after discontinuing GKX infusion, 30–40 minutes
			Recovery may be hastened by administration of yohimbine (0.125 mg/kg, IV) after infusion discontinued
Inhalation Agents			
Halothane	To effect[25]	Inhalation (face mask)	Recommended induction agent for young or sick pigs
			Endotracheal intubation possible
			Recovery more rapid than that from parenteral anesthetics
Isoflurane	To effect[25]	Inhalation (face mask)	Recommended induction agent for young or sick pigs
			Endotracheal intubation possible
			Recovery more rapid than that from parenteral anesthetics

[a]Make combination by reconstituting tiletamine HCL–zolazepam with 2.5 ml ketamine (100 mg/ml) and 2.5 ml xylazine (100 mg/ml). Each milliliter of the resultant combination will contain 50 mg tiletamine, 50 mg zolazepam, 50 mg ketamine, and 50 mg xylazine.
[b]Solution contains 50 mg/ml of glycerol guaiacolate, 2 mg/ml of ketamine, and 1 mg/ml of xylazine. The combination should be mixed in the desired quantity immediately before use because of the potential diminished potency of the mixture during storage. Concentration of drugs in this mixture varies among species.
IM = intramuscular, IV = intravenous.

cated pigs, the auricular vein is often used. The location of the auricular vein may vary by breed and presence of ear notching in both domesticated and miniature pigs, but the vein is usually found easily on the dorsal aspect of the pinna. Potbellied pigs have shorter and broader ears than domesticated farm breeds. Because of this, the auricular vein is often too small and fragile to use for administration of intravenous anesthetic agents. If attempts to induce anesthesia via the auricular vein are unsuccessful, it is best to wait and induce anesthesia by a different route, if possible. After induction, a venous catheter is inserted percutaneously for subsequent administration of drugs and fluids. When intravenous anesthetics are necessary to induce anesthesia, however, it is best to first secure an intravenous catheter into a superficial vein, such as the cephalic, saphenous (cranial or caudal branch of the medial or lateral saphenous), or plantar common digital vein. These vessels may be more easily located and identified in younger animals than in older ones.

A second method to induce deep sedation or anesthesia is by deep intramuscular injection of anesthetic drugs into cervical muscles or either the semimembranosus or semitendinosus muscle. This method is recommended because it does not seem to cause undue stress to the patient. Regardless of the drug chosen, a long needle (at least 3.8 cm) must be used for intramuscular administration because of the thick subcutaneous layer of fat. Absorption of the drug is slower from fat, thus the onset of action is prolonged and the effect is often less pronounced.

Lastly, induction of anesthesia by face mask administration of inhalant anesthetics is another option. The stress associated with the procedure can be minimized if the pig is petted and talked to softly during induction. This method of induction may be the best option in depressed or debilitated animals; however, sick animals that still resist this method can be given a low dose of xylazine–ketamine, tiletamine HCL–zolazepam, or fentanyl–droperidol intramuscularly before proceeding with mask induction. Isoflurane is

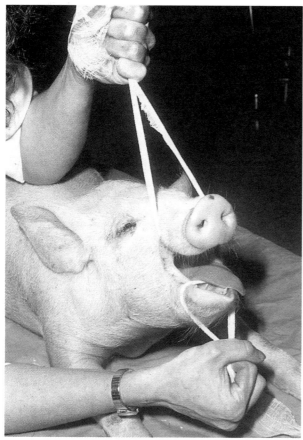

Figure 1—Use of gauze strips to hold the mouth open and maximize visualization of the laryngeal opening.

TABLE V
Suggested Endotracheal Tube Size[29]

Weight (kg)	Internal Diameter (mm)
5 to 10	3 to 4
10 to 20	5 to 6
20 to 50	7 to 9
Adult sow (> 50 kg)	14

recommended for this method of induction because it has a low blood–gas coefficient (1.41). An advantage of isoflurane is that induction is slightly more rapid. In addition, because anesthetic gases cannot be scavenged completely and leak from around the mask, contamination of room air with levels of anesthetic gases occurs. Although trace levels of inhalant anesthetics have not been proven to be harmful, it is best to minimize exposure to personnel and use a relatively inert anesthetic agent. Less than 0.2% isoflurane undergoes hepatic metabolism in isoflurane-anesthetized humans,[26] whereas approximately 20% of halothane[27] and 50% of methoxyflurane[28] undergo hepatic metabolism. Halothane (blood–gas coefficient, 2.36) can also be used to mask-induce pigs; this method may take slightly longer.

Methoxyflurane is not recommended for mask induction because it is highly lipid soluble (blood–gas coefficient, 13.0). As a result, induction is prolonged and stormy.

Tracheal Intubation

After induction of anesthesia, tracheal intubation is recommended to protect the airway and allow a means of ventilation, if necessary. When thiobarbiturates are used for anesthetic induction, apnea may occur and rapid intubation becomes necessary; however, for selected short procedures, endotracheal intubation may not be necessary.

There are several anatomic characteristics that are unique to pigs that must be taken into account for tracheal intubation. First, the mouth of a pig does not open wide, especially when compared with that of a dog or a cat. This, in addition to a long soft palate, makes it difficult to visualize the laryngeal opening. Therefore, the mouth is opened as wide as possible using two strips of gauze—one to hold the maxilla up, the other to pull the mandible down (Figure 1). This technique allows more complete visualization than if a person's hands were used to hold the jaws open. The distal tip of the endotracheal tube is used to gently manipulate the soft palate and epiglottis, enabling visualization of the larynx. In adult pigs, the laryngoscope blade may not be long enough to adequately visualize the larynx. In this situation, a tongue depressor can be taped to the laryngoscope blade, extending the blade to the desired length.

Pigs tend to develop laryngospasm during light planes of anesthesia. Assuming that sufficient induction drug has been given to produce an adequate depth of anesthesia for intubation, it is beneficial to desensitize the larynx with topically applied lidocaine before intubation. The laryngeal opening (rima glottis) and trachea of the pig are small in proportion to the pig's overall size. Several endotracheal tubes of graduated sizes should be available (Table V[29]) to maximize success and prevent laryngeal trauma and edema caused by repeated attempts at intubation.

Before attempting intubation, one should be aware of the unique anatomy of the pharynx and larynx of a pig. The larynx of a pig slopes somewhat ventrally, and the trachea does not follow in the same direction. Instead, the trachea goes in a more dorsal direction (Figure 2); when an endotracheal tube is being inserted, the angle of the tube must be changed according-

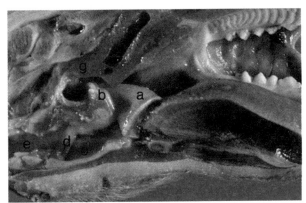

Figure 2—Sagittal cross-section of the head of a pig. *a* = epiglottis, *b* = arytenoid cartilage, *c* = posterior floor of the larynx, *d* = lateral laryngeal ventricle, *e* = trachea, *f* = esophagus (esophageal opening), *g* = approximate location of pharyngeal recess (not clearly identified in this specimen).

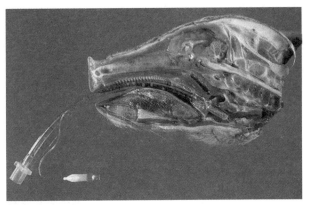

Figure 3A

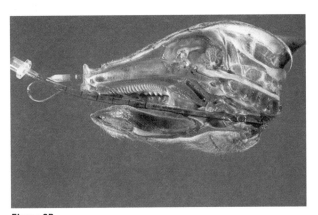

Figure 3B
Figure 3—Endotracheal intubation in the pig. (**A**) The endotracheal tube is inserted between the arytenoid cartilages with the concave side of the endotracheal tube ventral. (**B**) After it is passed between the arytenoid cartilages, the endotracheal tube is rotated 180 degrees to facilitate passage into the trachea.

ly. Once the tip of the endotracheal tube has been placed between the arytenoid cartilages (Figure 3A), the tube must be rotated approximately 180 degrees so the tip is directed somewhat dorsally to allow advancement of the tube through the cricoid cartilage and into the trachea (Figure 3B). After this adjustment has been made, the tube can be advanced easily.

Another difference in pigs is the presence of a blind pouch, the pharyngeal recess, located immediately dorsal to the esophagus (Figure 2). Intubation is ineffective if the endotracheal tube is mistakenly placed in this location. If it does not advance easily, the endotracheal tube is either located in the pharyngeal recess or is too large for the trachea. If the tube is too large, a smaller tube should be reinserted.

Correct placement of the endotracheal tube in pigs can be confirmed by (1) visualization of the tube passing through the arytenoid cartilages, (2) clearing and condensation within the endotracheal tube as the pig inhales and exhales, (3) feeling movement of air at the distal end of the endotracheal tube with each exhalation, (4) lack of gurgling sounds, and (5) movement of the rebreathing bag when the tube is connected to the anesthetic breathing circuit. Measurement of the end-tidal concentration of carbon dioxide (ETCO2) and observation of the resultant waveform (capnogram) can be used to correctly identify tracheal tube placement when a capnograph is available. Monitoring mucous membrane color and observing improvement in color (i.e., pinking-up) is another parameter that may suggest correct placement. Conversely, muddy-colored mucous membranes or respiratory movements without movement of air from the tube may indicate an improperly placed endotracheal tube. For obvious reasons, palpation of the trachea and esophagus is difficult to perform in pigs.

Maintenance

Depending on the method of induction, caution must be taken to avoid over-anesthesia during maintenance. For example, when anesthesia is induced by intramuscular injection of atropine, xylazine, and tiletamine HCL–zolazepam and is maintained with methoxyflurane, halothane, or isoflurane, the anesthetic vaporizer must be set fairly low because of the basal anesthesia produced by the parenteral agents already present. Throughout the procedure, as the effect from the parenteral drugs decreases, the vaporizer setting may need to be increased to maintain an appropriate depth of anesthesia.

For comparison, when anesthesia is induced and maintained with an inhalation agent (without premedication), the vaporizer setting needs to be higher to maintain an appropriate depth of anesthesia. This is due to the absence of a basal level of anesthesia produced by parenteral agents. All of the currently available inhalant anesthetic agents (methoxyflurane, halothane, or isoflurane) may be used to maintain anesthesia in potbellied pigs. Because the depth of anesthesia may need to be changed during the procedure, it is recommended that anesthetic depth be monitored.

Support and Monitoring

Eye signs during anesthesia are difficult to interpret in pigs. As the depth of anesthesia changes, a pattern of ocular movement is not as readily apparent in pigs as it is in dogs and cats. Eye signs may be further complicated when a dissociative anesthetic (e.g., ketamine or tiletamine HCL–zolazepam) has been administered. The eye becomes centrally located after administration of either agent and will remain so until the effect of the dissociative drug wanes.

Both cardiac and respiratory function should be monitored during anesthesia. Monitoring should be performed to identify possible problems before a disaster occurs. An esophageal stethoscope to monitor both heart rate and rhythm may be inserted into the esophagus, similar to the method used for dogs and cats; however, this can be a challenge because of the pharyngeal recess. Insertion can be achieved when the stethoscope is placed into the esophagus immediately after intubation; the pig must be in sternal recumbency and the laryngoscope is used for guidance. The stethoscope can be attached to an auditory monitor if available. An electrocardiogram may be attached to the pig using leads with alligator clips, or an esophageal electrocardiogram may be used to monitor both heart rate and rhythm.

Breathing during anesthesia is shallow and rapid. Pigs seem to breathe better when placed in either lateral or dorsal recumbency; breathing is more labored when in sternal recumbency. If a sternal position is necessary for the procedure, endotracheal intubation is recommended so ventilation may be assisted or controlled if necessary.

During general anesthesia, especially in sick or hypovolemic patients, a balanced electrolyte solution (e.g., lactated Ringer's solution) should be administered intravenously through a venous catheter. Intravenous catheters are secured easily with cyanoacrylate glue and then taped. The recommended rate for fluid administration during anesthesia is 10 ml/kg/hr.

Body temperature should be monitored throughout anesthesia and during recovery. A warm circulating-water blanket is recommended to help maintain body temperature during these periods because pigs have poor ability to thermoregulate. It should be remembered that hypothermia decreases the MAC of the inhalant anesthetic necessary to produce the required depth of anesthesia.

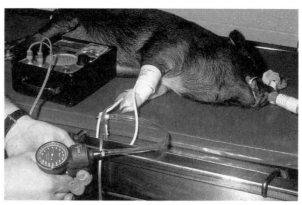

Figure 4—Placement of the Doppler crystal over the median artery of the medial palmar aspect of the metacarpus for indirect blood pressure measurement.

Arterial blood pressure can be monitored indirectly using a Doppler ultrasonographic device with a cuff placed proximal to the Doppler crystal. This method only measures systolic blood pressure. The crystal is positioned over a superficial artery. Suggested arteries include the coccygeal artery at the ventral base of the tail or the median artery on the medial palmar aspect of the metacarpus (Figure 4). The indirect method is imprecise but allows the practitioner to follow trends. Because the limb of a pig is more conical than cylindrical in shape, it is sometimes difficult to measure blood pressure with this device; however, the continuous audible signal assures blood flow, and changes in sound intensity (when the amplifier has not been altered) reflect possible changes in blood flow.

Blood pressure can be measured directly by cannulating a superficial artery. The auricular, femoral, or medial saphenous artery are the easiest arteries to locate and catheterize. The arterial line is connected to either a commercial pressure transducer or to an aneroid manometer, depending on available equipment. Monitoring arterial blood pressure with an aneroid manometer offers an inexpensive method to monitor blood pressure directly.

Ideally, the adequacy of ventilation is assessed by measuring the partial pressure of carbon dioxide in arterial blood ($PaCO_2$); however, this is an invasive procedure that requires specialized equipment. Alternately, a capnograph may be used as a noninvasive method for measuring carbon dioxide. A port for sampling the exhaled gases is attached between the endotracheal tube and Y-piece of the breathing circuit, and continuous sampling of carbon dioxide occurs. The $ETCO_2$ value is always less than that of the $PaCO_2$. The gradient between the two values varies due to ventilation–perfusion imbalances. The gradient is determined by simultaneously sampling of arterial blood $PaCO_2$ and $ETCO_2$. In healthy dogs anesthetized with halothane in oxygen, this difference is less than 5 mm Hg.[30] Because carbon dioxide must first be brought to the lungs for elimination, ETCO2 measurement provides additional information regarding the circulation.

Pulse oximetry provides a noninvasive technique for continuous measurement of hemoglobin saturation with oxygen. A small probe is placed on the tongue, ear, or lip, and, using two wavelengths of light (infrared and red), hemoglobin saturation is determined. Pulse oximetry readily helps identify possible hypoxemia, which alerts the practitioner to signs of early complications. These units, however, tend to underread oxygen saturation.

Recovery

To facilitate a smooth recovery from anesthesia, pigs should be placed in lateral recumbency in a warm, dimly lit cage. The body temperature should be taken, and hypothermia should be treated if present. Hypothermia prolongs recovery from general anesthesia. Ideally, the cage floor should provide good footing so the pig does not slip in the cage when attempting to stand. The endotracheal tube should remain in place until the pig has a strong swallowing reflex. At that time, the cuff is deflated and the endotracheal tube is removed.

Recovery from anesthesia may be improved by adding xylazine to the initial anesthetic protocol, and small intramuscular doses (0.5 mg/kg) of the drug should be repeated during recovery. Swindle recommends buprenorphine (0.05 to 0.1 mg/kg intramuscularly or intravenously every eight hours) or butorphanol (0.1 to 0.3 mg/kg either intramuscularly or intravenously every eight hours) for treatment of postsurgical pain.[31] Phenylbutazone (4 to 8 mg/kg orally twice daily) or enteric-coated aspirin (10 to 20 mg/kg orally four times daily) can be administered for musculoskeletal pain. We have treated pigs for postsurgical pain after abdominal surgery with small doses of xylazine (0.5 mg/kg intravenously). One dose seemed to improve the comfort of the pig for approximately 1.5 to 2 hours, at which time the dose was repeated.

Recovery from anesthesia is usually of short duration when only inhalation agents have been used. When parenteral agents have been used for induction, the recovery time is generally prolonged because the drugs must be metabolized and eliminated.

Complications

Compromised ventilation, including hypoventilation or apnea, may occur during anesthesia. First, the cause should be identified (body position, airway obstruction, excessive depth of anesthesia) and correct-

ed. Intubated patients maintained under anesthesia with inhalant anesthetics are treated by instituting intermittent positive-pressure ventilation. To prevent deeper levels of anesthesia, the vaporizer setting must be decreased. If an excessive depth of anesthesia has been identified, the vaporizer is turned off and the breathing circuit is flushed with 100% oxygen. If an anesthetic circuit is not available, an ambu bag is used.

If tracheal intubation has not been accomplished, doxapram, a centrally acting respiratory stimulant, is administered intravenously (0.5 to 0.9 mg/kg, which is the small animal dose). Because doxapram is absorbed through mucous membranes, several drops can be administered sublingually when intravenous administration is not possible. Doxapram increases tidal volume, and higher doses increase respiratory rate. Ventilation should be supported until the pig is able to breathe adequately.

Malignant hyperthermia syndrome, which is a genetic condition most commonly reported in humans and domesticated pigs, may occur during anesthesia. The incidence is higher in pig breeds with light skin coloration (Pietrain, spotted swine, Landrace, and Poland China breeds). The duroc breed seems to be less affected. To date, only one case of malignant hyperthermia syndrome during isoflurane anesthesia in a potbellied pig has been reported.[32] It is believed that the genetic composition of the potbellied pig probably minimizes the syndrome in this breed.

About the Authors

Drs. Wertz and Wagner, who are Diplomates of the American College of Veterinary Anesthesiology, are affiliated with the Department of Clinical Sciences, College of Veterinary Medicine and Biomedical Sciences, Colorado State University, Fort Collins, Colorado. Dr. Wagner is also a Diplomate of the American College of Veterinary Pathologists.

REFERENCES

1. Bradford JR: Caring for potbellied pigs. *Vet Med* 86:1173–1181, 1991.
2. Braun W: Petite porcine pets. *Proc CVMA*, 1992.
3. Westercamp D: Physical examination of miniature pet pigs, in Reeves DE (ed): *Guidelines for the Veterinary Practitioner—Care and Management of Miniature Pigs.* Santa Barbara, Veterinary Practice Publishing Co, 1993, pp 47–50.
4. Reece WO: Respiration in mammals, in Swenson MJ (ed): *Duke's Physiology of Domestic Animals.* Ithaca, NY, Cornell University Press, 1984, p 231.
5. Forney S: Formulary. Colorado State University Veterinary Teaching Hospital, 1990–1991, pp 102–104.
6. Johnson LR: Physical and chemical restraint of miniature pigs, in Reeves DE (ed): *Guidelines for the Veterinary Practitioner—Care and Management of Miniature Pet Pigs.* Santa Barbara, Veterinary Practice Publishing Co, 1993, pp 59–66.

7. Radin MJ, Weiser MG, Fettman MJ: Hematologic and serum biochemical values for Yucatan miniature swine. *Lab Anim Sci* 36(4):425–427, 1986.

8. Carle BN, Dewhirst WH Jr: A method for bleeding swine. *JAVMA* 101:495–496, 1942.

9. Lawhorn B: A new approach for obtaining blood samples from pigs. *JAVMA* 192:781–782, 1988.

10. Thurmon JC, Benson GJ: Anesthesia in ruminants and swine, in Howard JL (ed): *Current Veterinary Therapy. III. Food Animal Practice.* Philadelphia, WB Saunders Co, 1993, 58–76.

11. Nishimura R, Kim H, Matsunaga S, et al: Comparison of sedative and analgesic/anesthetic effects induced by meteto-mide, acepromazine, azaperone, dropenidol and midazolam in laboratory pigs. *J Vet Med Sci* 55:687–690, 1993.

12. McGrath CV, Rempel WE, Addis PB, et al: Acepromazine and droperidol inhibition of halothane-induced malignant hyperthermia (porcine stress syndrome) in swine. *Am J Vet Res* 42:195–198, 1981.

13. Muir WW, Hubbell JAE: Drugs used for preanesthetic anesthetic. *Handbook of Veterinary Anesthesia.* St Louis, CV Mosby Co, 1989, pp l5–28.

14. Ragan HA, Gillis MF: Restraint, venipuncture, endotracheal intubation, and anesthesia of miniature swine. *Lab Anim Sci* 25:409–419, 1975.

15. Benson GV, Hartsfield SM, Thurmon JC: A method for anesthetizing pigs using small animal inhalation equipment. *Pract Vet* (Spring-Summer):20–25, 1977.

16. Cantor GH, Brunson DB, Reibold TW: A comparison of four short-acting anesthetic combinations for swine. *VM SAC* 76(5):715–720, 1981.

17. Benson GJ, Thurmon JC: Anesthesia of swine under field conditions. *JAVMA* 174:594–596, 1979.

18. Ko JCH, Williams BL, Smith VL, et al: Comparison of Telazol, Telazol-xylazine, and Telazol-ketamine-xylazine as chemical restraint and anesthetic induction combination in swine. *Lab Anim Sci* 43:476–480, 1993.

19. Thurmon JC: Injectable anesthetic agents and techniques in ruminants and swine. *Vet Clin North Am Small Anim Pract* 2(3):567–591, 1986.

20. Lumb WV, Jones EW: Anesthesia of laboratory and zoo animals. *Veterinary Anesthesia*, ed 2. Philadelphia, Lea & Febiger, 1984, pp 458–460.

21. Gray KN, Raulston GL, Flow BL, et al: Repeated immobilization of miniature swine with an acepromazine-ketamine combination. *Southwest Vet* 31:27–30, 1978.

22. Ko JCH, Thurmon JC, Benson JG, et al: "Potbellied" pigs anesthetic management and anesthetics (abstr). *Proc V-MAC* 8, University of Illinois, 1992.

23. Breese CE, Dodman NH: Xylazine-ketamine-oxymorphone: An injectable anesthetic combination in swine. *JAVMA* 184: 182–183, 1984.

24. Thurmon JC, Tranquilli WJ, Benson GB: Glyceryl guaiacolate, ketamine and xylazine: Balanced anesthesia by intravenous infusion in swine. *Proc ACVA Sci Meet*, New Orleans, 1984.

25. Tranquilli WJ: Techniques of inhalation anesthesia in ruminants and swine. *Vet Clin North Am Small Anim Pract* 2(3): 593–619, 1986.

26. Holaday DA, Fiserova-Bergerova V, Latto IP, et al: Resistance of isoflurane to biotransformation in man. *Anesthesiology* 43:325–332, 1975.

27. Rehder K, Forbes J, Allen H, et al: Halothane biotransformation in man: A quantitative study. *Anesthesiology* 28:711–715, 1967.

28. Holaday DA, Rudofsky S, Treuhaft PS: The metabolic degradation of methoxyflurane in man. *Anesthesiology* 33: 579–593, 1970.

29. Thurmon JC, Benson GJ: Special anesthesia considerations in swine, in Short CE (ed): *Principles and Practice of Veterinary Anesthesia.* Baltimore, Williams & Wilkins, 1987, p 312.

30. Hightower CE, Kiorpes AL, Butler HC: End-tidal partial pressure of CO_2 as an estimate of arterial partial pressure of CO_2 during various ventilatory regimens in halothane-anesthetized dogs. *Am J Vet Res* 41:610–612, 1980.

31. Swindle MM: Mini pigs as pets. *Proc TNAVC*:648–649, 1993.

32. Claxton-Gill MS, Cornick-Seahorn JL, Gamboa JC: Suspected malignant hyperthermia syndrome in a miniature potbellied pig anesthetized with isoflurane. *JAVMA* 203: 1434–1436, 1993.

A Clinical Guide to the Pet Ferret

Lennox M. Ryland, DVM
Washington State Department of Health
Olympia, Washington

Susan L. Bernard, MS
John R. Gorham, DVM, PhD

Animal Disease Research Unit
Agricultural Research Service, USDA
Washington State University
Pullman, Washington

Man's association with ferrets can be traced back as far as the fourth century BC, when the long-bodied, supple descendants of the European polecat were first domesticated and used for exterminating snakes and rodents, and later, for hunting rabbits. The domestic ferret (*Mustela putorius furo*) should not be confused with the native North American black-footed ferret (*Mustela nigripes*), now nearly extinct.[1] Unlike its fellow Mustelidae (e.g., skunks, otters, mink, weasels, badgers), the domestic ferret is not a wild animal, and it has survived for generations only in captivity. Long raised as a laboratory animal for studies in reproductive physiology, pharmacology, and virology, the ferret is becoming increasingly popular today as a household pet. For the veterinary practitioner unfamiliar with the care and management of a pet ferret, the following is intended to be a guide to routine prophylactic, diagnostic, and therapeutic procedures.

Species Characteristics

There are two varieties of ferrets, based on coloration: fitch ferrets are buff with black masks, feet, and tails (Figure 1); albino ferrets are white with pink eyes. The albino phenotype and color mutants (e.g., Siamese, silver, and silver mitt) are recessive to the fitch. Female ferrets are called *jills* and males, *hobs*. Baby ferrets are *kits*.[2]

Kits are born deaf and blind after 42 days gestation. The average litter size is 8 (range, 2 to 17). Their eyes and ears open at 21 to 37 days of age, and their deciduous teeth begin to erupt at 14 days, at which time kits begin to eat solid food. Their permanent canines erupt at 47 to 52 days of age, and kits are weaned by the time they are 8 weeks old. They reach their adult weight at 4 months of age.[3] Males are typically twice as large as females (range, 600 to 2000 g), but both sexes undergo photoperiodic weight fluctuations of 30 to 40% of their body weight, adding subcutaneous fat in the fall and losing this fat in the spring.[4]

Ferrets reach sexual maturity in the spring following their birth (or at 9 to 12 months of age).[3] The female is seasonally polyestrous, with a normal breeding season from March to August, though females may remain in heat for up to 6 months if copulation does not occur. Onset of estrus can be recognized by enlargement of the vulva (Figure 2), which

Originally published in Volume 5, Number 1, January 1983
Updated from reprint in *Exotic Animal Medicine in Practice*. Volume 1, 1991

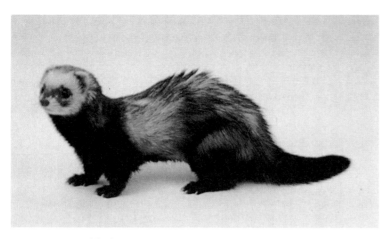

Figure 1—Typical fitch ferret.

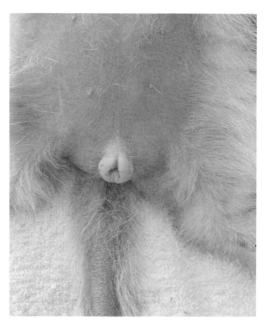

Figure 2—*(Right)* Swollen vulva indicative of estrus. Note alopecia of ventral abdomen and tail.

regresses to normal size within 2 to 3 weeks after coitus. Ovulation is induced by copulation, and if fertilization fails to occur, a pseudopregnancy of 42 days will ensue. Male ferrets' breeding readiness is signaled by descent of the testes into the scrotum. Two litters per year can be obtained if the females are bred early in the breeding season.

Gross anatomic features of the ferret include the absence of a cecum, appendix, and prostate gland (male).[5] Ferrets have a vertebral formula of $C_7T_{14}L_6S_3Cd_{14-18}$ with 14 pairs of ribs.[6] The ferret's permanent dental formula is $2(I^3/_3 \ C^1/_1 \ P^4/_3 \ M^1/_2)$.[7] Supernumerary incisors are common in adults.[8] Ferrets do not have well-developed sweat glands and are prone to heat prostration at a temperature approaching 32°C (90°F). The average life span in laboratory colonies is 5 to 6 years, but pet ferrets commonly live 9 or 10 years.

Ferrets typically have genial personalities and adapt well to human companionship, particularly if they are raised from infancy in close human contact. They are inquisitive and playful animals by nature, and when given supervised freedom in which to satisfy their innate curiosity and inclination to burrow, they need no special exercise equipment. Because they tend to urinate and defecate in habitual places, they can be easily trained to use a litter box. Some pet ferrets have even been trained to walk on a leash and harness. There is no natural animosity between ferrets and cats or dogs.

Diet

The nutritional requirements of ferrets have not been determined. For more than 25 years at Washington State University (WSU), ferrets have been maintained adequately on a standard wet feed mink diet (30% fat, 35% protein, 5 to 6% ash). Pet ferrets are maintained with commercial cat food supplemented with table scraps. At WSU, because nutritional deficiencies have never been recognized in the colony and because there

are few reports in the literature, the nutritional requirements of ferrets are assumed to be similar to those of cats and mink. The National Research Council requirements for mink and cats are listed in Table I.[9,10] Since ferrets will eat to their caloric requirement, they can eventually get into a situation of low protein intake on cat food. This can result in poor reproductive performance.[38] Milk is a good source of supplemental calcium, but may cause loose feces. The ferret has little, if any, capacity to digest fiber. Small bones should be withheld from the diet to prevent their becoming lodged in the mouth or gastrointestinal tract. Ferrets do not need to eat mice or other rodents. Fresh water, in either a cup or drinking bottle, should be available at all times.

Restraint

The ferret is best restrained when grasped above the shoulders, with one hand gently squeezing the forelimbs together, the thumb under the animal's chin. A handler may choose to wear a leather glove, as even the best trained ferret becomes apprehensive in strange surroundings.

The drugs and dosages commonly used to provide chemical restraint and sedation in ferrets are summarized in Table II. At WSU, a simultaneous intramuscular injection of xylazine HCl (1 to 4 mg/kg) and ketamine HCl (20 to 30 mg/kg) is used routinely for short periods of chemical restraint (10 to 20 minutes). If longer periods of anesthesia are needed, gas anesthesia (methoxyflurane or halothane) delivered by mask works well. The use of barbiturates is limited due to the relative inaccessibility of peripheral veins. Intramuscular and subcutaneous injections are given as with the cat or dog, with due regard to the increased fat layer present in autumn or winter.

Vaccinations

Ferrets must be protected against canine distemper by

TABLE I
RECOMMENDED NUTRIENT ALLOWANCES FOR CATS AND MINK[9,10]
(PERCENTAGE OR AMOUNT/KG DIET, DRY BASIS[a])

Nutrient	Unit	Amount Mink	Amount Cat
Protein	%	25–32	28
Fat	%	6–20	9
Linoleic acid	%	ND[b]	1
Minerals			
Calcium	%	0.3	1.0
Phosphorus	%	0.3	0.8
Potassium	%	ND	0.3
Sodium chloride	%	0.5	0.5
Magnesium	%	ND	0.05
Iron	mg	114	100
Copper	mg	ND	5
Manganese	mg	ND	10
Zinc	mg	ND	30
Iodine	mg	ND	1
Selenium	mg	ND	0.1
Vitamins			
Vitamin A	IU	10,000	10,000
Vitamin D	IU	ND	1,000
Vitamin E	IU	25	80
Thiamine	mg	1.2	5
Riboflavin	mg	1.5	5
Pantothenic acid	mg	4–8	10
Niacin	mg	20	45
Pyridoxine	mg	1.1	4
Folic acid	mg	0.5	1.0
Biotin	mg	ND	0.05
Vitamin B_{12}	mg	30	0.02
Choline	mg	1,000	2,000

[a]Based on a diet with metabolizable energy concentration of 4 kcal/g of dry matter (cat) and 4.25 kcal/g of dry matter (mink).
[b]Not determined.

TABLE II
DRUGS USED FOR CHEMICAL RESTRAINT AND SEDATION IN FERRETS

Drug	Dosage	Route
Sedatives		
Acepromazine	0.2–0.5 mg/kg	IM, SQ
Xylazine	1.0 mg/kg	IM, SQ
Preanesthetics		
Atropine	0.05 mg/kg	IM, SQ
Acepromazine	0.1–0.25 mg/kg	IM, SQ
Anesthetics		
Ketamine	20–35 mg/kg	IM, SQ
(9 parts:1 part	(ketamine)	
acepromazine)	0.2–0.35 mg/kg	
	(acepromazine)	
Xylazine	1–4 mg/kg	SQ
(followed by ketamine)	(xylazine)	
	20–30 mg/kg	
	(ketamine)	
Halothane		Mask
Methoxyflurane		Mask
Pentobarbital	30 mg/kg	IP

hepatitis, feline rhinotracheitis, or feline calicivirus, and do not require vaccination against these diseases. There is no definitive evidence that ferrets are susceptible to disease produced by canine parvovirus; therefore, vaccination is probably not warranted. Because clinical trials have never been conducted on the safety or efficacy of the commonly used four- and five-way canine vaccines, the authors are hesitant to recommend them for use in ferrets. A schedule of vaccinations and prophylactic procedures is outlined in Table III.

Routine Surgical Procedures
Female ferrets not intended for breeding purposes should be spayed at six to eight months of age. Estrous

TABLE III
SCHEDULE OF VACCINATIONS AND ROUTINE PROPHYLACTIC CARE

Age	Plan
6–8 weeks (4–6 weeks if dam unvaccinated)	First CDV;[a] fecal
9–12 weeks	Second CDV; fecal
12 weeks	Rabies[b] vaccination
6–8 months	Spay/castrate; fecal Remove musk glands (optional)
1 year	Rabies booster (annual)
3 years	CDV booster (triennial)

[a]CDV = canine distemper vaccine (nonferret origin).
[b]Killed.

vaccination with modified live virus of chick embryo tissue culture origin. The first dose of vaccine should be administered at six to eight weeks of age (four to six weeks if kits are from unvaccinated dams) and a booster given two weeks later; thereafter, boosters should be given every three years. Killed vaccine provides only short-term immunity that is slow to develop and that is not effective in all ferrets.[11] Distemper vaccine prepared from ferret cell culture should not be used, because attenuated virus may possibly retain its virulence for its natural host.

Rabies vaccine, killed only, should be administered annually, beginning at three months of age. The ferret is assumed to be highly susceptible to rabies and capable of transmitting the virus. Two cases of ferret rabies have been reported in the United States since 1954, and in one of those, the possibility exists that clinical disease followed vaccination with modified live rabies virus.[12]

Ferrets are not susceptible to disease produced by feline panleukopenia, mink virus enteritis, canine females have high endogenous estrogen levels which cause a greater than 50% prevalence of fatal bone marrow depression (see *metabolic diseases*).[13] The use of one intramuscular injection of 100 IU of human chorionic gonadotropin (HCG) 10 or more days after onset of estrus will cause ovulation. Females will cycle out of heat in 20 to 25 days and remain in anestrus for 40 to 50 days.[13] The use of megestrol acetate to delay or prevent estrus in ferrets greatly increases the risk of subsequent pyometra and should be avoided.

Male ferrets not intended for breeding should be castrated at six to eight months of age to reduce their aggressiveness and desire to roam and to remove some of the musky odor resulting from sebaceous secretions. The testes are present in the scrotum only during the breeding season; from July to December, they are located in the subcutis of the caudoventral abdomen.

Ferrets have paired musk-producing glands lateral to the anus which secrete when the animal is angry, excited, or in estrus. These may be removed at the time of neutering or spaying. Standard procedures for canine anal sac excision may be followed. A modified protocol designed specifically for ferret musk gland resection has been published.[14] Excision of these paired glands will reduce, but cannot eliminate, the ferret's musky odor.

Physiologic and Laboratory Data

Blood samples for clinical laboratory procedures may be obtained by toenail clipping ($\leq$0.5 ml), caudal tail venipuncture, or by jugular venipuncture. Cardiac puncture is possible by both transthoracic and transdiaphragmatic approaches but represents additional risk.

Hematological values for ferrets are presented in Table IV[5] and are generally similar to those of the cat. Notable exceptions include the ferret's higher hematocrit (mean, 52.3%), more numerous erythrocytes (mean, $9.17 \times 10^6/mm^3$), and higher percentage of reticulocytes (mean, 4.6%). Estrous females will tend to have lower platelet and leukocyte counts.

Normal serum chemistry values for ferrets are given in Table V. No major differences between these values and those of the cat or dog are apparent. Mild to moderate proteinuria is a consistent finding in normal ferrets and is postulated to result from the ferret's relatively high systolic blood pressure.[5] The naturally dark urine of the male may give false positive values for ketonuria when colorimetric determinations are used.

The ferret's normal heart rate approximates 250 beats/minute.[5] Electrocardiographic (ECG) measurements of wave amplitude are similar to those of the normal feline ECG, although the height of the ferret's R wave may approach but should not exceed 2.0 mV. Radiographically, the cardiac silhouette may be interpreted incorrectly as having dilatation of the left ventricle.

The ferret's normal respiratory rate is 33 to 36 breaths/minute and its body temperature varies between 38 and 40°C (100.8 to 104°F).

Common Parasites and Fungi

Ferrets are subject to most of the external parasites of domestic dogs and cats. Infestation with *Sarcoptes scabiei* may take two forms. In cases in which skin lesions predominate, focal to generalized alopecia and intense

TABLE IV

HEMATOLOGIC VALUES OF NORMAL FERRETS OF BOTH SEXES[a]

Hematology	Mean	Range
Hematocrit (%)	52.3	42–61
Hemoglobin (g/dl)	17.0	15–18
Erythrocytes ($10^6/mm^3$)	9.17	6.8–12.2
Leukocytes ($10^3/mm^3$)	10.1	4.0–19
Leukocytes		
Lymphocytes (%)	34.5	12–54
Neutrophils (%)	58.3	11–84
Monocytes (%)	4.4	0–9.0
Eosinophils (%)	2.5	0–7.0
Basophils (%)	0.1	0–2.0
Reticulocytes (%)	4.6	1–14
Platelets ($10^3/mm^3$)	499	297–910
Total protein (g/dl)	6.0	5.1–7.4

[a]Adapted from Thornton PC, Wright PA, et al: The ferret, *Mustela putorius furo*, as a new species in toxicology, on behalf of Laboratory Animals Ltd. 13:119–124, 1979. Adapted with permission.

TABLE V

SERUM CHEMISTRY VALUES OF NORMAL FERRETS OF BOTH SEXES[a]

Parameter	Unit	Mean	Range
Glucose	mg/dl	136	94–207
BUN	mg/dl	22	10–45
Albumin	mg/dl	3.2	2.3–3.8
Alkaline phosphatase	IU/L	23	9–84
Aspartate aminotransferase (SAST; SGOT)	IU/L	65	28–120
Total bilirubin	mg/dl	<1.0	
Cholesterol	mg/dl	165	64–296
Creatinine	mg/dl	0.6	0.4–0.9
Sodium	mmol/L	148	137–162
Potassium	mmol/L	5.9	4.5–7.7
Chloride	mmol/L	116	106–125
Calcium	mg/dl	9.2	8.0–11.8
Phosphorus	mg/dl	5.9	4.0–9.1

[a]Adapted from Thornton PC, Wright PA, et al: The ferret, *Mustela putorius furo*, as a new species in toxicology, on behalf of Laboratory Animals Ltd. 13:119–124, 1979. Adapted with permission.

pruritus are associated with the mite, which can be found in a skin scraping. In cases in which sarcoptic lesions are confined to the toes and feet, the feet are swollen, scabby, and if untreated, clawless. Treatment consists of cutting back the claws and removing the scabs after softening them in warm water. The mites may be eliminated by application of sulfur ointment or lime and sulfur dips and washes. Organophosphates and carbamates should be used with caution, as safe levels for ferrets have not been established. However, at WSU, sarcoptic mange has been treated successfully with carbaryl (0.5%) shampoos applied weekly for three weeks. Pruritus may be reduced by concomitant administration of corticosteroids (2 mg/kg prednisone). Ferrets may also be infested with fleas (*Ctenocephalides* spp.) and ear mites (*Otodectes cyanotis*) which may be treated with rotenone or pyrethrin products.[15]

Less is known about the susceptibility of the ferret to the common internal parasites of the dog and cat, although coccidiosis and toxoplasmosis have been reported. The ferret is undoubtedly also susceptible to a variety of gastrointestinal helminths (including *Toxascaris leonina*) and protozoa (including *Giardia* spp.[39]). Guidelines for cats should be followed whenever treatment is initiated. Natural infections with *Dirofilaria immitis* have been reported in ferrets.[16] Because of the small size of its heart, 6 to 10 adult worms are sufficient to produce severe respiratory distress, ascites, and death. Avermectins are very effective against *Dirofilaria* in ferrets.[17]

Ringworm (*Microsporum canis*) has been reported in young ferrets and may be transmitted by cats. Lesions are similar to those in other species (Figure 3). Affected ferrets may be treated orally with griseofulvin (25 mg/kg), although clinical signs often regress without treatment.

Bacterial Diseases

Ferrets are moderately susceptible to botulism (*Clostridium botulinum*) types A and B, and they are highly

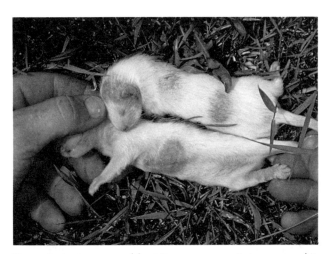

Figure 3—Lesions caused by *Microsporum canis* in a young kit. These lesions regressed without treatment.

susceptible to botulism type C. Signs of dysphagia, ataxia, and paresis appear 12 to 96 hours after eating contaminated foods. Death follows with paralysis of respiratory muscles. There is no successful treatment, although the disease can be prevented by excluding from the diet ingredients of questionable origin or freshness, or by prophylactic annual use of type C toxoid.

Avian, bovine, and human strains of mycobacteria cause tuberculosis in ferrets. Lesions are seen primarily in the alimentary tract and abdominal lymph nodes. Signs may not appear until the late stages of active infection, when the animal becomes emaciated and may exhibit paralysis of the pelvic adductor muscles. Paralysis later affects all four limbs.[18] Massive accumulations of histiocytes in abdominal organs and intracellular acid-fast bacilli are diagnostic. Tuberculosis may be suspected if the animal gives a thermal response to the subcutaneous tuberculin test or if it has palpably enlarged mesenteric lymph nodes.

Staphylococcal, streptococcal, and corynebacterial abscesses and localized infections of the mammary glands (in nursing jills), uterus, vulva, infected bite wounds incurred during mating, and oral injuries caused by ingested bones are common. Group C streptococcal pneumonia and septicemia may lead to valvular endocarditis. Treatment should be similar to that used in cats, based on results of culture and antibiotic susceptibility testing. However, ferrets should be given no more than 50 mg of streptomycin at 12-hour intervals, because it is toxic in higher doses.[15]

Campylobacter fetus subsp. *jejuni* has been isolated from six of nine ferrets with proliferative colitis. Clinical signs of proliferative colitis included green mucohemorrhagic feces, rectal prolapse, anorexia, and dehydration.[19] Supportive fluid therapy combined with broad-spectrum antibiotics (chloramphenicol or gentamicin) did not alleviate the condition. All affected ferrets died or were euthanatized when moribund.[19]

Viral Diseases

Ferrets are highly susceptible to canine distemper. Moreover, because the case fatality rate approaches 100%, ferrets are used as test animals for the detection of the virus. The initial signs of disease appear 7 to 10 days after exposure and include anorexia and mucopurulent ocular and nasal discharges (Figure 4). A rash appears commonly under the chin and in the inguinal area 10 to 12 days following exposure (Figure 5). The foot pads may swell and become hyperkeratotic. The animal continues to deteriorate until death, 12 to 16 days after exposure with ferret-adapted strains (21 to 25 days with canine strains). Ferrets that survive the catarrhal phase may die during a central nervous system phase of distemper, signs of which include hyperexcitability, excess salivation, muscular tremor, convulsions, and coma. Because the signs of distemper are so typical, the disease is rarely confused with other conditions. Clinical diagnosis can be confirmed with fluorescent antibody techniques or histopathology. In the authors' experience with over 1000 cases of distemper, not a single ferret has survived, suggesting that euthanasia is a practical alternative to symptomatic, supportive treatment.

Ferrets are susceptible to infection with several strains of human influenza virus, which may cause initial signs similar to those of distemper. Within 48 hours of exposure, the affected ferret becomes listless, febrile, and anorectic, and its nose becomes moist. Sneezing attacks may develop, accompanied by a purulent nasal discharge. Congestion may be relieved by antihistamines suitable for use in other small animals. Recovery usually occurs within five days of onset of signs and the ferret is immune for at least five weeks against the homologous influenza strain. Vaccination with attenuated live virus affords protection of a similar duration, but it is not recommended routinely.[20]

Aleutian disease is usually subclinical in ferrets, but affected animals may become hypergammaglobulinemic and cachectic, with black, tarry feces. They may eventually succumb as long as 200 days after infection. Stressed animals may die unexpectedly even though in good flesh.[21] The disease may be differentiated from acute episodes of nonspecific enteritis and should be suspected if the ferret's gamma globulin fraction exceeds 20% of total serum protein. The diagnosis can be confirmed by counter immunoelectrophoresis. Lesions include lymphocytic and plasmacytic infiltration of liver, spleen, lungs, and kidneys, and follicular hyperplasia of lymph nodes. There appears to be a biological difference between Aleutian disease virus of mink or ferret origin.[22]

Feline leukemia virus (FeLV) does not appear to produce clinical disease in ferrets. The authors have recognized FeLV-positive, clinically healthy, ferrets.[40] It is possible that ferrets have their own retrovirus which cross reacts with the FeLV assay.[a]

Ferrets are susceptible to pseudorabies and infectious bovine rhinotracheitis. However, natural outbreaks of these diseases have not been reported.

Metabolic Diseases

One of the most common clinical problems seen in pet ferrets is bone marrow depression associated with prolonged estrus.[13,23] There is a greater than 50% prevalence of this disorder during the months of April through July in intact nonbred females. Bone marrow depression is due to high endogenous estrogen levels during estrus, producing pancytopenia. Clinical signs include pale mucous membranes, bilaterally symmetrical alopecia, melena, petechial hemorrhages, anorexia, and depression (Figure 6). Pale (fatty) bone marrow which floats in formalin is the most consistent finding. Pancytopenia predisposes animals to secondary bacterial infections and bleeding disorders. Treatment of bone marrow depression is difficult, as most animals have a packed-cell volume (PCV) of less than 10% and a platelet

count under 20,000/mm². Two animals are known to have survived this condition using two different treatment regimens. One female was ovariohysterectomized despite a PCV of 6%.[41] The other ferret was treated successfully with ovariohysterectomy and 15 intravenous blood transfusions (10 ml each) over a five-month period, coupled with anabolic steroids, corticosteroids, force feeding, and oral vitamin supplementation.[24] A bone marrow transplant was also done but is of questionable value. The use of whole blood transfusions (if available) and surgery may be the most logical treatment. If surgery is not elected, the animal can be cycled out of heat with HCG, as described previously. During this period, anabolic steroids, vitamins, and transfusions are recommended.

Posterior paralysis accompanied by incontinence may appear in an otherwise healthy animal. This paralysis may be due to hemivertebrae, vertebral fractures, intervertebral disk disease, hematomyelia, or myelitis.[13,25,26] Ferrets with no radiographic lesions and ferrets with intervertebral disk problems have responded favorably to steroid therapy. This condition can recur.

Urolithiasis is fairly common in ferrets. It is manifested by urinary incontinence and malaise and can be fatal.[27] Males and females are affected equally. Renal and cystic calculi composed of magnesium ammonium phosphate (struvite) have been reported. Therapy is similar to that for feline urolithiasis and cystitis. Limiting dietary ash and providing adequate water may aid in decreasing the recurrence of uroliths.

Pregnant and postparturient females are predisposed to several nutrition-dependent diseases, such as eclamptogenic toxemia and *nursing sickness*. Vitamin and mineral supplementation suitable for use in cats should be instituted during pregnancy and lactation. Insuring that the dam's dietary needs are met during these critical times will help reduce preweaning deaths among kits due to lactational failure or cannibalism. Cannibalism is more pronounced in certain families and may be an undesirable genetic trait, though normally most dams or kits will consume a dead neonate.

Ferrets are subject to a variety of spontaneous and congenital malformations that may be hereditary. These include anencephaly, neuroschisis, gastroschisis, cryptorchidism, amelia, corneal dermoids, and cataracts.[28,29]

Endocrine imbalances similar to those of dogs and cats have been reported in ferrets. At least one ferret has been treated satisfactorily for diabetes mellitus with insulin[b] (1 to 2 units/kg).[30]

A bilaterally symmetrical alopecia of the tail and/or ventral abdomen is common in estrous females and has been observed in males during the normal breeding season (Figure 2). The cause of the alopecia is unknown but a hormonal basis is suspected. Hair returns to normal once the breeding season ends or if the female goes out of heat (either by breeding or HCG injection). Avidin

[a]Leukassay F®, Pitman-Moore, Inc., Washington Crossing, NJ 08560.

[b]NPH Iletin®, Eli Lilly and Co., Indianapolis, IN 46285.

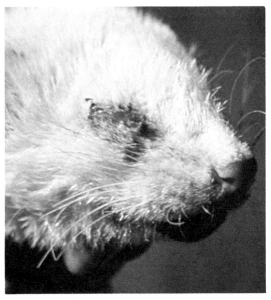

Figure 4—Nasal and ocular discharge associated with canine distemper in ferrets.

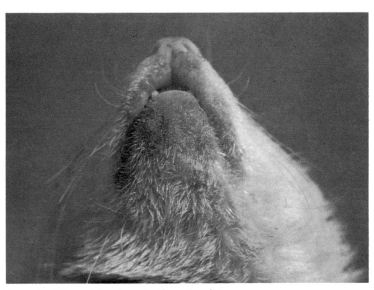

Figure 5—Chin rash in a ferret with canine distemper.

(present in raw eggs) binds up biotin and can cause alopecia.[15] Biotin deficiency can be avoided by decreasing the number of raw eggs in the diet, by boiling the eggs for 15 minutes, or by supplementing the feed with additional biotin.

Zinc toxicity in ferrets causes a diffuse nephrosis manifested by cachexia and macrocytic, hypochromic anemia.[31] Diets contaminated with high levels of zinc are associated with these toxic signs.[32] Treatment includes removal of the cause and supportive therapy.

Neoplastic Diseases

A variety of spontaneous epithelial and mesenchymal neoplasms have been reported in ferrets. Two cases of lymphosarcoma have been reported.[8,33] Affected animals were not tested for FeLV; therefore, the relationship between FeLV and ferret lymphosarcoma is not known.

Ovarian leiomyomas are common in ferrets. These neoplasms do not appear to interfere with ovulation and pregnancy and are incidental findings at necropsy.[34] Bilateral ovarian thecomas with endometrial hyperplasia have been reported in one ferret as an incidental finding.[33] An estrogen-secreting adrenal adenoma reportedly caused an ovariectomized female to exhibit signs of estrus.[33] No other apparent hormonal imbalance was recognized in this female.

Cutaneous squamous cell carcinomas have been reported in ferrets. One tumor was removed successfully, with no evidence of metastasis four months later.[33,35] Cutaneous collections of mast cells have been reported. These mast cell tumors are not considered aggressive.[36]

Adenocarcinoma in two ferrets has been described. One was pancreatic and was considered an incidental postmortem finding.[33] The second was hepatocellular and was from a cachectic ferret with a chronic draining abdominal fistula.[8]

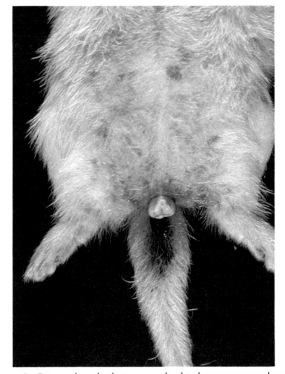

Figure 6—Estrous female that succumbed to bone marrow depression. Cutaneous petechiae, melena (staining tail), and alopecia are common.

Malignant megakaryocytic myelosis was reported in a lethargic, anorectic four-year-old female ferret.[37] Systemic metastases were reported.

These examples of confirmed diagnoses are given to underscore the similarities between ferrets and more familiar companion animal species. Judicious use of diagnostic tools (history, physical examination, clinical pathology, radiology) is as relevant to ferrets as to the dog or cat. Once a diagnosis has been reached, medical therapy, where appropriate, should follow guidelines established for cats unless experience dictates otherwise.

Acknowledgment

The authors wish to thank Dr. C. W. Leathers for his critical review of this article.

REFERENCES

1. *Threatened Wildlife of the United States*, Publication 114, US Government Printing Office, Washington, DC, US Dept. of the Interior, Bureau of Sport Fisheries and Wildlife, 1973, p 289.
2. Roberts MF: *All about Ferrets.* Neptune City, NJ, TFH Public Inc, Ltd, 1977.
3. Shump AV, Shump KA: Growth and development of the European fitch (*Mustela putorius*). *Lab Anim Sci* 28:89-91, 1978.
4. Hammond J. *The Ferret: Some Observations on Photoperiod and Gonadal Activity, and Their Role in Seasonal Pelt and Bodyweight Changes.* Cambridge, Heffer & Sons Ltd, 1974, pp 3-11.
5. Thornton PC, Wright PA, et al: The ferret, *Mustela putorius furo*, as a new species in toxicology. *Lab Anim* 13:119-124, 1979.
6. Owen R: *On the Anatomy of Vertebrates*, vol 2. New York, AMS Press, 1973.
7. Owen R: *On the Anatomy of Vertebrates*, vol 3. New York, AMS Press, 1973.
8. Andrews PL, Illman O, et al: Some observations of anatomical abnormalities and disease states in a population of 350 ferrets (*Mustela furo L.*) *Z Versuchstierkd* 21:346-353, 1979.
9. *Nutrient Requirements of Cats*, vol 13. Washington, DC, National Academy of Sciences, 1978.
10. *Nutrient Requirements of Mink and Foxes*, vol 7. Washington, DC, National Academy of Sciences, 1968.
11. Ott RL, Svehag SE, et al: Resistance to experimental distemper in ferrets following the use of killed tissue vaccine. *West Vet* 6:107-111, 1959.
12. *Veterinary Public Health Notes*, US Dept. of Health and Human Services. Public Health Service, Centers for Disease Control, Atlanta, GA, 30333. Oct. 1980.
13. Bernard SL, Leathers CW, et al: Estrogen induced bone marrow depression in ferrets. *Am J Vet Res*, in press.
14. Creed JE, Kainer RA: Surgical extirpation and related anatomy of anal sacs of the ferret. *JAVMA* 179:575-577, 1981.
15. Ryland LM, Gorham JR: The ferret and its diseases. *JAVMA* 173:1154-1158, 1978.
16. Miller WR, Merton DA: Dirofilariasis in a ferret. *JAVMA* 180:1103-1104, 1982.
17. Blair LS, Campbell WC: Trial of Avermectin B₁a, mebendazole and Melarsoprol against pre-cardiac *Dirofilaria immitis* in the ferret (*Mustela putorius furo*). *J Parasitol* 64:1032-1034, 1978.
18. Symmers WS, Symmers C, et al: Observations on tuberculosis in ferrets (*Mustela furo L.*). *J Comp Pathol* 63:20-30, 1953.
19. Fox JG, Murphy JC, et al: Proliferative colitis in ferrets. *Am J Vet Res* 43:858-864, 1982.
20. Potter CW, Oxford JS, et al: Immunity to influenza in ferrets. I. Responses to live and killed virus. *Br J Exp Pathol* 53:153-167, 1972.
21. Ohshima K, Shen DT, et al: Comparison of the lesions of Aleutian disease of mink and hypergammaglobulinemia in ferrets. *Am J Vet Res* 39:653-657, 1978.
22. Porter HG, Porter DD, et al: Aleutian disease in ferrets. *Infect Immun* 36:379-386, 1982.
23. Kociba GJ, Caputo CA: Aplastic anemia associated with estrus in pet ferrets. *JAVMA* 178:1293-1294, 1981.
24. Ryland LM: Remission of estrus-associated anemia following ovariohysterectomy and multiple blood transfusion in a ferret. *JAVMA* 181:820-822, 1982.
25. Fredrick MA: Intervertebral disc syndrome in a domestic ferret. *VM SAC* 76:835, 1981.
26. Padgett GA, Alexander JE: Posterior paralysis in mink. *Northeastern Mink Farms* 110:20-21, 1966.
27. Nguyen HT, Moreland AF, et al: Urolithiasis in ferrets (*Mustela putorius*). *Lab Anim Sci* 29:342-345, 1979.
28. Willis LS, Barrow MV: The ferret (*Mustela putorius furo L.*) as a laboratory animal. *Lab Anim Sci* 21:712-716, 1971.
29. Utroska B, Austin AL: Bilateral cataracts in a ferret. *VM SAC* 74:1176, 1979.
30. Carpenter JW, Novilla MN: Diabetes mellitus in a black footed ferret. *JAVMA* 171:890-893, 1977.
31. Straube EF, Schuster NH, et al: Zinc toxicity in the ferret. *J Comp Pathol* 90:355-361, 1980.
32. Straube EF, Walden NB: Zinc poisoning in ferrets (*Mustela Putorius furo*). *Lab Anim* 15:45-47, 1981.
33. Chesterman FC, Pomerance A: Spontaneous neoplasms in ferrets and polecats. *J Pathol Bacteriol* 89:529-533, 1965.
34. Cotchin E: Smooth-muscle hyperplasia and neoplasia in the ovaries of domestic ferrets (*Mustela putorius furo*). *J Pathol* 130:169-179, 1980.
35. Zwicker GM, Carlton WW: Spontaneous squamous cell carcinoma in a ferret. *J Wildl Dis* 10:213-216, 1974.
36. Symmers SC, Thomson APD: Multiple carcinomata and focal mast cell accumulations in the skin of a ferret (*Mustela furo L.*) with a note on other tumors in ferrets. *J Pathol Bacteriol* 65:481-492, 1953.
37. Chaudhung KA, Shilinger RB: Spontaneous megakaryocytic myelosis in a four-year-old domestic ferret (*Mustela furo*). *Vet Pathol* 19:561-564, 1982.
38. Evans RH: Personal communication, Ralston Purina Co, St. Louis, MO.
39. Kaufman J: Personal communication, Fort Collins, CO.
40. Strother M: Personal communication, Washington State Univ.
41. Ranta L: Personal communication, Desert Veterinary Clinic, Richland, WA.

UPDATE

Since the original publication of this article in 1983, numerous reports describing various clinical disease syndromes have appeared in the literature. The reader is advised to consult a comprehensive review of material published through 1993.[1]

NEOPLASTIC DISEASES

Pancreatic islet cell tumors (insulinomas) are commonly reported in middle-aged and older ferrets. Clinical signs reflect hypoglycemia and include generalized or hindlimb weakness, ptyalism, or seizures. A blood glucose concentration of < 60 mg/dl, with or without an elevated insulin level, is suggestive of insulinoma. The diagnosis is confirmed at surgery. Surgical excision of benign tumors may be curative, but malignant tumors often micrometastasize early. Medical management consists of increasing the blood glucose concentration by administration of prednisone, diazoxide, and frequent feedings.

Lymphosarcoma in ferrets may present as acute mediastinal neoplasia with pleural effusion or as chronic peripheral lymphadenopathy. Ferrets of any age may be affected; however, mediastinal disease is more common in younger animals. Diagnostic methods are identical to those in other species and include radiography, ultrasound, hematology, biochemical profile, cytology, and histopathology of biopsied tissues. Treatment protocols are similar to those recommended for dogs and cats. These tumors in ferrets have not been associated with feline leukemia virus infection.

(continues on page 155)

An Introduction to Chinchillas*

Carol J. Merry, RVT, MS, PhD

Department of Health and

   Human Services

Public Health Service

Centers for Disease Control and Prevention

National Institute for Occupational

   Safety and Health

Division of Biomedical and

   Behavioral Science

Physical Agents Effects Branch

Cincinnati, Ohio

*The use of trade names in this article is for reference only and does not imply endorsement by the author, the Public Health Service, the National Institute for Occupational Safety and Health, or the publisher.

Wild chinchillas were originally native to the South American countries of Peru, Bolivia, Chile, and Argentina. The animals were primarily found on the western slope of the Andes Mountains from sea level to 15,000 feet. The climate of the region is generally cool and

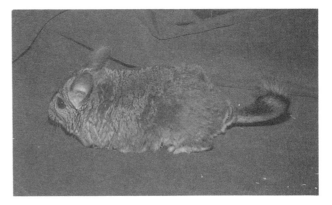

semiarid. Chinchillas were prized by the local Indian tribe, the Chinchas, who used the soft fur to

Originally published in *Veterinary Technician* Volume 11, Number 5, June 1990 adorn ceremonial apparel. The Chinchas were conquered by the Spaniards in the 1500s. The Spaniards coined the term *chinchilla*, or "little chincha."[1]

By the late 1800s, several million chinchilla pelts were being sent to Europe annually. The extensive hunting led to depletion of chinchillas in their native habitat; the animals are now practically extinct in the wild. As many as 90% of the remaining wild chinchillas exist on a 16-square-mile preserve in Chile.[2]

Chinchillas were brought to the United States by Mathias Chapman in February 1923.[3] Chapman established a small breeding colony; by the late 1940s, several ranchers were raising breeding stock descended from his original 11 animals. The first auction of pelts in the United States was held on June 21, 1954[4]; before this date, only breeding animals were marketed.

Today, there are chinchilla ranchers throughout the United States and Canada. Some ranchers raise a few individuals for breeding stock or the pet market; other ranchers manage thousands of animals, primarily for the fur trade. There are two generally recognized species: *Chinchilla brevicaudata* and *C. lanigera*. The latter species is raised in the United States.

Chinchillas are rodents with a single pair of incisors and four sets of molars. The teeth grow throughout life. The animals are most closely related to porcupines, guinea pigs (cavies), and agoutis. Chinchillas are described as resembling squirrels or giant gerbils; they have compact bodies, bushy tails, large eyes and ears, and long whiskers.

Adults weigh from 450 to 800 grams and are 25 to 35 centimeters long. Females are generally larger than males. The standard color is gray and ranges from very light to very dark. Selective breeding has produced mutant strains with beige, white, black, brown, silver, violet, or multicolored fur. Two common colors are pictured in Figure 1.

Chinchillas are herbivores. The young are precocial at birth. Breeders anecdotally report that the life span approaches 20 years. Chinchillas are gregarious, curious, and active. Although normally nocturnal, the animals are responsive to training and handling during the day. Vocalization includes a soft cooing sound of contentment, a bark of alarm or aggression, a spitting growl when very upset, and a doleful babylike cry when frightened or injured.

In recent years, the population of chinchillas in the United States has multiplied as a result of several developments. Fur ranchers that work cooperatively in large marketing groups have expanded production and stimulated demand for chinchilla as a luxury, ranch-raised fur. In addition, chinchillas are increasingly valuable as research subjects, particularly in otologic investigations.

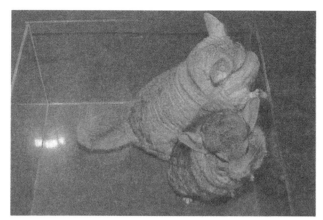

Figure 1—Beige and standard gray chinchillas.

Researchers can obtain inexpensive fur-chewing chinchillas from ranchers. The animals are hardy and convenient to house and work with in the laboratory. They are virtually odorless, and their dietary needs are easily fulfilled. Chinchillas have a charming, inquisitive temperament if handled gently. Their longevity makes them useful for long-term studies.

Of significance in auditory research, chinchillas have large bullae surrounded by thin bone that allows easy surgical access to the middle ear. The cochlea and surrounding structures are similarly accessible. Chinchillas have auditory sensitivity remarkably similar to that of humans.[5] Especially in studies of noise exposure and chemical ototoxicity, chinchillas offer a reasonable alternative to species that are more expensive or difficult to manage.

A new and burgeoning market for chinchillas as pets has also recently surfaced. The temperament and easy maintenance that make chinchillas attractive laboratory animals also endear them to the public.

Research chinchillas usually are fur chewers that are worthless to ranchers; discriminating pet owners, however, pay a premium for beautiful animals. In the midwestern United States, current pet prices for standard grays average $60 for males and more than $80 for females. The public is particularly attracted to the exotic mutant colors, which are rare and expensive. Veterinarians and technicians are increasingly asked to treat chinchillas and to offer advice on their care.

Care Feeding

The natural diet of wild chinchillas comprises grasses and seeds. The animals have extremely large ceca, which assist in the digestion of roughage. Captive chinchillas should be fed high-quality pellets (e.g., ChinChow®—Ralston Purina or Provico®—Provico Feeds). Hay is given ad libitum. Loose timothy or similar grass is preferable, but cubed alfalfa is acceptable (Figure 2). Hay must be free of mold and insecticides.

Many chinchillas enjoy small supplemental feedings a few times a week. Such feedings can include one-quarter teaspoon (1 cc) of dry oatmeal, one or two raisins, a thin apple slice, a few sunflower seeds, or a carrot sliver. Excessive supplements can cause obesity, bloat, diarrhea, or other digestive upsets. Mineralized salt spools can be offered but are not necessary (Figure 2).

Chinchillas should be provided with objects on which they can gnaw and wear down their teeth. Suitable objects include a piece of white pine board, an untreated fruit-tree branch, or a commercially available chew block (blocks can be obtained from Blue Cloud Mineral Company, Saugus, California, or from Nutritional Research Associates, South Whitley, Indiana).

Water

Water, which should be always available, is best supplied by hanging bottles or continuous-drip systems. A chinchilla that has never accessed its drinking water this way should be closely observed to ensure that it is drinking from the bottle or drip outlet. It might be advisable to offer a water dish in addition to the bottle until the animal is secure in the new surroundings and is drinking well from the bottle.

Housing

In the wild, chinchillas live in burrows and rock crevices with a constant temperature of 10° to 13°C (50° to 55°F). Pet owners therefore should consider chinchillas to be caged indoor house pets. Adults can tolerate temperatures just above freezing but cannot survive in stagnant or drafty quarters. The animals are sensitive to heat and are stressed by temperatures hotter than 27°C (80°F). During moderate weather, owners can provide an outdoor hutch or run into which the pet is placed for a few hours each evening. Chinchillas seem to enjoy this outside exercise.

The ideal environment is a well-ventilated room with a temperature of 16° to 21°C (60° to 70°F), a humidity of 40% to 60%, and a 12-hour light-and-dark cycle. Cages with wire mesh bottoms are easy to clean, but some breeders and animal care personnel prefer solid-bottom cages bedded with white pine or hardwood chips (not cedar chips or sawdust). Solid bottoms are better for females with young; infants can be injured if their legs are caught in a mesh floor.

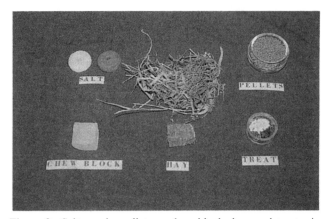

Figure 2—Salt spools, pellets, a chew block, hay, and treat mix are suitable dietary components.

Commercial cages vary in size. A cage that is 41 × 46 × 31 centimeters (16 × 18 × 12 inches) is adequate for a single chinchilla. A self-feeder for pellets and a water bottle should be attached to the cage. Cubed hay can be placed on the floor of the cage; if loose hay is provided, a hay rack is recommended. Exercise wheels are unnecessary.

Dusting

Chinchillas in the wild take frequent dust baths to help absorb skin oils before grooming. In captivity, periodic (several times weekly) dustings are required to maintain a good appearance. Sanitized chinchilla dust is available in grades ranging from extremely fine to slightly coarse (Blue Cloud Mineral Company). Talc and playground sand are not recommended. Cages can be equipped with custom dust bins that slide or tip in and out, or a pan filled with two to three centimeters of dust can be placed in the cage. Chinchillas will roll in the dust and fluff their fur for as long as an hour; the pan then can be removed (Figure 3).

Occasionally, dusting precipitates eye problems. In such cases, dust baths should be decreased or eliminated. Undusted chinchillas loose their fluffiness and develop matted fur; these conditions might not be significant, particularly in a research situation. Pet owners and breeders of show animals often offer dust daily.

Breeding

Chinchillas are mature at seven to nine months of age. Gestation is approximately 111 days, and the average litter contains two young (Figure 4).[6] The young are born precocial and fully furred. The eyes and ears are open, and teeth are present. Infants usually weigh 30 to 50 grams and are ready for weaning at six to eight weeks of age.

The external genitalia of males and females can be simi-

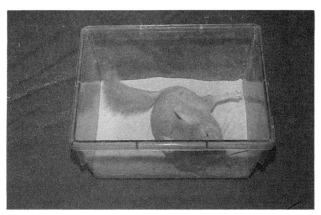

Figure 3—A chinchilla taking a dust bath.

lar in appearance. Male chinchillas have a larger genital papilla. Although there is no true scrotum, the abdominal testicles drop into the anal region during breeding. In females, the papilla is closer to the anus (Figure 5). In an anestrous or pregnant female, the vagina is tightly closed by a closure membrane; the anus and papilla thus appear to be adjacent.[7]

Commercial breeders use polygamous caging. One male has access to as many as five females. Adjacent pens of females have solid dividers and are interconnected in the back by a runway with adjustable doors into the pen of each female. When the doors are open, the male can come and go as it pleases. Each female wears a collar that prevents entry into the runway.

Chinchillas can be bred in pairs on a smaller scale. Animals should be introduced gradually because females can behave savagely toward strange males. Females discharge a vaginal plug after breeding. The plug can be a reliable indication that mating occurred.

Females undergo postpartum estrus within a few days after giving birth. Many breeders allow the male to have access to the mother and young for one week to encourage more breeding. A piece of polyvinyl chloride or metal pipe can be placed in the cage to allow the young to hide if the activity of the adults becomes too boisterous. In pair breeding, it might be unnecessary to remove the male from the cage. If the female continues to accept his presence, the male seldom bothers the offspring.

Common Ailments

Chinchillas are generally healthy. Poor husbandry and inadequate diet, however, are frequent sources of health problems. The following sections discuss common illnesses and offer recommended corrective actions.

Conjunctivitis

Conjunctivitis without clinical signs of upper respiratory infection is often caused by mechanical irritation of the

JAN.	1	2	3	4	5	6	7	8	9	10	11	12	13	14	15	16	17	18	19	20	21	22	23	24	25	26	27	28	29	30	31	
Apr.	21	22	23	24	25	26	27	28	29	30	1	2	3	4	5	6	7	8	9	10	11	12	13	14	15	16	17	18	19	20	21	May
FEB.	1	2	3	4	5	6	7	8	9	10	11	12	13	14	15	16	17	18	19	20	21	22	23	24	25	26	27	28	29	30	31	
May	22	23	24	25	26	27	28	29	30	31	1	2	3	4	5	6	7	8	9	10	11	12	13	14	15	16	17	18				June
MAR.	1	2	3	4	5	6	7	8	9	10	11	12	13	14	15	16	17	18	19	20	21	22	23	24	25	26	27	28	29	30	31	
June	19	20	21	22	23	24	25	26	27	28	29	30	1	2	3	4	5	6	7	8	9	10	11	12	13	14	15	16	17	18	19	July
APR.	1	2	3	4	5	6	7	8	9	10	11	12	13	14	15	16	17	18	19	20	21	22	23	24	25	26	27	28	29	30	31	
July	20	21	22	23	24	25	26	27	28	29	30	31	1	2	3	4	5	6	7	8	9	10	11	12	13	14	15	16	17	18		Aug.
MAY	1	2	3	4	5	6	7	8	9	10	11	12	13	14	15	16	17	18	19	20	21	22	23	24	25	26	27	28	29	30	31	
Aug.	19	20	21	22	23	24	25	26	27	28	29	30	31	1	2	3	4	5	6	7	8	9	10	11	12	13	14	15	16	17	18	Sept.
JUNE	1	2	3	4	5	6	7	8	9	10	11	12	13	14	15	16	17	18	19	20	21	22	23	24	25	26	27	28	29	30	31	
Sept.	19	20	21	22	23	24	25	26	27	28	29	30	1	2	3	4	5	6	7	8	9	10	11	12	13	14	15	16	17	18		Oct.
JULY	1	2	3	4	5	6	7	8	9	10	11	12	13	14	15	16	17	18	19	20	21	22	23	24	25	26	27	28	29	30	31	
Oct.	19	20	21	22	23	24	25	26	27	28	29	30	31	1	2	3	4	5	6	7	8	9	10	11	12	13	14	15	16	17	18	Nov.
AUG.	1	2	3	4	5	6	7	8	9	10	11	12	13	14	15	16	17	18	19	20	21	22	23	24	25	26	27	28	29	30	31	
Nov.	19	20	21	22	23	24	25	26	27	28	29	30	1	2	3	4	5	6	7	8	9	10	11	12	13	14	15	16	17	18	19	Dec.
SEPT.	1	2	3	4	5	6	7	8	9	10	11	12	13	14	15	16	17	18	19	20	21	22	23	24	25	26	27	28	29	30	31	
Dec.	20	21	22	23	24	25	26	27	28	29	30	31	1	2	3	4	5	6	7	8	9	10	11	12	13	14	15	16	17	18		Jan.
OCT.	1	2	3	4	5	6	7	8	9	10	11	12	13	14	15	16	17	18	19	20	21	22	23	24	25	26	27	28	29	30	31	
Jan.	19	20	21	22	23	24	25	26	27	28	29	30	31	1	2	3	4	5	6	7	8	9	10	11	12	13	14	15	16	17	18	Feb.
NOV.	1	2	3	4	5	6	7	8	9	10	11	12	13	14	15	16	17	18	19	20	21	22	23	24	25	26	27	28	29	30	31	
Feb.	19	20	21	22	23	24	25	26	27	28	29	1	2	3	4	5	6	7	8	9	10	11	12	13	14	15	16	17	18	19		Mar.
DEC.	1	2	3	4	5	6	7	8	9	10	11	12	13	14	15	16	17	18	19	20	21	22	23	24	25	26	27	28	29	30	31	
Mar.	20	21	22	23	24	25	26	27	28	29	30	31	1	2	3	4	5	6	7	8	9	10	11	12	13	14	15	16	17	18	19	Apr.

Figure 4—A gestation chart for chinchillas. The numbers in boldface represent the date of conception. The probable date of birth, 111 days later, is directly below. (From Houston JW, Presturich JP: *Chinchilla Care*, ed 4. Los Angeles, Borden Publishing Co, 1962, p 43. Reproduced with permission.)

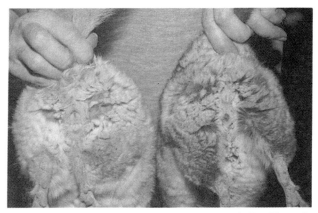

Figure 5—A comparison of male and female genitalia. The male is on the right.

eyes. Such irritation can result from dust baths, dirty bedding, or poorly ventilated quarters. Improved husbandry, cessation of dust baths for a few weeks, and brief therapy with ophthalmic ointment usually resolve the problem. Obtaining a culture from the affected eye might demonstrate a bacterial organism, which should be tested for sensitivity to appropriate antibiotic agents.

Enteritis

Enteritis usually can be traced to poor management. Soft or liquid feces or an abrupt absence of feces might be the first clinical sign. Patients can be listless and dehydrated. Occasionally, a chinchilla is found dead and the diagnosis is based on necropsy. Fecal cultures from affected animals often produce an overgrowth of such organisms as *Pseudomonas, Pasteurella, Proteus, Salmonella,* and *Escherichia coli*.[8] *Pseudomonas* infections evidently are particularly common.

Treatment is difficult because of the acute onset and rapid death associated with enteritis. Antibiotic therapy (based on sensitivity testing of cultured organisms) and fluid replacement are the primary forms of treatment. Oral sulfonamides and chloramphenicol palmitate are readily accepted by chinchillas but must be judiciously administered because the agents can suppress normal gut flora.

For patients that are undergoing antibiotic therapy, breeders often recommend daily feeding of one teaspoon of flavored yogurt (with active cultures) to help replenish favorable gut flora. Most chinchillas quickly learn to accept yogurt and eat it readily from a spoon. Providing a second water bottle filled with an oral electrolyte solution (e.g., Pedialyte®—Ross Laboratories) might be beneficial.

Less commonly reported gastrointestinal problems include parasitic infestation with *Giardia*, coccidia, or tape-worms.[9] These parasites are rare in properly managed herds.

Hair Rings

Male chinchillas can accumulate a ring of hair around the penis and under the prepuce. If not removed, this hair affects breeding ability and can lead to irritation, infection, and severe damage to the penis. Males should be checked for this condition at least four times per year. Hair rings are removed by applying a sterile lubricant to the penis and prepuce and gently rolling the ring off the penis.

Dental Problems

The incisors and molars of chinchillas grow throughout life. Severe dental problems can develop in animals that are deprived of chew blocks and other gnawing material or that have malocclusion. The teeth can curl outward into the cheek spaces or, in extreme cases, can grow inward and upward into the palate.

The tooth roots can penetrate the bony ocular orbits and produce so-called weepy eyes. Patients with this condition have difficulty eating and frequently are thin and untidy in appearance. Crooked incisors can be trimmed with guillotine-type nail trimmers. Malocclusion of the molar surfaces is difficult to treat. Affected chinchillas are unsuitable as pets and are usually pelted by fur ranchers as quickly as possible.

Fur Chewing

Fur chewing is the curse of the chinchilla industry. A lion's mane appearance is often produced when all of the fur within reach on the lower body has been chewed short (Figure 6). Fungal cultures and microscopic examinations are invariably negative.

There are many popular theories but scant documented research concerning the cause of fur chewing. It has been suggested that the vice is induced by boredom or stress. Loud noises, improper diet, stagnant quarters, and small or dirty cages have been incriminated. The fact that fur chewing sometimes seems to be transmitted from mother to offspring might indicate that the behavior is learned.

One theory suggests that the syndrome is caused by a fur-breakage fungus that has not yet been isolated. In the 1960s, this idea was promoted among breeders by Ethel M. Shaull. Dr. Shaull determined that "normal" chinchillas sometimes became fur chewers when housed in proximity to chewers.[10] In addition, chewers treated with captan or other fungicides frequently regrew their fur, at least temporarily. Some ranchers thus add fungicides to the dust

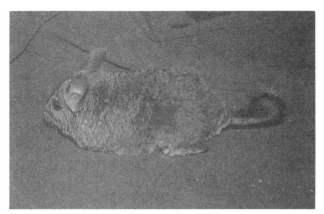

Figure 6—A fur chewer.

bath material at periodic intervals.

According to another hypothesis, fur chewers might have abnormal adrenal glands or hypophyses. One researcher used histologic examination to demonstrate hyperplasia of the hypophysis and fatty degeneration of the adrenal cortex in fur chewers.[11] Another study considered histologic indicators, isotope tracers, and plasma chemistry in fur chewers. There was evidence of increased thyroidal and adrenocortical activity, but it is unclear whether this activity was a cause or an effect of the syndrome.[12]

More documented research is needed. Ranchers rigorously cull fur chewers from their stock. Although such chinchillas might not be objectionable for research, the motley appearance makes them undesirable as pets.

Clinical Information
Anesthesia

In a clinical setting, chinchillas usually respond well to inhalation anesthesia via masking as well as to parenteral (intramuscular) anesthesia. Halothane, halothane combined with nitrous oxide, and methoxyflurane have been successfully used to maintain an adequate plane of anesthesia for surgery.

The head of the patient can be inserted into a small cone to facilitate delivery of the gas. The animal can also be placed in a small induction chamber until sedation is sufficient to allow masking. Application of an appropriate eye ointment is recommended to prevent drying of the ocular membranes by the air and gas flow. As an alternative, anesthesia can be induced with an injectable agent, such as ketamine hydrochloride (10 mg/kg); the patient can then be masked until a stable plane of anesthesia is achieved.

For the sake of quick immobilization, short procedures, or convenience, it might be preferable to achieve anesthesia via intramuscular injection. Ketamine hydrochloride

combined with acepromazine maleate or with xylazine hydrochloride has been noted to be safe and effective.[13] Ketamine hydrochloride can be administered alone for short (20-minute) procedures. For longer procedures, a mixture of ketamine hydrochloride and xylazine hydrochloride is useful. A dose of 20 to 30 mg/kg of ketamine hydrochloride and 1.5 mg/kg of xylazine hydrochloride can be administered intramuscularly. This dose provides as much as two hours of adequate anesthesia and requires a four- to six-hour recovery period.

A stock bottle containing 10 cc of ketamine hydrochloride (100 mg/ml) plus 2.5 cc of xylazine hydrochloride (20 mg/ml) can be prepared in advance. The dose can be calculated by multiplying the weight of the patient (in kilograms) by 0.375 for 30 mg/kg or by 0.275 for 20 mg/kg. For a one-hour procedure, a 600-gram chinchilla can thus be given 0.600 kg × 0.275 mg/kg, or 0.17 cc, of the mixture. The dose is best administered in the upper thigh muscle with a 25-gauge needle mounted on a 1-cc tuberculin syringe. If necessary, anesthesia can be prolonged by giving ketamine hydrochloride at 25% to 50% of the original dose.

To dry mucous secretions, atropine (at 0.05 mg/kg, or weight [in kg] × 0.1) can be administered 15 minutes before the induction of anesthesia. When ketamine hydrochloride is used, eye ointment is applied because the patient's eyes will remain open and unblinking. The use of a warming pad is recommended to maintain the body temperature of sedated patients. A convenient pad that requires no power supply is the Deltaphase® Isothermal Pad (Braintree Scientific). Such pads are activated by immersion in warm water or by heating in a microwave oven.

Hematology

It is difficult to draw blood from chinchillas. For anesthetized patients, especially those undergoing terminal procedures, cardiac puncture is effective. In diagnosing an animal that is awake, toe clipping or foot puncture (with a lancet or sterile needle) provides enough blood for a microhematocrit, differential slide, or Unipet® (Becton Dickinson) white blood cell count. The femoral vein can be used. The leg veins, tail veins, and ear veins are generally difficult to use.

The cranial sinus of a chinchilla is located at the confluence of the sagittal cranial suture and the two bullae. This sinus is an accessible site for obtaining large quantities of blood (0.5 to 1.0 cc) during chronic procedures.[a]

[a]Boettcher FA, Bancroft BR, Salvi RJ: Personal communication, State University of New York at Buffalo, 1989.

TABLE I
Reported Chinchilla Blood Values[a]

Parameter	Newberne[14]	Casella[15]		Kraft[16]		Strike[17]	
Number of animals	12	—	8	10	5	41	52
Sex	—	Male	Female	Male	Female	Male	Female
Age (years)	—	1	1	1.5 to 4.0	1.5 to 4.0	1.8	1.8
Red blood cells ($\times 10^6/\mu$l)	6.93	8.75	7.69	9.45	10.67	7.25	6.60
White blood cells (/μl)	9,300	9,633	9,633	11,539	11,300	7,610	7,990
Percentage of total white blood cells (%)							
Neutrophils	45.0	30.0	23.0	27.3	37.1	42.2	44.6
Lymphocytes	51.0	64.0	73.0	68.5	59.0	54.7	53.6
Monocytes	1.0	4.0	2.0	1.6	1.4	1.3	1.2
Eosinophils	2.0	1.0	1.0	2.6	2.3	0.9	0.5
Basophils	0	1.0	1.0	0.0	0.0	0.9	0.4
Hemoglobin (g/dl)	13.2	13.0	13.0	12.8	13.5	11.7	11.7
Platelets ($\times 10^3/\mu$l)	—	—	—	—	—	254	298
Blood sampling	Ear Vein	—	—	Ear Vein	Ear Vein	Cardiac Puncture	Cardiac Puncture

[a]Data compiled by Douglas W. Stone, DVM, Department of Animal Laboratories, Ohio State University.

Simple Averages from Data

Red blood cells	8.19
White blood cells	9,572
Neutrophils	36%
Lymphocytes	60%
Monocytes	2%
Eosinophils	1%
Basophils	1%
Hemoglobin	12.7

TABLE II
Chinchilla Serum Chemistry Values[18]

Parameter	Range
Blood glucose (mg/dl)	60 to 120
Serum urea nitrogen (mg/dl)	10 to 25
Cholesterol (mg/dl)	40 to 100
Total plasma protein (g/dl)	5 to 6
Albumin plasma protein (g/dl)	2.5 to 4.2
Aspartate transferase (units/dl)	15 to 45
Alanine transferase (units/dl)	10 to 35
Alkaline phosphatase (units/dl)	3 to 12
Calcium (mg/dl)	10 to 25
Phosphorus (mg/dl)	4 to 8
Sodium (mEq/L)	130 to 155
Potassium (mEq/L)	5.0 to 6.5
Chloride (mEq/L)	105 to 115

The normal packed cell volume of a chinchilla is approximately 40%. The blood volume ranges from 40 to 65 ml/kg. Other standard blood values appear in Table I. Table II lists serum chemistry values. Additional normal values for chinchillas include the following: the rectal temperature is 37° to 38°C (99° to 100°F); the resting respiratory rate is 45 to 65 breaths/min; and the resting heart rate is 150 beats/min.

Urinalysis

The urine of chinchillas, like that of other herbivorous animals, is normally alkaline and contains varying amounts of calcium carbonate crystals. The results of a typical urinalysis using a dipstick (N-Multistix®—Miles Laboratories) are depicted in the box, "Normal Chinchilla Urinalysis."

The microscopic examination can demonstrate varying amounts of amorphous debris and tiny crystals. White and red blood cells are not normally present. Casts are rare. In a clean-catch sample, few bacteria should be present. A few squamous epithelial cells are normal; the presence of cells is especially likely in females, which occasionally shed many epithelial cells.

Normal Chinchilla Urinalysis

Color	Yellow to slightly amber
Turbidity	Usually cloudy
pH	8.5
Protein	Negative to trace
Glucose	Negative
Nitrates	Negative
Ketones	Negative
Bilirubin	Negative
Urobilinogen	0.1 to 1.0 mg/dl
Blood	Negative
Specific gravity	Often exceeds 1.045

Conclusion

Chinchillas have become animals that veterinarians and technicians can expect to encounter. The ranch-raised fur market, the pet industry, and research institutions recognize that chinchillas are valuable and desirable. Veterinarians and technicians therefore can benefit from a familiarity with the basic characteristics, husbandry, and medical management of these animals. Such information is particularly useful to veterinary personnel in private pet practices and research laboratories.

Acknowledgments

The author thanks Douglas W. Stone, DVM, of the Department of Animal Laboratories, Ohio State University, for supplying written and verbal information that was valuable in the preparation of this article. Unpublished general data concerning chinchillas were provided by Michael Rudnick, PhD, MD. Special appreciation is expressed to Linda Carr and Judy Curless for typing and proofreading the manuscript.

■

REFERENCES

1. Houston JW, Presturich JP: *Chinchilla Care*, ed 4. Los Angeles, Borden Publishing Co, 1962, p 15.
2. Cubberly P: Last refuge for wild chinchilla protected. *Focus* 10(6):5, 1988.
3. Zeinert K: *All About Chinchillas*. Neptune City, NJ, TFH Publications, 1986, pp 11–16.
4. Bowen EG, Jenkins RW: *Chinchilla: History, Husbandry, Marketing*. Westerville, OH, Shoots Chinchilla Ranch, 1988, p 10.
5. Henderson D, Hamernik RP: Evoked-response audibility curve of the chinchilla. *J Acoust Soc Am* 54(4):1099–1101, 1973.
6. Houston JW, Presturich JP: *Chinchilla Care*, ed 4. Los Angeles, Borden Publishing Co, 1962, p 43.
7. Hafez ESE: *Reproduction and Breeding Techniques for Laboratory Animals*. Philadelphia, Lea & Febiger, 1970, pp 209–223.
8. Kraft H: *Diseases of Chinchillas*. Neptune City, NJ, TFH Publications, 1987, pp 106–107.
9. Stampa S, Hobson NK: Control of some internal parasites of chinchillas. *JAVMA* 149:929–932, 1966.
10. Shaull EM: Fur quality and fur breakage in the chinchilla. *Chinchilla World* 37(2):9, 1988.
11. Kraft H: *Diseases of Chinchillas*. Neptune City, NJ, TFH Publications, 1987, p 127.
12. Vanjonack WJ, Johnson HD: Relationship of thyroid and adrenal function to "fur chewing" in the chinchilla. *Comp Biochem Physiol [A]* 45:115–120, 1973.
13. Hargett CE, Gautier IM: *Comparison of Three Anesthetics for Chinchilla*. Fort Rucker, AL, Army Aeromedical Research Laboratory, 1988, pp 1–22.
14. Newberne PM: A preliminary report on the blood picture of the South American chinchilla. *JAVMA* 122:221–222, 1953.
15. Casella RL: The peripheral hemogram in the chinchilla. *Mod Vet Pract* 44:51, 1963.
16. Kraft VH: The morphological blood picture of the chinchilla villigera. *Blut* 6:386–387, 1959.
17. Strike TA: Hemogram and bone marrow differential of the chinchilla. *Lab Anim Care* 20:30–38, 1970.
18. *The Care of Experimental Animals: A Guide for Canada*. Ottawa, Ontario, Canadian Council on Animal Care, 1969, p 438.

Husbandry and Medical Management of Rodents and Hedgehogs

All Wild Things Exotic Animal Hospital
Indianapolis, Indiana
Beth Ann Breitweiser, DVM

HAMSTERS

Mesocricetus auratus is a desert, tunnel-dwelling hamster from Syria (Figure 1). The standard habitat of the hamster in captivity, typically a plastic home, wheel, and water bottle, frequently provides an endless stream of patients for the average veterinarian willing to see hamsters. These tubular dwellings, especially when they are filled with cedar shavings, often contribute to ill health and disease.

Habitat-related Illness

The limited air circulation in the typical rodent dwelling, assuming it is kept relatively clean, may not be as big a problem for hamsters as it is for other small mammals. Hamsters have the ability to handle larger amounts of carbon dioxide by excreting it through their urine in a salt or crystalline form, which allows the hamster in the wild to last comfortably in its home for longer periods (e.g., until a sandstorm ends.) Mucin glands in the hamster's urinary tract process these crystals to prevent damage. When excreted, the crystallized carbon dioxide is frequently mistaken for pus. The hamster can produce up to 10 cc of a crystalline urine per day under normal conditions and in the presence of unlimited water. Problems occur when the hamster in captivity is unable to leave its "tunnel" for fresh air; the volatile oils in cedar and pine shavings irritate the mucus membranes and induce liver enzymes, creating an environment for disease. Infrequent cage changes lead to higher ammonia levels. In combination with cedar, these habitats become torture chambers that instigate many variations on upper respiratory disease. The tiny dwarf or Chinese hamsters seem to be even more intolerant of soft wood byproducts than do their Syrian or European cousins.

Cages that are kept too clean pose a different threat. Hamsters need to keep a constant stash of food around in order to feel secure. As nocturnal animals, they spend long nights storing food. If someone is constantly removing that stash, the hamster will then save the food in its huge cheek pouches. Seeds may begin to sprout or the food may spoil or meld together if left in the pouch too long. Impacted cheek pouches can be easily cleared and flushed. To prevent a recurrence, however, the stash must be returned to its storage site when the cage is cleaned.

Impacted cheek pouches must be distinguished from an all-too-common neoplasia of the cheek pouch. Expressing the pouch through the mouth is easy unless the mass inside is attached. Pituitary tumors are also common in hamsters and can manifest clinically through abnormal behavior. Excessive cheek stuffing is one such abnormal act and should be viewed with suspicion if the behavior persists.

Stress and Disease

Hamsters are also susceptible to stress, which is made worse by disease and poor nutrition. One common sequela of stress is infant cannibalism. Mothers should be left alone with an ample supply of food and water one week prior to and one week following parturition. If feeling exposed and vulnerable, she may try stuffing her babies in her cheek pouches in order to protect them or escape with them, thus appearing to eat them. Since she has no place to run or hide, she may keep them in there so long that they suffocate. Once the babies are dead, the mother will eat them in order to keep the nest disease free. Most motherly carnivorous episodes occur to newly purchased females under the stress of a new environment. Usually the new owners weren't even aware the hamster was pregnant when it was purchased.

Good quality rodent chow, supplemented with dried grass seeds and plants, should reduce some stresses and perhaps prevent the devastating diarrhea that may accompany newly acquired hamsters. Yogurt, lettuce, and broccoli are not native to the Syrian desert and could result in diarrhea or wet tail in hamsters. Many hamsters die from diarrhea induced by owners feeding such treats. Wet tail is a term used by pet shop merchants or pet owners to describe any condition in which the perianal region is moist or the fur in this area is matted down. Wet tail may result from an infection with

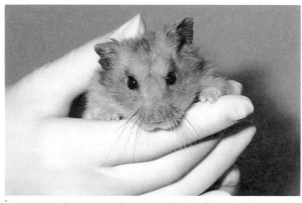

Figure 1—A hamster will remain docile if handled properly.

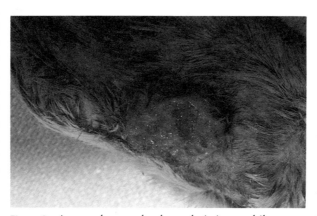

Figure 2—A ventral scent gland neoplasia in a gerbil.

campylobacter or similar organism that causes proliferative enteritis. It can also be caused by polyuria.

Cystic kidney disease, amyloidosis (of mainly female hamsters), or adrenal tumors are all common causes of polyuria/polydipsia in the hamster. Diagnostic evaluations, such as ultrasound and urinary analysis, should be performed to specify the cause of a disorder.[1]

Dermatologic conditions, such as alopecia, variable skin thickness, ear mites, *Demodex*, and nonhealing lesions, frequently are signs of a more serious condition. Dehydration may be from renal disease or simply from a clogged water bottle. The feet should be examined periodically in assessing overall health: Injuries can occur from the many miles logged on the wheel every night or from incompatible cage mates. String and threads can cause limb lesions in the young when they wrap around the appendage and cut off circulation. Inadequate humidity when combined with drying cage substrates like corn cob can dehydrate the pups and lead to ring constrictions, especially of the tail in pinkie rats. Finally, hamsters that cannot run in their environment will spend their time creating escape routes. In the event a pet hamster is successful in breaking out, owners should be mindful of temporarily moving mouse poisons and traps. Vitamin K therapy generally is effective in reducing toxicity in hamsters that have ingested such poisons. The cheek pouches also should be cleared after an escape or the hamster may continue to poison itself or its cage mates.

GERBILS

Meriones unguiculatus, a tunneling, desert-dwelling rodent from Mongolia, is a common visitor to veterinary offices, primarily because gerbils are frequently afflicted with neoplasias. These tumors are associated with both the male and female ventral scent glands (Figure 2) and are best managed through excisional biopsies.

Care and Handling

Handling of these small rodents is difficult due to

their size and anatomic frailties. Management is easiest using a small, cloth towel to pick up the animal. A technique that works well for most small rodentia is to immobilize the head and neck with the first finger and thumb, then rest the body in the palm. Teeth, eyes, abdomens, etc. can then be easily examined with little movement. This method also prevents proctosed globes that may arise from the animal's scruffing techniques, but which are more of a problem in hamsters.

Before examining a gerbil, it is important to know that gerbils' tails deglove easily, so they should be grasped near the base only. Amputation of the exposed tail tip is frequently the consequence of tail injuries. A gerbil's back legs are its primary means of ambulation, similar to a rabbit or macropod (e.g., wallaby), and are also used to express displeasure or to give warning to others of impending danger. This stamping of the hind limbs against the floor may easily lead to fractures, which are a challenge to repair. Stylets from 22-gauge spinal needles will just barely fit down the medullary canals of the larger bones. "Melt & mold" casting material can then be put around the leg to prevent rotation and protect the pin. If the cast is perfectly smooth, the gerbil will be less likely to chew it, assuming the animal has been distracted for a period of time following anesthesia as it gets used to the weight of the cast.

Grooming Problems

The claws on gerbil feet, like those of rabbits, tend to become rapidly overgrown. Nail trimming should be a regular part of a routine examination, especially since most clients are reluctant to restrain their pets sufficiently to accomplish this task. A gerbil will groom its face with its front paws, which can result in eye trauma when the nails are not sufficiently trimmed. Excessive facial grooming that leads to the loss of fur from the front paws may indicate infection in the harderian gland. This lacrimal gland is common to many rodentia and normally excretes porphyrin pigments, which increase with stress, debilitation, or disease. The gerbil seems to be more sensitive than other rodents to excessive harderian gland excretions. The condition, exacerbated by the gerbil scratching and grooming the area in an attempt to relieve the irritation, can progress to staphylococcus or streptococcus infections. As a result, nasal dermatitis in the gerbil may lead to complete facial alopecia, accompanied by dermal scabs and crusts. The eyes become matted shut, and the gerbil gets very depressed and may stop eating due to the loss of sight and smell. Nasal dermatitis can be treated with topical soaps or scrubs, such as chlorhexidine, and with topical antibiotics.

The cause for the harderian gland discharges must be ascertained in order to effect a cure. Cedar or pine bedding, filthy conditions, tooth problems, as well as other medical conditions can result in excessive glandular discharges. Heavy smoking in the home also can aggravate the eye irritations and glandular inflammation, as well as lead to a scruffy, dirty coat.

All physical exams should include examinations of the teeth. Molars do not continue to erupt in the gerbil as they do in the rabbit and chinchilla, but should not be forgotten. Otoscope cones work well as oral speculums. Oral foreign bodies, such as plant material, bedding or seed hulls, can lodge in various places and create oral ulcers and necroses. Gerbils will sometimes lose their upper incisors, requiring monthly, lower-incisor trims, or simple extractions.

Gerbils are famous for their monogamous pair bonds, which are formed most tenaciously as young animals. However, when one animal has had even a short stay in the hospital, the owner must be cautioned about reintroducing the animals to each other. Generally, a female is the aggressor over the male, especially if an unknown male is introduced into her cage. Gerbils are just as sensitive to redecorating as they are to intruders. Their safety in the wild depends on escape routes that are well plotted and memorized. If their tunnels are rearranged, the gerbil may experience a seizure due to the stress.[2] Generally nervous creatures, a gerbil can have a seizure without provocation; it is best not to indelicately initiate anything.

RATS

Rattus norvegicus is almost everywhere on the planet. There is debate about which continent first started spreading this species. The most adaptable small mammal pet on the market today—both energetic and curious—domesticated rats are highly recommended as companions for children. They are more active during the night and prefer to bed down in a nest when they sleep. If enough time is given to the relationship, however, they can adjust to their owners' schedules. Many clients have reported rats that sleep with them at night and guard the house against intruders while they are away. Although it doesn't bark, a large rat running down the hall can be very intimidating to a would-be burglar.

Environmental Hazards

While appropriate as pets, rats are vulnerable to varying forms of distress when permitted to wander about the house. Anorexia, oral edema, dyspnea, and foul breath are all signs of electrical cord burns. Painful joints, blood in the urine, and sores on the bottoms of the feet may indicate recent poisoning from leftover mouse or rat bait laced with warfarin. Alternately, too much time in an aquarium, where the air circulation is poor, is also detrimental. Rats tend to urinate a lot, which elevates the level of ammonia in the cage. Ammonia build-up in enclosed cages displaces oxygen and can initiate the introduction of several bacteria that tend to shorten the life of the average house rat. These organisms take up residence in the compromised respiratory tract and lead to pneumonia, lung abscesses, etc. Harderian gland inflammation and secretions (Figure 3) are usually precursors or warning beacons to conditions of the lung and should be thoroughly investigated.

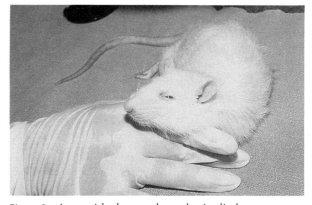

Figure 3—A rat with abnormal porphyrin discharge.

Pneumonia, generally treatable if it is bacterial in nature, is a frequent cause of death in rats and should be differentiated from the also common thoracic neoplasia. Several viral infections, such as sialodacryoadenitis and the rat corona virus, cause pneumonia and harderian gland inflammation that are not treatable. The viruses may run their course, sometimes killing the younger rats, usually causing permanent harderian gland damage and chronic porphyrin discharge called chromodacryorrhea.[3]

Simple overcrowding can lower the immune system of the rat, especially in males. As with other rodentia, these animals are very susceptible to the toxic effects of the volatile oils in cedar and pine shavings. Many rats present with anorexia when, in fact, they were unable to eat and breathe at the same time due to advanced respiratory disease. An open wire cage eliminates the problem of toxic gases as one cause of these diseases of the respiratory tract. The wires should be closer together than the thickness of the rat's head, or it may escape. Wash the rat in a soap designed to cut oil, such as certain dishwashing liquids, in order to remove any residual oils. Short-term, anti-inflammatory agents and oxygen may be necessary to keep the rat alive long enough to give antibiotics time to work. Most antibiotics pose little threat to the rat, unlike many other creatures that lack canine teeth.[4] Scruffy rats may be aging or they may be affected with fungal or bacterial dermatitis. Determine the etiology and then shampoo the rat with an appropriate medicated soap. Several washings may be required, or systemic medications may be needed for more tenacious infections. Chlorhexidine scrub, which can be used in conjunction with oral medications, is one treatment option that is very effective in reducing primary and secondary infections that impart a greasy appearance to the rat's fur.

Diet and Nutrition

As giant chain stores become the only shopping option in many small towns, food choices for small ani-

mals in these communities continue to diminish. As a result, malnutrition is on the rise. Rats will not do well on green hamster pellets and sunflower seeds. Yet, lack of selection can only account for part of the decline in nutrition. Clients too frequently think it's cute to see a rat sit up and beg for a potato chip; like children, rats generally take the junk food options offered them. There are some very good diets on the market for rats: Laboratory chows and processed rodent blocks should be given instead of dog food or other historical choices. If these foods are not available, balanced ratios of the same foods that people eat may be offered; i.e. carbohydrates, grains and nuts, and fruits and vegetables, including corn and plant proteins such as beans. When overfed, rats have a tendency to easily become obese; their weight should be monitored and corrected through dietary manipulation.

The biggest problem with rats as pets is that they don't live very long. Age differs with specific varieties and breeds but, for the most part, rats live only two to three years. Mammary cancer is a common killer, but can be virtually eliminated by spaying the rat.[5] A mammary mass can easily be removed to provide continued quality of life, but will not extend the average life of the rat. Other masses like hemangioma may present as a primary mammary neoplasia; however, surgery to remove these tumors is bloody and does not have a predictable outcome.[5] The client should be advised.

GUINEA PIGS

Cavia porcellus is a herding, terrestrial, cecal-fermenting creature of habit from various countries in South America. A guinea pig is susceptible to allergens and intolerant of pain. When its abdomen hurts, it will grind its teeth or make frequent soft cries even when not being touched. Diarrhea, anorexia, or lack of fecal production usually indicates an emergency condition. Because the lower molars often grow into or over the tongue in the guinea pig, an examination should initially focus on the molars, first for the presence of food in the mouth then for the appropriate occlusal surface. All the enrofloxacin in the world won't help the pig until its teeth are trimmed back. It should then be checked on a regular schedule for overgrown teeth (Figure 4). The exact schedule must be worked out for each pet; however, every three months is not unusual. Amoxicillan should not be used in a guinea pig. It kills normal cecal flora and can result in the death of the guinea pig. Anaphylactic reactions, seen in rabbits, are not commonly seen in guinea pigs.[6]

Environment and Hygiene

The guinea pig is appropriately named for the mess it creates of its bedding, food, and water. The guinea pig loves to play: If toys are not provided, it will amuse itself with its sipper bottle or do laps around its cage, spreading litter as it goes. The large

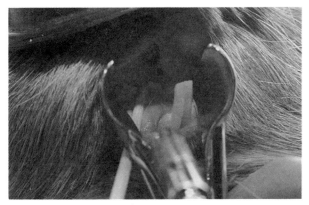

Figure 4—Overgrown molars in a guinea pig.

volumes of urine a guinea pig creates, in combination with its naturally sensitive feet, mandate that especially clean, dry conditions be maintained in its habitat. Good quality bedding should be changed more regularly than is done for other small mammals kept as pets.

Some safe toys include wadded paper balls, hard plastic cat toys with bells, or large PVC pipe to run through. Good bedding options include aspen shavings, recycled paper pellets, grass pellets, or other processed inert, odor-free products. Pet product producers are notorious for overextending their market by putting the picture of a guinea pig on packages of cedar shavings, rabbit food, or fish aquariums, all of which can be detrimental to the health of the animal. Rabbit food contains no vitamin C and too much vitamin D for a guinea pig.[7] Cedar shavings contaminate the air from its volatile oils (i.e. thujone) that induce liver enzymes and erode the mucus membranes, allowing bacterial and viral invasions. The use of fish aquariums for housing keeps air from circulating and usually confines a guinea pig to a very small space and limits exercise. In unsanitary cages and without any activity, guinea pigs can develop ulcerative pododermatitis, abscesses, or abnormal pedal calluses that affect proximal joint health and function and lead to pigs that are reluctant to move. Septic arthritis is a common sequela. A child's swimming pool makes a much better home for guinea pigs. The pool needs to be deep enough to allow a few inches for bedding, plus 10 inches for confining the pig.[8] Wire bottom cages are acceptable if a pig was born on wire and is thus conditioned to the environment; however, it is difficult to track that type of history for pigs bought at pet shops. Guinea pigs not familiar with maneuvering on wire frequently injure their legs, feet, and nails. If startled or scared, they may scream and run violently through and around the cage. This type of fright is especially dangerous if there are babies with mothers or if the animal is being kept on the upper level of a cage. The mother or other pigs in the cage may stampede the babies or dive from the cage like a lemming when the door is opened.

Guinea pig lice, common findings that may or may not cause itching, are usually visible to the naked eye. Lice are killed easily with a pyrethrin dip. Sarcoptic mites are a lot more difficult to deal with in pigs. Regardless of clinical signs, multiple scrapings may yield nothing because even low populations of mites can cause the animal to severely damage itself. Ivermectin 0.3 mg/kg subcutaneously every 10 days for three cycles, plus repeated dips, are sometimes necessary to kill the zoonotic pests. Contaminated bedding must be removed, and the animal should be treated for secondary bacterial dermatitis and lacerations if present. Bandaging the back legs may be necessary to prevent self-mutilation until the parasite and hypersensitive reaction can be resolved.

Nutrition

Most owners do not know how to handle food containing vitamin C so that even if the food is appropriate for guinea pigs, it rapidly loses its nutritional value. Packages of pellets should not be transparent and should only be purchased when a milling date is clearly visible. Vitamin C dissipates in the presence of light and within 90 days of milling. One easy recommendation is to purchase the food within 30 days of the milling date, buy only one month's supply, and keep it in an air-tight, light resistant, plastic container. Since guinea pigs are fussy about changes in their lives, a new brand or even a new bag of food can initiate anorexia. For this reason, it is a good idea to stick with a brand name (devoid of seeds and colored mystery puffs) of plain guinea pig pellets. Purchase the new food a week before the old bag runs out. Over the course of the week, slowly mix in the new food with the old food so that the pig isn't shocked by the change of taste. Every milling will be slightly different so that even the same brand may taste different to the pig. It is also a good idea to keep hay available within the guinea pig's enclosure, as well as to supplement the diet with kale, parsley, citrus and other vegetables that contain vitamin C. Introduce vegetables slowly so that pig doesn't "pig out" on them: Too much fresh vegetation can be a shock to the normal gut flora and cause irreversible diarrhea, resulting in death.

MICE

Mus musculus, one of the most widespread animals in the wild and one of the more rapidly reproducing, is commonly raised as food for other animals (e.g. snakes, monitors, etc.) rather than as pets. Concern for their health usually involves questions regarding their ingestion by something else. For instance, most conditions that plague mice do not seem to affect the reptiles that eat them. But the nutritional quality of the mouse does decrease with disease. Warfarin toxicity is a critical exception and no wild mouse should be used for pet food. Mice treated with ivermectin for mites should not be fed to turtles, and possibly many other reptiles and amphibians.

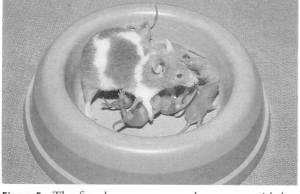

Figure 5—The female mouse covers her young with her body when nursing.

Reproduction and Breeding

Maximizing mouse reproduction for research and profit is a well-studied science. Mountains of information are readily available on increasing rapid mouse growth and reproduction.[9] There are some basic principles, however, of which the veterinarian should be aware. For example, although the male frequently is removed before or just after the babies are born, the male is very involved in the care of the young. He will clean and protect the babies, sometimes covering them with his body, just as the female does when nursing (Figure 5). If the female is lax in her duties or dies, the male will increase his mothering. Mice are group nesters. In other words, several mothers put all their young in one group and all mothers will nurse all the babies. During informal research I conducted of not more than ten litters, all the runts survived that were in the cages with several females and other litters. In the cages with only one female and one litter, not only did the runts often die, but the next weakest pup in the litter became the runt and also died.

Parasites and Disease

The mouse often presents with various tumors and parasites. The mouse will shred its ears and upper torso or even enucleate itself scratching from mites. Mouse mites, which tend to affect dark-colored or spotted, brown mice more severely than the rest, even in the same cage,[10] can be treated with ivermectin subcutaneously every two weeks for three treatments. Treatment that doesn't resolve the itching may be impeded by a hypersensitive reaction. Trimming the nails and removing the mouse from organic, nonprocessed bedding should be part of the therapy. Wild mice are common pests of factories, warehouses, etc. Shavings can become contaminated and then serve as fomites for the wild mice parasites to infest a pet mouse. Processed pellets, such as rabbit pellets or aspen pellets for bedding, may be more beneficial because these are usually packaged immediately following production, thereby providing less chance for contamination.

Neoplasias in mice are almost too numerous to mention. Tumor-producing viruses that are passed to the young transplacentally perpetuate these masses. Mammary tumors in mice are more risky to remove than in rats.[11] The tumors generally tend to bleed and break apart easily. Even taking a biopsy can cause severe hemorrhage. Excisions of masses that grow into the thoracic wall can cause sudden loss of negative pressure to the chest and subsequent death. Owners should be informed of the risks prior to any attempts at removal.

HEDGEHOG

Atelerix albiventris is one of a few species that inhabits the African continent. Though larger than most rodents, these hedgehogs are smaller than their European cousins. Omnivorous in their eating habits, they can eat and tolerate animals that would kill other mammals—thereby providing a viable option in pest control. (The problem in Australia of overpopulation by large, poisonous toads (*Bufo marinus*) theoretically could be helped by hedgehogs.) They actually utilize the toxins in these animals by smearing the toads' skin over their own spines, rendering them toxic as well.[12] Without exposure to toxic amphibians, hedgehog spines are virtually harmless to most people. Natural irritants in their saliva, however, can be spread over their spines with licking and can cause mild reactions in some individuals.

Diet and Nutrition

Dietary requirements for hedgehogs in captivity are relatively anecdotal to date. The cat food versus dog food debate rages on; whether to supplement or not to supplement is also in question. I had a case involving an animal with symptoms of severe heart failure that previously had been fed only a soft, dog food diet. The symptoms were resolved with taurine supplementation. The conclusion in this case was that cat food should be the suggested base food.

As with any "grubbing" species that has a tendency for obesity (i.e. skunks, bears, raccoons), the hedgehog may gorge itself if high-calorie foods are left in the cage at all times. If food is only provided on occasion, the animals may develop undesirable habits, such as endlessly clawing the floor of the enclosure. Grubs, pinkies, night crawlers, and small fruits should therefore be offered in addition to the cat food. The foods should be arranged in the cage under logs or plants so that the animal can search for them.

Environmental Management

The psychological well-being of hedgehogs is further enhanced by the addition of hiding areas in the cage. They may feel less exposed and may hide in them during the day. Large PVC pipes or terracotta flower pots are good choices. Hedgehogs do better behind smooth surfaces (i.e. no wire sidings). Again, kiddy pools are preferable to aquariums.

Hedgehogs chill easily and should be kept in warm temperatures of around 80°Fahrenheit, especially when ill. If the animals get too hot, they will flatten out on their bellies and pant. Continued heat may cause heat stress or create a state of torpor in the hedgehog. As with other small mammals and rodents, unclean conditions can contribute to the presence of parasites. Giardia, Coccidia, and nematodes are easily seen on direct smears or floats. There is never a limited supply of fecal material with these animals. Hedgehogs can be treated with conventional therapies for the parasites: fenbendazole, metronidazole, sulfa compounds, etc. Hedgehog mites are even more common. Unlike the guinea pig, a hedgehog will exhibit relatively little itching even with large numbers of mites. Mites are large and can be seen with the naked eye as they pass over the backs of the ears, sometimes in sheets of thousands like blankets of fireants crossing a river. Children's eyes are better detectors, but everyone should be able to see the piles of white cellular debris left between the spines. Hogs without mites have nice clean skin between their spines. The mites are *Chorioptes* that look similar to *Sarcoptes scabiei* but have a much shorter stalk or pedicel before the caruncle, an appendage of the legs that looks like a suction cup.

Handling

The physical exam is a challenge. Leather gloves would seem to be more appropriate than rubber gloves to manage these spiny creatures, especially for hands that have no calluses. Animals accustomed to being handled will keep their spines down and tolerate a full physical; however, isoflurane may be needed with others. Small towel barriers work well for the average animal, but a hands-off approach often is more productive. Place the critter in an aquarium and then hold it above eye level. Left alone, they relax. Much can be learned about the underside of the animal by observing through glass. A common source of difficulty, the feet also can be scrutinized in this manner. Soft nails are an

indication that the owner is not keeping the cage clean and dry. Swollen, red feet are not normal and may indicate anything from abrasive substrata to fungal infections. Fat hogs will get cellulitis in their skin rolls and abnormal wear to the sides of their feet. Long nails should be trimmed. Different species may have a different number of toes, so don't forget any. A slight overbite is normal. Tartar build-up may indicate a poor diet. Hard cat food is better than soft, but A/D® in a can from Hills™ will entice any picky eater in the hospital.

Touching the underside of a hedgehog with a stethoscope can stimulate their very sensitive coil reflex. The result often is a huffing, jumping spiny ball dangling from the instrument's cord. Taking a temperature on an awake animal can be equally tricky. The thumb and middle finger should be used to slowly and firmly lift the muscle skirt on each side of the body until it is over the hips. Then close the hand slightly over the back. The animal's legs and head are forced out. This position can be held comfortably by both parties for a while, until the handler relaxes the grip even slightly. The hedgehog can feel the change, and a clinched hand will be holding an expanded spine ball in a split second. Some handlers recommend scruffing with similar results. Overall, patience and persistence are the main keys to a stress-free physical examination for both the hedgehog and the veterinarian.

REFERENCES

1. Breitweiser B: Practical approach to hamster urinary analysis. *Jrnl Small Exot Anim Med* 3:104–105, 1992.
2. Harkness JE, Wagner JE: *The Biology and Medicine of Rabbits and Rodents.* Media, PA, Williams & Wilkins, 1995, p 50.
3. Williams D: Three Blind Mice... *Proc North Am Vet Conf,* 7:805–806, 1993.
4. Dixon LW: Antibiotic toxicosis in the guinea pig. *JAVMA* 12:1436, 1986.
5. Lermayer RM: African pygmy hedgehogs latest pet sensation! The economics of raising hedgehogs. *Live Animal Trade and Transport Magazine,* pp 45–48, December 1992.
6. Dixon LW: Antibiotic toxicosis in the guinea pig. *JAVMA* 12:1436, 1986.
7. Harkness JE, Wagner JE: *The Biology and Medicine of Rabbits and Rodents.* Media, PA, Williams & Wilkins, 1995, p 33.
8. Ibid. p 32.
9. Vandenbergh JG: Social interactions and the coordination of reproductive behavior in rodents and nonhuman primates. *JAVMA* 9:1161–1164, 1998.
10. Bauck L: Common problems of the small rodent. *Small Mammal-Reptile Medicine and Surgery for the Practitioner.* Fifth Annual Conference, 1993.
11. Harkness JE, Wagner JE: *The Biology and Medicine of Rabbits and Rodents.* Media, PA, Williams & Wilkins, 1995, p 256.
12. Smith, Anthony J.: Husbandry and medicine of African hedgehogs (*Atelerix albiventris*). *Jrnl Small Exot Anim Med* 1:21–28, 1992.

(continues on page 215)

The Biology, Care, and Diseases
of the Syrian Hamster*

August H. Battles, DVM
Diplomate, American College of Laboratory Animal Medicine
Albany Medical College
Albany, New York

Hamsters are rodents with anatomic, physiologic, and clinical peculiarities that have made them useful as research animals. They are not native to the United States but were brought there for research purposes.[1] Although there are many species of hamsters, the Syrian (golden) hamster is the most common.[2]

The hamster is relatively resistant to diseases compared with other rodents. Proliferative ileitis, thought to be a bacterial disease, is the most frequently seen disease. Viral infections have been reported often, but most cause few clinical diseases. Protozoa, nematodes, cestodes, and mites are capable of parasitizing a hamster.[2] The incidence of neoplasms is low in hamsters, with lymphomas being the most common.[3] In aged hamsters, amyloidosis and atrial thrombosis are frequently seen and are responsible for the death of a large percentage of the aged.[3,4] Hamsters with dental disease, although not often reported, are seen by clinical veterinarians. Reproductive problems also occur and are frequently related to management, which plays an important part in disease prevention in hamsters.

This article reviews the biology and care of hamsters as well as the common problems presented to veterinary practitioners.

History

Hamsters were introduced into the United States in 1938. The Syrian hamster ranges in the wild from Rumania and Bulgaria southeastward through Asia Minor, Israel, and northwestern Iran. They were first used as laboratory research animals in 1930, at which time a litter of eight was brought to what is now Israel. All present domesticated strains of Syrian hamsters developed from this stock.[1]

Chinese hamsters were brought to the United States in 1948. From 1949 to 1952, they were domesticated and reproduction in captivity began. This species is useful in research because it offers a unique morphologic feature of having the lowest number of chromosomes of the common laboratory animal and is susceptible to diabetes mellitus and other diseases of public health significance. Chinese hamsters, however, are more difficult to breed in captivity than Syrian hamsters are.[5]

*This work was supported in part by the National Institute of Health Grant RR07001.

Characteristics

Hamsters are rodents in the family Cricetidae, Cricetidae are characterized by having large cheek pouches, short tails, and thick bodies.[6] The two most common genera of hamsters in the Cricetidae are the Syrian (*Mesocricetus auratus*) and the Chinese (*Cricetulus griseus*).[2] The Syrian hamster has 22 pairs of chromosomes and the Chinese hamster has 11.[5,7]

Varieties of Syrian hamsters include the wild type or reddish brown, cinnamon, cream, white piebald, and longhaired "teddy bear." Reddish golden brown is the most common. Chinese hamsters are smaller than Syrian hamsters and are dark brown.

Rodents are remarkably uniform in characteristics, especially in dentition. Like other rodents, hamsters have four incisors—two upper and two lower. The incisors grow throughout life, and there is no nerve in the incisor teeth except at the base. The outer surface of incisor teeth is to some extent self-sharpening. Rodents lack canine and premolar teeth.

The radius and ulna are distinct bones of the lower arm, and the elbow joint allows free rotation of the forearm. The hand has five fingers and the foot three to five toes. The penis of rodents has a baculum (os penis). The brain has a smooth cerebrum and large olfactory bulbs. The functions of the areas of the cerebrum are generalized rather than specialized.[6]

Adult Syrian hamsters weigh between 85 to 150 g, with the female being larger and maturing earlier. Newborn hamsters (pups) weigh approximately 2 to 4 g, with the male being slightly larger. The maximum weight is attained by six months of age.[8]

Hamsters have well-developed cheek pouches that are used to transport and store food and to conceal a newborn litter when danger is present (Figure 1). The cheek pouch, an evagination of the lateral buccal wall, is devoid of glands, highly distensible, lined with stratified squamous epithelium, and well vascularized.[7,8]

The stomach is divided into two distinct regions that are separated by a constriction and are described as the *squamous* and *glandular stomachs*.[8] The nonglandular forestomach is characteristic of ruminants in that it contains microorganisms and a high pH suggestive of a fermentation process.[9]

Adult male and female hamsters can be differentiated easily; the caudal area of a male is elongated because the testicles are carried caudally and well outside and behind the body. The vesicular gland and testes appear large in relation to the body size. The abdominal cavity of males may seem to be filled with the vesicular gland, which is an outpouching of the vas deferens with branching tubules. In addition to the vesicular gland, there are two additional accessory sex glands—the coagulating gland and the prostate. The sex of younger hamsters can be determined by measuring the distance between the anus and the genitals, which is greater in males. In the perineal area of females, there are three openings: the anus, the vulva, and the urethra. The uterus is bicornuate, with each uterine horn having a separate opening into the vagina. The female generally has 12 to 14 nipples.[7]

The anatomic and functional peculiarities of hamsters are noted in some of the glands. Sebaceous glands, referred to as *hip glands*, are located on either flank in both males and females (Figure 2) and are used as sex

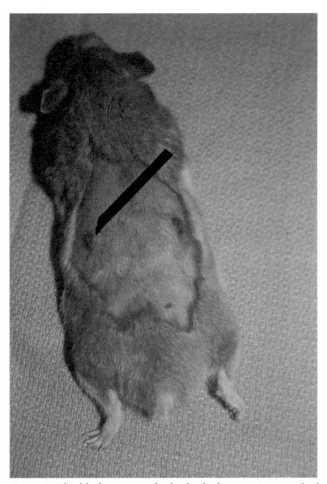

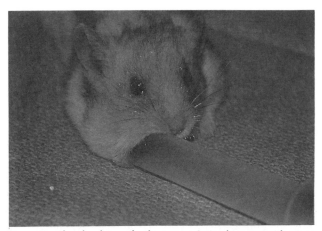

Figure 1—The cheek pouch of a mature Syrian hamster with a 3-cc syringe case inserted to demonstrate the size of the pouch.

Figure 2—The black spots on the back of a hamster (one marked with an arrow) are called the *hip glands*.

glands and for olfactory marking of territory. They can be visualized if the hair is clipped over the flank. In sexually aroused males, these glands become matted from secretions and are readily visible.[8] Hamsters will scratch themselves, as if the area was pruritic. The harderian glands have also been shown to secrete sexually attractive substances.[10] The adrenal glands of male hamsters are larger than those of females. In other rodents, the size of the adrenal glands does not differ between the sexes.[11]

Syrian hamsters have a relatively short life span, usually 18 to 24 months; unlike many other mammals, females have a shorter life span than males. Old-age lesions, such as cardiac thrombosis and amyloidosis, that affect the life span occur earlier in the females.[12] Female Syrian hamsters have a reproductive life span of one year, while males have a reproductive life span of two years.[13]

Sexual maturity of Syrian hamsters occurs around two months and is two weeks earlier in females than in males. The estrous cycle is four days.[13] Estrus usually begins in the evening hours, with ovulation occurring between 12:00 midnight and 1:00 AM. Females demonstrate lordosis. On the morning after estrus, a characteristic thick, white, opaque, smelly discharge may be expressed from the vagina. On Day 3, a waxy discharge may be present. On Day 4, there is a translucent mucous discharge. If bred, sperm may be seen in the vaginal smear. A copulation plug may be found in the cage the morning after breeding. The plug is a white, waxy mass extruded in the form of a cast of the vaginal cavity and is composed of secretions from the male's accessory sex glands and secretions and cells from the female's vaginal wall.[14] Estrus occurs one to eight days after parturition.[13]

The average duration of pregnancy is 15½ days; it is characterized by a series of changes in the vaginal excretions. When correlated with weight changes, these excretions can be used to distinguish pregnant from nonpregnant individuals as early as 10 days of gestation. On Day 4 of pregnancy, the vagina contains a stringy transparent fluid that may appear to have many bubbles; and on Day 5 or 6 it may contain white flakes. The flocculent content continues to increase until Day 9 or 10, at which time the discharge becomes white and waxy, similar to the discharge after the evening of estrus.[14]

Pseudopregnancy can occur in a nonfertile mating and lasts from 8 to 12 days. A pseudopregnant female resembles a pregnant female until termination of the pseudopregnancy. During the final two days of pseudopregnancy, there is a decrease in body weight. At the end of pseudopregnancy, a normal estrous cycle is resumed.[14]

The average litter size is six to eight pups. Before parturition, a female is restless and exhibits excessive grooming and nest-building tasks. A bloody discharge may be present before the first fetus is born. Newborns are hairless, blind, and have closed ears and undeveloped limbs. Teeth are evident at birth. Hair growth begins at nine days of age.[15] Pups are capable of eating hard food at 7 to 10 days of age and open their eyes at 14 to 15 days of age. Weaning occurs at 21 to 25 days of age.[8]

Unlike seasonal hibernators, Syrian hamsters may hibernate in response to lowered environmental temperatures (below 40° F [4.4°C]). All will not hibernate spontaneously, but instead hibernation depends on such variables as food supply. The duration of hibernation is short, usually two to three days, but may be as long as five to seven days. Hibernation is not a continuous state, with arousal and return to hibernation occurring within a 12-hour period or less.[16]

Basic physiologic norms of hamsters are listed in Table I.[7,8,17]

Husbandry

Hamsters are nocturnal, burrow-dwelling animals with brief periods of diurnal activity. They may develop a pugnacious disposition if they are aroused during their rest period. Food and water consumption take place mainly during the evening hours. Females (when larger than the males) are the dominant individuals; a female can be very aggressive toward a smaller male, especially during anestrus, and has been known to inflict serious injury. Frequent, gentle handling of hamsters will keep them tame and easy to handle. Hamsters have a tendency to seek dark, protected areas.[6]

The nutritional requirements of omnivorous hamsters have not been determined specifically, but a pelleted rodent diet containing 15% to 20% protein is currently recommended.[18] Hamsters eat approximately 12 g of

TABLE I
Physiologic Data[7,8,17]

Body temperature	37° to 38°C (98° to 99°F)
Respiratory rate	35–135 breaths/min
Blood volume	0.078 ml/g body weight
Heart rate	250–500 beats/min
Packed cell volume	36% to 55%
Red blood cells	6 to 10 × 10^6/mm^3
White blood cells	3 to 11 × 10^3/mm^3
Neutrophils	10% to 42%
Lymphocytes	50% to 95%
Eosinophils	0% to 4.5%
Monocytes	0% to 3%
Basophils	0% to 10%
Platelets	200 to 500 × 10^3/mm^3
Urine	Crystalluria, cream-colored, turbid, pH 8.0
Serum protein	4.5–7.5 g/dl
Albumin	2.6–4.1 g/dl
Globulin	2.7–4.2 g/dl
Serum glucose	60–150 mg/dl
Blood urea nitrogen	12–25 mg/dl
Creatinine	0.91–0.99 mg/dl
Total bilirubin	0.25–0.60 mg/dl
Cholesterol	25–135 mg/dl
Serum calcium	5–12 mg/dl
Serum phosphorus	3.4–8.2 mg/dl

feed and drink 10 ml of water/100 g of body weight/day and, like rabbits and many other rodents, are coprophagic.[8] Lesions often develop around the nares when hamsters are fed from narrow, slotted food hoppers in a shoe-box–style cage often used for other rodents. Hoppers with slots 7/16 of an inch wide are recommended to allow easy removal of food pellets.[19] A pregnant hamster at 13 days of gestation should have a one-week supply of food (about 50% more feed than the normal adult diet) placed in the cage to minimize daily disturbance. A newborn hamster begins to eat at 7 to 10 days of age. Food for a lactating female should be placed on the cage floor; otherwise she will become preoccupied with removing feed from the hopper and neglect the pups. The food on the floor will also allow the young easy access.

Housing

Several types of cages are available for housing hamsters. Because hamsters chew plastic, wood, and soft metals, the cage should have only rounded corners with no areas available for the hamster to chew. A dark place to hide, such as a can, and sufficient litter material in which to burrow are desirable. The recommended temperature for hamsters is 65° to 70°F (18.3° to 21.1°C), but adult hamsters can tolerate lower environmental temperatures; a temperature of 71° to 75°F (21.6° to 23.8°C), however, is recommended for pups.[8] An adult hamster requires a floor space of at least 122.6 cm² (19 in.²) and a cage height of 15.2 cm (6 in.). A 12-hour light cycle is preferred.[20]

Clinical Techniques

A hamster can be handled by cupping the hands gently under it or by picking it up in a small can. It is very important not to surprise a hamster because a startled hamster often bites. After placing the hamster onto a smooth surface, slowly close one hand to allow the loose skin to bunch and then grasp the skin (not the body). The hamster then should be immobilized sufficiently to allow injections to be given (Figure 3).

Several techniques can be used to obtain blood samples. After applying a rubber band tourniquet (Figure 4), the cephalic vein can be used to collect a sample of blood with a 27-gauge needle and a capillary tube (Figure 5). A sample can also be collected with a capillary tube after trimming a toenail. Blood also can be collected through the periorbital sinus by using a microhematocrit tube or directly from the heart by using a 23- to 25-gauge needle on a syringe. Up to 2 ml of blood can be removed safely from a 100-g hamster.[21]

Fecal and urinary samples usually can be obtained readily when a hamster is initially handled. Thus, it is wise to have a collection cup, such as a cap from a syringe case, available before handling the hamster.

Medication can be administered orally, intramuscularly, intravenously, or intraperitoneally. The intraperitoneal route is used most often. A 16-gauge, one and

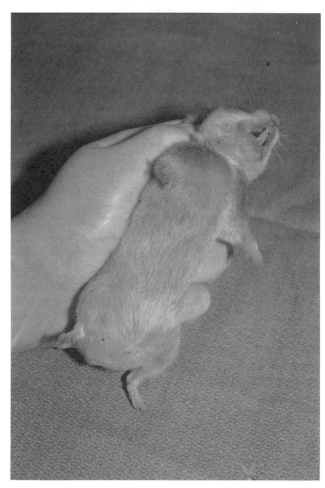

Figure 3—This hamster has been immobilized so that an injection can be given.

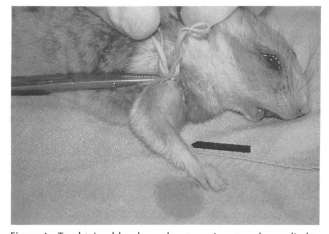

Figure 4—To obtain a blood sample, a tourniquet can be applied to the arm of the hamster. The cephalic vein (arrow) then becomes readily apparent.

one-half to two and one-half–inch, blunt, stainless steel gastric–feeding needle can be used for oral administration. The cephalic or sublingual vein can be used for intravenous injections.[22] Intramuscular injections can be given in the gluteal or lumbar area.

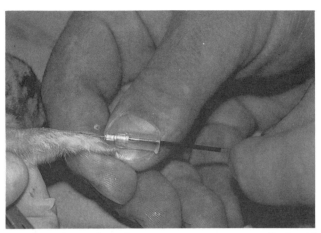

Figure 5—After applying the tourniquet, a 27-gauge needle should be inserted into the cephalic vein and blood collected into a capillary tube.

Pharmaceutic Agents

Antibiotics should be used with caution when treating hamsters because several antibiotics have been associated with induced enterocolitis. Hamsters can develop anorexia, a ruffled haircoat, and diarrhea. There is a reduction of gram-positive flora and a proliferation of gram-negative organisms. *Clostridium difficile* was shown to be a toxin-producing organism that was responsible for lethal enterocolitis.[23]

The use of penicillin, ampicillin, vancomycin hydrochloride, erythromycin, cephalosporin, lincomycin, and oral gentamicin are reported to induce enterocolitis and death in hamsters.[23-25] Other antibiotics also have been reported to induce enterocolitis, but dosage and route may determine whether they are capable of inducing disease. Tetracycline produced no disease when given at an oral dosage of 5 mg every eight hours for five days to hamsters weighing 70 to 90 g. Metronidazole also was reported to produce no disease when it was given at an oral dosage of 7.5 mg every eight hours for five days to hamsters weighing 70 to 90 g.[23] Chloramphenicol palmitate when given at a dose less than or equal to 300 mg/kg did not produce disease.[26]

Chloramphenicol palmitate (50 mg/kg orally) is the antibiotic of choice for treating hamsters. Tetracycline (400 mg/L of water) is also used, but sucrose may need to be added to improve palatability.

The use of ketamine hydrochloride alone has produced variable anesthetic results; however, when combined with xylazine hydrochloride, it has produced satisfactory muscle relaxation and analgesia for abdominal surgical anesthesia. Ketamine (50 to 200 mg/kg) and xylazine (10 mg/kg) produced a longer duration of anesthesia when given intraperitoneally versus intramuscularly. The duration of anesthesia was also dose related. Ketamine (50 mg/kg) and xylazine (10 mg/kg) given intraperitoneally produced anesthesia with a mean duration of 227.3 ± 6.7 minutes. By increasing the dose of ketamine (200 mg/kg), the duration of anesthesia

was extended, with a mean of 71.1 ± 4.2 minutes.[27]

Sodium pentobarbital given intraperitoneally at a dose of 50 to 90 mg/kg at a concentration of 10 mg/ml has been suggested for surgical anesthesia lasting 15 to 17 minutes. The minimum lethal dose of pentobarbital is 135 to 150 mg/kg.[28]

Volatile anesthetics, such as methoxyflurane or halothane, when placed on a sponge in a covered container, can anesthetize hamsters for a short period of time. The use of atropine (0.2 to 0.5 mg/kg subcutaneously) is recommended before giving halothane.[28]

Morphine at high doses (150 mg/kg) by intramuscular, subcutaneous, or intraperitoneal injection reportedly results in analgesia without apparent narcosis or respiratory depression. The large volume needed to produce analgesia would limit its clinical usefulness, however. The use of droperidol and fentanyl citrate is not recommended in hamsters because of the effects on the central nervous system.[28]

For short procedures, the use of methoxyflurane has the advantages of safety and speed of recovery. The use of ketamine at a high dose (200 mg/kg) and xylazine for prolonged surgical procedures potentiates the risk of death from anesthesia. Minimal time under anesthesia should be obtained to minimize risk of death.

Infectious Diseases

Proliferative ileitis is the bacterial infection encountered most often in hamsters. It has also been referred to as *wet tail*, *regional enteritis*, *terminal ileitis*, and *atypical ileal hyperplasia*. The cause(s) of the disease is not known. *Campylobacter fetus* subspecies *jejuni* has been isolated from hamsters with proliferative ileitis.[29] Pure cultures of *Campylobacter fetus* subspecies *jejuni* did not produce disease when given to healthy hamsters. Ileal extracts from hamsters with proliferative ileitis did produce disease, however, suggesting unknown synergisms or predisposing factors. Stress from a variety of causes may serve as an important factor.[29] Improper diet or change of diet, overcrowding, and familial predisposition are also considered contributory factors. Long-haired and teddy bear hamsters, along with recently weaned hamsters, seem to be highly susceptible.[8]

The infectious agents are spread by a fecal to oral route. Fomites may play a role in transmission. The agent may be passed from weanling to weanling or adult to weanling. The ubiquitous nature of *C. fetus* subspecies *jejuni* has raised the possibility of other animal species being involved as a source of infection. Hamsters have been considered a potential reservoir of human campylobacterosis.[30]

Proliferative ileitis may cause death within one to seven days of onset of clinical signs of watery diarrhea. Signs include matting of fur on the tail or other areas of the body, a hunched stance, irritability, dehydration, and emaciation. If the patient survives the acute attack, ileal obstruction, intussusception, peritonitis, or impaction may occur. Intussusception may be manifested as bloody diarrhea or a prolapsed rectum.

Gross lesions at necropsy include thickening and reddening of the walls of the lower portion of the small intestine. The ileum, jejunum, colon, and rectum contain semifluid yellow material and some gas. In some instances, the bowel mucosa is necrotic and ulcerated. Microscopically there is hyperplasia of crypt epithelium; this results in widening and elongation of the villi. As the disease progresses, abscesses extend through the entire thickness of the gut. Peyer's patches are often obliterated.[29] A silver stain will demonstrate slightly curved bacilli, which are the *Campylobacter* organisms.

Treatment by adding tetracycline to the drinking water at 400 mg/L for 10 days has been used successfully to offset mortality.[31] Prevention is best obtained through selection of hamsters with no familial history of this disease. Avoidance of stress and good husbandry are essential.

Bacterial pneumonia has been reported to be the second most prominent cause of death in hamsters and to be caused by *Pasteurella pneumotropica, Streptococcus pneumoniae*, or other *Streptococcus* spp. Clinical signs are depression, anorexia, and nasal and ocular discharge with respiratory distress. *Mycoplasma pulmonis* has been isolated from the lungs of hamsters, but its role as a pathogen is unknown.[32]

Other bacteria have been reported to produce disease only on rare occasions. Tyzzer's disease caused by *Bacillus piliformis* has been reported; it produced diarrhea and death. Observations at necropsy included white nodules in the heart, dilated cecum and colon containing semiliquid feces, and occasional white spots on the liver.[33] *Escherichia coli* has been reported to produce enteritis without epithelial cell hyperplasia of the villi of the ileum.[34] Bacterial lymphadenitis occurs in the hamster and is similar to that seen in the guinea pig. *Staphylococcus aureus*, β-hemolytic *Streptococcus* Lancefield Group C, and *Streptobacillus moniliformis* have been associated with lymphadenitis. Surgical drainage and antibiotic treatment are indicated. Treatment of well-encapsulated abscesses may be unrewarding.[2,35] Salmonellosis occurs in hamsters but only has been reported rarely. Affected hamsters are depressed and have a rough haircoat. At necropsy, there may be enlargement of the liver, spleen, and lymph nodes as well as patchy hemorrhage of the lungs. Enteritis usually is not present. Prevention is based on good management to minimize introduction of contaminated food or bedding.[36]

Viral infections creating overt clinical signs in hamsters have been reported infrequently. Most viral diseases present as a complicating factor in a production colony or in experimental conditions. Of the viral diseases, lymphocytic choriomeningitis is important because of its zoonotic implications; it is caused by an arenavirus, which is an RNA virus. Clinical signs are rare and depend on the age of the hamster when infected, the strain of the hamster and the virus, the route and dose of infection, and the immunologic competence of the host. If infection occurs congenitally or neonatally, the hamster may show retardation, unthriftiness, weakness, tremors, and prostration. Reproductive impairment has been reported in chronically infected females. Transmission occurs through direct contact, fomites, and aerosols. Findings at necropsy include glomerulonephritis, vasculitis, and lymphocytic infiltration in various organs, including the meninges and brain.[3,37] Prevention and control are based on regular testing of colonies for antibodies.[2]

Sendai virus (parainfluenza I), an RNA virus of the paramyxovirus group, has been reported to result in occasional death of suckling hamsters. Sendai virus is believed to suppress the immunity system.[38] Separate housing from mice, rats, and guinea pigs is suggested for prevention and control.

Parasitic Infections

Protozoa, nematodes, and cestodes are found in the intestinal tract of hamsters. The role of protozoa as a pathogen has not been determined. Protozoa have been found in normal and diseased animals. Both the mouse pinworm, *Syphacia obvelata*, and the rat pinworm, *Syphacia muris*, are capable of infecting hamsters.[39,40] Either can be diagnosed easily by using clear cellophane tape to make an impression smear from the rectum. Both parasites are predominantly located in the cecum. Treatment consists of using piperazine citrate at a dosage of 10 mg/ml of drinking water for seven days, then off for five days, then retreat for an additional seven days.[41]

Hymenolepis nana, a cestode, is an important internal parasite of the hamster because of its zoonotic capabilities.[2] Severe infections may cause intestinal occlusion, impaction, and death. It has a direct or indirect cycle, with flour beetles or fleas as the intermediate host. Diagnosis is made by confirming eggs in the feces or finding them in the adult on postmortem examination. Ground feed containing 0.33% active niclosamide fed ad libitum to hamsters for seven days is safe and effective for eliminating this parasite.[42]

Acariasis is predominantly associated in hamsters with two species of *Demodex* (*D. criceti* and *D. auratus*). Clinically, alopecia of the rump and back with dry scaly skin is present. Pruritus is not usually present.[43] Predisposing factors of malnutrition, concurrent systemic disease, and age are believed necessary for the development of demodectic mange.[44] Mites can be demonstrated by skin scrapings.

Infestation with ear mites (*Notoedres* sp.) also occurs. In females, it usually occurs in the ears only. In males, it occurs on the ears, nose, genitalia, tail, and feet.[8]

Neoplasms

The incidence of spontaneous neoplasms occurring in hamsters is reported to be low (3.7%) compared with the incidence in other rodents. Age, sex, and strain influence the distribution of tumors.[45] The incidence of neoplasms increases in certain strains and in males, which have a longer life span.

Most tumors have been observed after one year of age. Polyps of the intestine, adenomas of the adrenal cortex and thyroid, papillomas of the stomach, and hemangiomas of the spleen are reported to occur. Lymphomas are the most frequently occurring neoplasms in Syrian hamsters and consist predominantly of lymphosarcomas of the lymph gland and small intestine and reticulum cell sarcomas of the lymph nodes.[3] Epizootics of diffuse, poorly differentiated lymphocytic, immunoblastic, or plasmacytoid lymphoma induced by an infectious, horizontally transmitting viroid agent have been reported.[46]

Spontaneous Geriatric Lesions

Compared with other species, Syrian hamsters have a short life span; thus, spontaneous aging diseases are frequently seen. Two of the most common geriatric diseases are amyloidosis and thrombosis. Amyloidosis is frequently associated with thrombosis. Treatment of these geriatric lesions consists of managing clinical signs. A diagnosis of amyloidosis or thrombosis carries a poor prognosis.

Amyloidosis occurs earlier in females and more frequently in certain strains, with an incidence as high as 86%.[47] It occurs in all organs but most often involves the kidneys, spleen, adrenal glands, and liver.[12] Amyloid is produced by reticuloendothelial cells, plasma cells, and histiocytes. The pathogenesis of amyloidosis in hamsters is not understood completely. Amyloid is a protein; three systemic forms presently are recognized. The classification of amyloidosis in hamsters is unclear and needs further study.[48]

A nephrotic syndrome is frequently associated with amyloidosis. Edema, ascites, proteinuria, decreased serum albumin, and increased total globulin are frequently seen in hamsters with amyloidosis.[49,50] Renal failure results from deposits of amyloid. Grossly, the kidneys may appear red-brown, slightly pitted to pale, and misshapened, depending on the degree of involvement.[3]

Microscopically, the renal glomerular capillary tufts may be enlarged and contain amyloid, an amorphous hyaline material (Figure 6). In the liver, amyloid is located adjacent to blood vessels and in portal areas and to a lesser extent around the central veins. Congestion and centrolobular hepatocytic atrophy can occur in a severely affected liver. In the spleen, amyloid replaces the sinusoids, the reticuloendothelial cells, and the macrophages of the red pulp. Replacement of these areas with amyloid causes wide avascular areas. In the adrenal glands, extensive accumulation results in atrophy of cortical cells.[3]

Cardiac thrombosis has been reported to occur as frequently as 73%.[4] The left atrium is the most frequent location, but thrombi may occur in all chambers of the heart (Figure 7). The incidence of thrombosis is equal in both sexes, with females developing lesions earlier in

life than males. Consumption coagulopathy and increased fibrinolytic activity have been reported in conjunction with thrombotic disease. Laboratory findings include reduction of activities of factors II, VII, VIII, and X; reduced plasminogen; elevated fibrinogen-fibrin degradation products; and thrombocytopenia.

The process of formation of thrombi in a hamster's

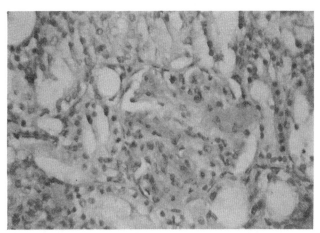

Figure 6—A glomerulus containing amyloid. (Congo red, ×40)

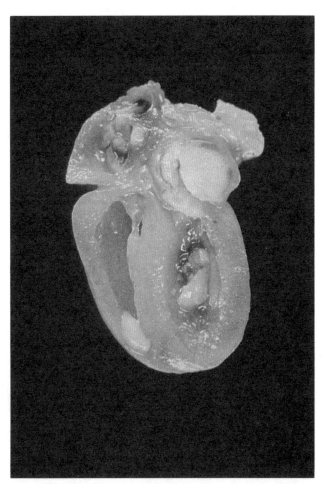

Figure 7—A hamster's heart with thrombi present in all four chambers.

heart is believed to occur not in one stage but with many repetitions of the thrombotic process.[51] Thrombi appear histologically to have varying degrees of organization, suggesting they are formed from more than one episode. The outer fibrotic portion of the older thrombi often contains lymphocyte infiltrates; white, foamy macrophages are found more centrally. Heart failure, vascular injury, septic infections, and amyloidosis have been considered to be inciting factors in the formation of thrombi in hamsters.

Polycystic disease is a developmental or congenital defect seen in hamsters older than one year of age. Cysts are grossly visible and are most often seen in the liver. In the liver, the cysts arise from the biliary duct; histologically the cells resemble biliary epithelium. Grossly, the cysts in the liver can be single or multiple. The wall of the cyst is thin and filled with light-colored fluid. Cystic structures in other organs are histologically similar in that they are dilated and lined with flattened cuboidal epithelium.[52] The condition has not been associated with clinical signs.

Miscellaneous Geriatric Diseases

A calcifying vasculopathy reported to be very common in hamsters is characterized by mild or severe calcification of the vascular walls. The aorta as well as the cardiac, renal, and gastric arteries are affected most often. In advanced cases, the basal laminae of the respiratory epithelium are involved as well as the walls of the alveoli, bronchi, and basal membranes of the renal tubules.[53]

Gastric ulcers occur in older hamsters—more frequently in the glandular stomach than in the forestomach.[54] Liver disease, such as cholangitis, as well as cysts are commonly seen. Cholangitis can be associated with focal or multifocal abscesses.[45] Pyelonephritis and nephrocalcinosis also have been reported in older hamsters.[55] In males, spermatic granuloma, orchitis, prostatitis, prostatic calcification, and seminal vesicular inflam-

mation have been reported in hamsters 62 weeks of age and older. In females, ovarian cysts and endometritis occur. Myocardial fibrosis, myocarditis, pericarditis, and vascular calcinosis have been reported.[56] In the skeletal system, chondrosis (especially of the vertebral joints) is common. The lesions have shown marked extensions toward surrounding soft tissue and resulted in cartilaginous metaplasia of tendons and fascia. These lesions occurred more often in females than in males.[45]

Dental diseases occur more frequently in aged hamsters. In one study, dental caries and periodontitis were the most common nonneoplastic diseases of the digestive system, with an incidence as high as 88%.[45] Periodontitis is associated with abscessation and necrosis extending into the facial region (Figure 8) and involving the harderian glands and brain. The associated vascular thrombosis, especially of the orbital veins, can result in pulmonary emboli.[45] Hamsters have been used experimentally in the study of caries and periodontal disease, both of which can be induced by a finely ground diet or high-carbohydrate concentration. Bacteria play a role in developing plaque that adheres and progressively overgrows the tooth surfaces.[57] The yellowing of the teeth is a normal process of aging and is not related to disease.[7] Malocclusions of the incisors may be a cause of weight loss from inability to eat properly. There is no nerve in the incisor; if overgrowth occurs, the incisors can be trimmed with an instrument (e.g., a canine nail clipper).

Reproductive Problems

Reproductive failures most often are related to errors in management. In one study, starvation for more than one estrous cycle blocked normal follicular development but was reversed by feeding for five days.[58] In another study, exposure to cold temperature (45.5°F [7.5°C]) for two weeks produced anestrus.[59] Male Syrian hamsters, through a pineal-mediated response, developed atrophy of the gonads and accessory sex glands when exposed to a cycle of 22 hours of darkness and 2 hours of light.[60] Sexual receptivity can be blocked when a female hamster is placed in an all-female group.[61] Senescence occurs once the female reaches 15 months of age.[62] Mate incompatibility may also be a cause of mating failures.

Cannibalism resulting from lack of maternal experience and environmental disturbances is a frequent cause of loss of newborn. It is essential that the female not be disturbed 2 days before or 10 days after delivery. If disturbing becomes necessary, feeding the female fresh foods will decrease the probability of cannibalism.[2]

Pregnancy toxemia has been described and was characterized by disseminated thrombi in the kidneys, liver, intestines, and placenta. No pathogenic organisms were found, but stress from shipping was considered a contributing factor. The histologic lesions resembled those seen in guinea pig pregnancy toxemia associated with uteroplacental ischemia.[63]

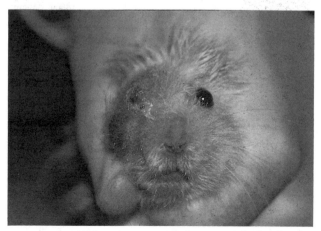

Figure 8—A teddy bear hamster with abscesses of the facial region from periodontitis.

REFERENCES

1. Hill BF: The Syrian hamster: Its utility in research. *Charles River Digest*: 3(2), 1969.
2. Van Hoosier GL, Ladiges WC: Biology and disease of hamsters, in Fox JG, Cohen BJ, Loew FM (eds): *Laboratory Animal Medicine*. Orlando, FL, Academic Press Inc, 1984, pp 123-147.
3. Schmidt RE, Eason RL, Hubbard GE, et al: *Pathology of Aging Syrian Hamsters*. Boca Raton, FL, CRC Press Inc, 1983.
4. McMartin DM, Dodds WJ: Atrial thrombosis. *Am J Pathol* 107(2):277-279, 1982.
5. Willington M: Observations on the breeding and care of the Chinese hamster. *Lab Anim Care* 15(1):94-101, 1965.
6. Walker EP, Warnick F, Lange KI, et al: *Mammals of the World*, vol 2. Baltimore, The John Hopkins Press, 1964, p 665.
7. Williams CSF: *Practical Guide to Lab Animals*. St. Louis, The CV Mosby Co, 1976, pp 26-34.
8. Harkness JE, Wagner JE: *The Biology and Medicine of Rabbits and Rodents*. Philadelphia, Lea & Febiger, 1983.
9. Warner RG, Ehle FR: Nutritional idiosyncrasies of the golden hamster (*Mesocricetus auratus*). *Lab Anim Sci* 26(4):670-673, 1976.
10. Payne HP: The attractiveness of harderian gland smears to sexually naive and experienced male golden hamsters. *Anim Behav* 27:897-904, 1979.
11. Ohtaki S: Conspicuous sex differences in zona reticularis of the adrenal cortex of Syrian hamsters. *Lab Anim Sci* 29(6):765-789, 1979.
12. McMartin DM: Morphologic lesions in aging Syrian hamsters. *J Gerontol* 34(4):502-511, 1979.
13. Hafez ESE: *Reproduction and Breeding Techniques for Laboratory Animals*. Philadelphia, Lea & Febiger, 1970, p 3.
14. Orsini MW: The external vaginal phenomena characterizing the stages of estrus cycle, pregnancy, pseudopregnancy, lactation, and the anestrus hamster, *Mesocricetus auratus*. *Proc Anim Care Panel*:193-205, 1961.
15. Musser TK, Silverman J: The hair cycle of the Syrian golden hamster (*Mesocricetus auratus*). *Lab Anim Sci* 30(4):681-683, 1980.
16. Hoffman RA: Hibernation and effects of low temperature, in Hoffman RA, Robinson PF, Magalhaes H (eds): *The Golden Hamster*. Ames, IA, Iowa State University Press, 1968, pp 25-40.
17. Altman PL, Dittmer DS: *Biology Data Book*, vol 3. Bethesda, MD, Federation of the American Association for Experimental Biology, 1974, p 1785.
18. Banta CA, Warner RG, Robertson JB: Protein nutrition of the golden hamster. *J Nutr* 105:38-45, 1975.
19. Harkness JE, Wagner JE, Kusewitt DF, et al: Weight loss and impaired reproduction in the hamster attributable to an unsuitable feeding apparatus. *Lab Anim Sci* 27(1):117-118, 1977.
20. Moreland AF, Barkley WE, Bottigliere NG, et al: *Guide for the Care and Use of Laboratory Animals*. Bethesda, MD, U.S. Department of Health, Education, and Welfare, 1980, p 34.
21. Desai RG: Hematology and microcirculation, in Hoffman RA, Robinson PF, Magalhaes H (eds): *The Golden Hamster*. Ames, IA, Iowa State University Press, 1968, p 185.
22. Ransom JH: Intravenous injection of unanesthetized hamsters. *Lab Anim Sci* 34(2):200, 1984.
23. Bartlett JG, Chang T, Moon N, et al: Antibiotic induced lethal enterocolitis in hamsters: Studies with eleven agents and evidence to support the pathogenic role of toxin. *Am J Vet Res* 39(9):1525-1530, 1978.
24. Ebright IR, Fekety R, Silva J, et al: Evaluation of eight cephalosporins in hamster colitis model. *Antimicrob Agents Chemother* 19(6):980-986, 1981.
25. Small JD: Fatal enterocolitis in hamsters given lincomycin hydrochloride. *Lab Anim Care* 18(4):411-419, 1968.
26. Fekety R, Silva J, Toshniwal R, et al: Antibiotic-associated colitis effects of antibiotics on *Clostridium difficile* and the disease in hamsters. *Rev Infect Dis* 1(2):386, 1979.
27. Curl JL, Peters LL: Ketamine hydrochloride and xylazine hydrochloride anesthesia in the golden hamster (*Mesocricetus auratus*). *Lab Anim Sci* 17:290-293, 1983.
28. Clifford DH: Preanesthesia, anesthesia, analgesia and euthanasia, in Fox JG, Cohen BJ, Loew FM (eds): *Laboratory Animal Medicine*. Orlando, FL, Academic Press Inc, 1984, pp 538-539.
29. Lentsch RH, McLaughlin RM, Wagner JE, Day TJ: *Campylobacter fetus* subspecies *jejuni* isolated from Syrian hamsters with proliferative ileitis. *Lab Anim Sci* 32(5):511-513, 1982.
30. Fox JG, Ackerman JI, Taylor NS: The hamster as a potential reservoir of human campylobacterosis. *J Infect Dis* 147(4):784, 1983.
31. Regina ML, Fales WH, Wagner JE: Effects of antibiotic treatment on the occurrence of experimentally induced proliferative ileitis of hamsters. *Lab Anim Sci* 30(1):38-41, 1980.
32. Renshaw HW, Van Hoosier GL, Amend NK: A survey of naturally occurring diseases of the Syrian hamster. *Lab Anim* 9:179-191, 1975.
33. Zook BC, Huang K, Rhorer RG: *Tyzzer's disease in Syrian hamsters*. *JAVMA* 171(9):833-836, 1977.
34. Frisk CS, Wagner JE, Owens DR: Hamster (*Mesocricetus auratus*) enteritis caused by epithelial cell-invasive *Escherichia coli*. *Infect Immun* 31(3):1232-1238, 1981.
35. Ganawy JR: Bacterial, mycoplasma, and rickettsial diseases, in Wagner JE, Manning PJ (eds): *Biology of the Guinea Pig*. New York, Academic Press, 1976, pp 121-135.
36. Innes JRM, Wilson C, Ross MA: Epizootic *Salmonella enteritidis* infection causing septic pulmonary phlebothrombosis in hamsters. *J Infect Dis* 98:133-144, 1956.
37. Parker JC, Igel HJ, Reynolds RK, et al: Lymphocytic choriomeningitis virus infection in fetal, newborn, and young adult Syrian hamsters. *Infect Immun* 13(3):967-981, 1976.
38. Garlinghouse LE, Van Hoosier GL: Studies on adjuvant-induced arthritis, tumor transplantability and serologic response to bovine serum albumin in sendai virus infected rats. *Am J Vet Res* 39(2):297-300, 1978.
39. Taffs LF: Pinworm infections in laboratory rodents: A review. *Lab Anim* 10:1-13, 1976.
40. Ross CR, Wagner JE, Wightman SR, et al: Experimental transmission of *Syphacia muris* among rats, mice, hamsters, and gerbils. *Lab Anim Sci* 30(1):35-37, 1980.
41. Anay ES, Davis BJ: Treatment of *Syphacia obvelata* in the Syrian hamster (*Mesocricetus auratus*) with piperazine citrate. *Am J Vet Res* 41(11):1899-1900, 1980.
42. Ronald NC, Wagner JE: Treatment of *Hymenolepis nana* in hamsters with yomesan (niclosamide). *Lab Anim Sci* 25(2):219-220, 1975.
43. Silveman J, Chavannes J: Balding. *Lab Anim* 12(3):14-15, 1983.
44. Estes PC, Richter CB, Franklin JA: Demodectic mange in the golden hamster. *Lab Anim Sci* 21(6):825-828, 1971.
45. Pour P, Althoff J, Salmasi SZ, Stephan K: Spontaneous tumors and common diseases in three types of hamsters. *J Natl Cancer Inst* 63(3):797-809, 1979.
46. Coggin JH, Bellomy BB, Thomas KO, et al: B-cell and T-cell lymphomas and other associated diseases induced by an infectious DNA viroid-like agent in hamsters (*Mesocricetus auratus*). *Am J Pathol* 110:254-256, 1983.
47. Pour P, Knoch N, Greiser E, et al: Spontaneous tumors and common diseases in two colonies of Syrian hamsters. I. Incidence and sites. *J Natl Cancer Inst* 56(5):931-935, 1976.
48. Mezza LE, Quimby FW, Darham SK, et al: Characterization of spontaneous amyloidosis of Syrian hamsters using the potassium permanganate method. *Lab Anim Sci* 34(4)376-380, 1984.
49. Gleiser CA, Van Hoosier GL, Sheldon WG, et al: Amyloidosis and renal paramyloid in a closed hamster colony. *Lab Anim Sci* 21(3):197-202, 1971.
50. Murphy JC, Fox JG: Nephrotic syndrome in Syrian hamsters. *Abstract of Papers Presented at the Scientific Sessions at the 31st Annual Session of Am Assoc Lab Anim Sci*:80-84, 1980.
51. Dodds JW, Raymond SK, Moynihan AC, et al: Spontaneous atrial thrombosis in ages Syrian hamsters. II. Hemostasis. *Thrombos Haemost* 38:457-465, 1977.
52. Gleiser CA, Van Hoosier GL, Sheldon WG: A polycystic disease of hamsters in a closed colony. *Lab Anim Care* 20(5):923-929, 1970.
53. Pour P, Birt D: Spontaneous diseases of Syrian hamsters—Their implications in toxicological research. Facts, thoughts, and suggestions. *Proj Exp Tumor Res* 24:145-156, 1979.
54. Pour P, Mohr U, Cardesa A, et al: Spontaneous tumors and common diseases in two colonies of Syrian hamsters. II. Respriatory tract and digestive system. *J Natl Cancer Inst* 56:937-949, 1976.
55. Pour P, Mohr U, Cardesa A, et al: Spontaneous tumors and common diseases in two colonies of Syrian hamsters. III. Urogenital system and endocrine glands. *J Natl Cancer Inst* 56:949-961, 1976.

56. Pour P, Mohr U, Cardesa A, et al: Spontaneous tumors and common diseases in two colonies of Syrian hamsters. IV. Vascular and lymphatic systems and lesions of other sites. *J Natl Cancer Inst* 56:963-974, 1976.
57. Keyes PH: Odontopathic infections, in Hoffman RA, Robinson PF, Magalhaes H (eds): *The Golden Hamster*. Ames, IA, Iowa State University Press, 1968, pp 253-282.
58. Printz RH, Greenwald GS: A neural mechanism regulating follicular development in the hamster. *Neuroendocrinology* 7:171-182, 1971.
59. Grineland RE, Folk GE: Effects of cold exposure on the oestrus cycle of the golden hamster (*Mesocricetus auratus*). *J Reprod Fertil* 4:1-6, 1966.
60. Rudeen PK, Rector RJ: Influence of a skeleton photoperiod on the reproductive organ atrophy in the male golden hamster. *J Reprod Fertil* 60:279-283, 1980.
61. Lisk RD, Langenberg KK, Banta JD: Blocked sexual receptivity in grouped female hamsters: Independence from ovarian function and continuous group maintenance. *Biol Reprod* 22:237-242, 1980.
62. Soderwall AL, Britenbaker AL: Reproductive capacities of different age hamsters (*Cricetus auratus*, Waterhouse). *J Gerontol* 10:469-470, 1955.
63. Richter A, Lausen NC, Lage AL: Pregnancy toxemia (eclampsia) in Syrian golden hamsters. *JAVMA* 185(11):1357-1358, 1984.

UPDATE

INFECTIOUS DISEASES

The pathogenesis of proliferative enteritis, frequently referred to as proliferative ileitis, has been further defined since publication of the original article. The disease is characterized by the presence of comma-shaped organisms within the apical parts of the columnar epithelium.[1] Stills produced the disease experimentally with the oral inoculation of intestinal tissue containing intracellular Campylobacter-like organisms (ICLO).[2] A 16S rRNA sequence analysis is used to detect intracellular *Desulfovibrio* organisms (IDO) in hamsters with ICL0-associated disease.[3] *Desulfovibrio* species are gram-negative organisms of the class *Proeobacteria*, a group perceived to contain mostly free-living sulfate reducing bacteria.[4] Intracellular *Desulfovibrio* organisms are clearly the Campylobacter-like organisms associated with proliferative ileitis. However, they may not have the ability to produce the disease without other agents, such as *Escherichia coli*, or insult.[3] The role of *E. coli* in the pathogenesis of proliferative ileitis in the hamster is uncertain; however, it may be involved synergistically with ICLO.[5]

PHARMACEUTICAL AGENTS

Since the original printing of this article, additional antibiotics and anesthetic regimes have been advocated for use in the hamster. An antibiotic of particular interest is enrofloxacin because of its broad-spectrum activity against both negative and positive organisms. The suggested dose in the hamster is 5 to 10 mg body weight per os or 100 mg/l of drinking water.[6] Other additional antimicrobial agents not associated with enterocolitis include oxytetracycline, administered at 20 mg/kg body weight (BW) subcutaneously (SC)[7]; trimethoprim and sulfadiazine (30 mg/kg BW, SC);[8] trimethoprim and sulfamethoxazole (15 mg/kg BW, orally twice daily);[8] tylosin (100 mg/kg BW per os once daily);[7] and vancomycin (20 mg/kg BW per os by gavage).[9]

The use of tiletamine/zolazepam at 30 mg/kg BW, administered intraperitoneally (IP) in combination with xylazine at 10 mg/kg IP has been suggested as an effective anesthetic regime. The mean surgical time with this combination was 30.0 ± 2.4 minutes. The mean surgical time for an intramuscular injection at the same dose was not significantly different from the administration. Therefore, the intraperitoneal route would be the preferred choice because of the minimal tissue damage, as compared to the intramuscular route.[10]

The administration of inhalant anesthetic agents such as isoflurane or halothane can be accomplished with anesthetic chambers, face masks, or intubation. Intubation of the hamster can be accomplished with the use of a customized laryngoscope. Intravenous over-the-needle catheters (16 to 20 gauge, depending on the size of the hamster) are suitable for intubation. The stylet should be filed down to decrease the possibility of oropharyngeal or tracheal trauma.[11]

REFERENCES

1. Lawson GHK, Rowland, AC, MacIntyre N: Demonstration of a new intracellular antigen in porcine intestinal adenomatosis and hamster proliferative ileitis. *Vet Microbiol* 10:303–313, 1985.
2. Stills HF: Isolation of an intracellular bacterium from hamsters (*Mesocricetus auratus*) with proliferative ileitis and reproduction of the disease with pure culture. *Infect Immun* 59:3227–3236, 1991.
3. Fox JG, Dewhirst FE, Fraser GL, Paster BJ, Shames B, Murphy JC: Intracellular Campylobacter-like organism from ferrets and hamsters with proliferative bowel disease is a *Desulfovibrio* sp. *Jour Clin Microbiol* 32(5):1229–37, 1994.
4. Oyaizu H, Woese CR: Phylogenetic relationship among the sulfate respiring bacteria, myxobacteria, and purple bacteria. *Sys Appl Microbiol* 6:257–263, 1985.
5. Dillehay DL, Paul KS, Boosinger TR, Fox G: Enterocecocolitis associated Campylobacter-like organisms in a hamster (*Mesocricetus auratus*) colony. *Lab Anim Sci* 44(1):12–16, 1994.
6. Dorrestein GM: Enrofloxacin in pet avian and exotic animal therapy, in *Proceedings of the 1st International Baytril Symposium*. Bonn, Germany, AG Bayer, 1992, pp 63–70.
7. McKellar QA: Drug dosages for small mammals. *Practice* (March):57–61, 1989.
8. Bauck L: Ophthalmic conditions in rabbits and rodents. *Compend Contin Edu Pract Vet* 11(3):258–268, 1989.
9. Boss SM, Gries CL, Kirchner BK, Smith and Francis: Use of vancomycin hydrochloride for treatment of *Clostridium difficile* enteritis in Syrian hamsters. *Lab Anim Sci* 44:31–37, 1994.
10. Forsythe DB, Payton AJ, Dixon PH, et al: Evaluation of Telazol-xylazine as an anesthetic combination for use in Syrian hamsters. *Lab Anim Sci* 42:497–502, 1992.
11. Wixson, SK: Current trends in rodent anesthesia and analgesia. Anesthesia and Analgesia in Laboratory Animals, *American College of Laboratory Animal Medicine Proceedings-1990 Forum*. Columbia, Maryland, 1990.

The Pet Ferret *(continued from page 129)*

HYPERADRENOCORTICISM

Adrenocortical tumors or nodular hyperplasia is common in middle-aged ferrets. Clinical signs include bilaterally symmetric alopecia of the caudal femoral region, abdomen, and tail. Spayed females may exhibit vulvar swelling. Hematologic and biochemical tests, including cortisol concentration and response to adrenocorticotropic hormone, are unreliable for diagnosis. Abdominal ultrasonography may disclose adrenal enlargement, but the diagnosis is most often confirmed at surgery. Tumors are usually unilateral and adrenalectomy of the affected gland may be curative.

BACTERIAL AND PARASITIC DISEASES

Recent studies suggest that almost all adult ferrets are infected with *Helicobacter mustelae* and that infected ferrets may develop gastric ulcers and gastric carcinomas.[2] Clinical signs include vomiting, emaciation, and abdominal distension. *Helicobacter pylori*, a similar organism, has been implicated in the pathogenesis of peptic ulcers and gastric neoplasias in humans. Diagnosis is by endoscopy and/or biopsy of suspicious lesions. While there are currently no reported guidelines for medical treatment of gastric ulcers in ferrets, therapy similar to that for human patients may be beneficial. The prognosis for gastric carcinomas in ferrets is poor.

Ferrets may also be asymptomatic carriers of *Cryptosporidia*, a single-celled intestinal parasite that is a sporadic cause of diarrhea in young animals. While disease is rarely seen in adult ferrets, the organism may be pathogenic for immunocompromised persons, including those with longstanding HIV infection. Persons at risk should be scrupulous about handwashing after all contact with ferrets and should avoid direct exposure to ferret feces and litterboxes.

CONDITIONS OF UNKNOWN ETIOLOGY

Hypertrophic and dilative cardiomyopathies are frequently diagnosed in ferrets. Clinical signs may include respiratory distress, pallor, cyanosis, inappetence, lethargy, exercise intolerance, and ascites. Physical findings may include muffled heart sounds, heart murmurs, gallop rhythms, and moist rales. Diagnosis and treatment are similar to those in the cat, and the prognosis is good for prolonging life when appropriate therapy is started early.

Megaesophagus has been reported in nine adult ferrets with signs of regurgitation, difficulty in swallowing, partial anorexia, and ptyalism.[3] Radiography revealed esophageal distension in the cervical and thoracic regions. Medical treatment directed against possible primary causes of megaesophagus in other species was unsuccessful and all ferrets died. The etiopathogenesis of this disorder has not yet been determined.

REFERENCES

1. Rosenthal K: Ferrets. *Vet Clin North Am Small Anim Pract* 24:1–23, 1994.
2. Fox JG, Otto G, Murphy JC, et al: Gastric colonization of the ferret with *Helicobacter* species: Natural and experimental infections. *Rev Infect Dis* (Suppl 8):S671–680, 1991.
3. Blanco MC, Fox JG, Rosenthal K, et al: Megaesophagus in nine ferrets. *JAVMA* 205:444–447, 1994.

The Guinea Pig: An Overview Part I

Larry J. Peters, DVM
Post Doctoral Fellow
Division of Laboratory Animal and Wildlife Medicine
College of Veterinary Medicine
University of Florida
Gainesville, Florida

Cavia porcellus, the common guinea pig or cavy, is only rarely seen in private practice, but it is being presented with increasing frequency throughout the United States.

The following article is intended not to convey all details of the guinea pig and its problems, but rather to provide a general overview and a practical aid for the clinician presented with the occasional guinea pig in distress. The subject matter will encompass the most common maladies affecting guinea pigs as family pets, in small backyard breeding enterprises, or in pet shops, and will outline treatment protocols that are practical and economical for both the clinician and client.

The pet cavy differs substantially from its counterpart in the research world, necessitating an equally differing treatment philosophy. Although they are physiologically the same, the emotional value attached to the pet, which exceeds its monetary worth, its atypical environment and diet, and the client's expectations of the doctor all make it more than merely a statistical unit. The emphasis is on treatment of the individual animal rather than population medicine.

History

Today's common pet guinea pig, or *cavy* as it is commonly referred to in show circles, represents the domesticated form of a South American rodent. Grouped taxonomically with chinchillas and porcupines, the creatures exist in nature as vegetarians, living gregariously in burrows. Even now they are raised domestically in rural areas of South America for their tasty flesh. These animals gained recognition first for use in research, and they are still produced primarily for this purpose. They are also quite popular as pets, in which capacity they perform admirably, rarely biting or scratching. Their basic good health and low monetary value have contributed to their infrequent appearance as patients in private practices.

Breeds

The guinea pig exists in three basic varieties, although interbreeding makes possible any combination of characteristics. The three basic varieties, or breeds, are as follows:

1. Shorthair or English—These animals have uniformly short hair with a wide range of color patterns. Inbred strains of this type constitute the typical research animal.
2. Abyssinian—This type is very popular as pets; they have whorls or rosettes in their short rough fur. Many color patterns exist. Criteria for certain show standards are based upon various characteristics of these rosettes.
3. Peruvian—This is the rarest variety, but one of the types most often presented for treatment due to its uniqueness and show value. The hair on these animals often exceeds 6 inches in length.

All three breeds exist in a variety of mono-, bio-, and tri-color patterns.

Anatomy and Physiology

Adult guinea pigs may weigh over 2 lb; obesity is common. Newborns range in weight from 50 to 100 g, depending upon the number in the litter. There have been reported life spans of nine years, but three to six is more realistic as the average in the home environment. Guinea pigs have four toes on each front foot and three on each rear. A diastema is present in the upper lip. All teeth have open roots which grow throughout the life of the animal and must be worn down continually. The ears are moderately large and hairless. The females have only two nipples, one in each inguinal region. The vagina is completely covered by a vaginal membrane except during estrus and parturition. Basic physiological norms are listed in Table I.

TABLE I
PHYSIOLOGICAL NORMS
FOR CAVIAE PORCELLUS

Temperature	38°-39°C
Respiratory rate	70-130/minute
Heart rate	230-300/minute
PCV	40-50%
RBC	$4.5\text{-}7 \times 10^6$
WBC	$5\text{-}15 \times 10^3$ (neutrophils 20-60%) (lymphocytes 35-75%)

Normal urine is thick and white or yellow in color, and it contains many crystals and has an alkaline pH typical of herbivores. The intestinal tract resembles that of the horse, with a large and active cecum.

Neutrophils show red granules with eosin dyes, and mononuclear leukocytes may contain purple or purple-specked vacuoles called *Kurloff's bodies.* These are most noticeable during late pregnancy when estrogen levels are highest.

The cavy, like man, nonhuman primates, the fruit bat, and some other species, requires a dietary source of vitamin C, as it is incapable of endogenous production.

Husbandry

The average guinea pig is a strong, healthy creature capable of tolerating the extremes of weather, housing, and handling to which the normal family subjects it. Even so, it is not invincible, and a great many of the cases presented to the practitioner are the result, directly or indirectly, of improper husbandry or handling.

Handling

Guinea pigs should be grasped firmly and quickly around the thorax from above with one hand. This should be done gently but solidly. The other hand should support the rear limbs and total body weight. Although they seldom bite, guinea pigs will squeal and wiggle until they feel secure. It is difficult, at best, for the small hands of a child to properly restrain a fractious guinea pig. Children can best hold a docile pet supported in their arms next to their bodies.

Guinea pigs are very susceptible to unusually stressful situations. They may go off feed and lose weight when moved from one family to another or even to a new cage. Abortions are not uncommon in late pregnancy following movement or frightening events.

Housing

Housing accommodations provided for pet guinea pigs are limited only by the imagination, ingenuity, and budget of the owners. There is no one specific right way to accommodate the family cavy as long as the family's emotional needs are met without compromising the cavy's physiological needs.

Because of its relatively clean and social nature, the cavy is easily housed. It cannot jump or climb and thus can be kept in an open-topped enclosure at least 10 inches high. Outside hutch-type enclosures are acceptable, but they should provide access to shade and draft-free sleeping and hiding quarters. Temperature ranges of 55 to 90°F are easily tolerated with lower humidities preferred. If the guinea pig is kept outdoors, protection from sudden weather changes is necessary. Young guinea pigs are more susceptible to the cold and do not thrive at temperatures less than 55°F. Adults can tolerate cold better than heat, showing signs of heat stress at higher temperatures and humidity levels, especially if they are deprived of adequate air flow or sufficient shade. Excessive heat has been associated with premature parturition, death of young, and failure to lactate.

Adults do not require a lot of space. Flooring can be solid or wire. Wire flooring provides a cleaner environment and easier maintenance, but the mesh size must be sufficiently large to allow the hocks to be easily retracted should a foot slip through. Foot lesions and fractured hocks are seen more frequently with wire flooring (Figure 1). Solid floors require more effort to keep sanitary, but most people find them, with bedding, more esthetically acceptable. Many types of bedding are acceptable, for example, wood shavings, shredded paper, commercial pellets, and hay. Frequency of bedding changes depends upon the number of animals and type of food fed.

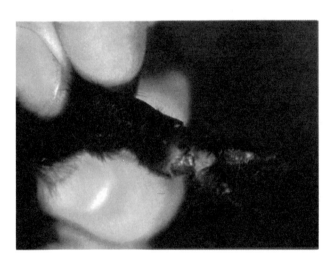

Figure 1—Foot lesion secondary to wire flooring.

Because of their sensitive nature and tendency to panic when frightened, guinea pigs should be housed in a quiet spot away from excitement and noise. Since they are nocturnal, they require periods of light for rest and do poorly if housed for long periods in dark closets or rooms.

More than one animal may be safely housed together and sexes may remain mixed indefinitely. New males may occasionally fight if there is a female nearby. Older, dominant animals may also chew on the ears and hair of subordinate ones.

Feeding and Watering

For a *pig,* the cavy is quite a finicky eater. It may turn up its nose because of changes in the taste or texture of its diet and refuse food or water that has become fouled. A favorite pastime of the cavy is to sit on the edge of its food or water bowl and excrete waste into it. Food should be supplied in hoppers or bins to minimize this occurrence.

The adult guinea pig consumes about 3 oz of water per day. If provided in an open container, the

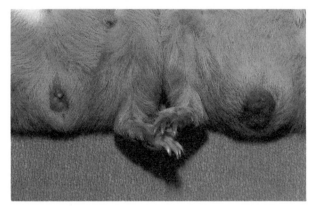

Figure 2—Genitalia of female guinea pig *(left)* and of male guinea pig *(right).*

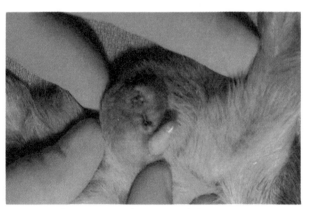

Figure 3—Male guinea pig with penis extruded.

water will be fouled with excreta quickly. Guinea pigs suck from sipper tubes rather than lap like rats; they chew on and blow food back up the tubes, fouling their water within hours. Thus water containers must be cleaned daily.

The most important factor of a guinea pig's diet is the need for vitamin C. This need can be met by feeding commercial guinea pig pellets specially formulated and manufactured to meet the guinea pig's nutritional requirements (with sufficient vitamin C added). However, even under optimum, dry, cool-storage conditions, vitamin C levels remain sufficient for only three months from date of milling. Therefore, unless a pet or feed store sells large volumes of guinea pig food, it may be difficult to obtain fresh, potent pellets, and vitamin C supplementation will still be necessary. The vitamin can be added to the drinking water at 20 mg/day/guinea pig; this solution should be prepared fresh daily, since 50% of the potency is lost within the first 24 hours. Probably the most common means of supplementation is by the addition of fresh greens to the diet. A handful of cabbage or kale or a carrot daily usually suffices. A thorough washing is necessary to insure that no harmful bacteria or pesticide is introduced to the pet. Guinea pigs will graze on lawns and grass clippings; large amounts of luscious greens may cause loose stools. Rabbit chow is often fed successfully instead of guinea pig pellets. Its physical appearance is similar and it is accepted by the cavy, but it is lower in protein and inadequate in vitamin C. The medicated type should never be used, as fatal disruption of the guinea pig's intestinal flora can result.

Roughage is not necessary if the guinea pig is on a good diet, but the animals enjoy burrowing into it, and a good-quality grass hay to nibble on appears to decrease barbering and hair pulling. It has also been reported to decrease hair thinning often associated with late pregnancy.[1]

Breeding

Only the basic essentials of guinea pig reproduction will be covered here since the majority of the clinical situations presented involve complications of pregnancy rather than lack of sufficient productivity.

The breeding age of males (boars) is four to six months and of females (sows) is three to five months, although puberty can occur as early as three to four weeks. Females have an estrous cycle of 14 to 19 days; estrus lasts for about 50 hours, during which time the vaginal membrane is open. The male is only accepted for about 15 hours during this time. A postpartum heat occurs about three to five hours following birth, and conception rates at this ovulation exceed 70%.

Although efficient, males are not particularly aggressive breeders. Copulation time is short and ejaculation is immediate. One to two days following copulation, a light-colored tubular mass of coagulated semen about an inch long called a *vaginal plug* falls from the vagina. This verifies that copulation, but not necessarily conception, has occurred.

Females should be bred, if pregnancy is desired, before nine months of age. In older virgin females the pubic symphysis becomes fused and fat has accumulated in the pelvic area, increasing chances of dystocia.

Guinea pigs may be bred in harems, as permanent pairs, or a male may be temporarily placed with the female during her estrus. Harems usually consist of one male and 10 to 12 females, with the animals left together continually. Problems are un-usual, and young will often nurse from other than their own dams. Care should be taken not to excite the group or the young may be trampled by the frightened herd as it stampedes in circular fashion around its pen. Rectangular rather than square enclosures help to lessen this tendency.

Sexing

The female displays a Y-shaped vaginal opening between the urethral orifice and the anus (Figure 2). This opening is closed by the vaginal membrane except during estrus and parturition. The urethral orifice in the female is external and ventral to the vaginal opening.

The male has no opening between the orifice at the tip of the penis and the anus (Figure 2). A slitlike structure, which is often mistaken for a vaginal opening, is evident in this area. It is merely the fold between the two halves of the scrotum following retraction of the testicles. The penis can be palpated just ventral to this slit and can be everted by gentle pressure (Figure 3). The ano-urethral distance is the same in both sexes. Internally the male possesses very large Y-shaped seminal vesicles. These structures, which resemble bicornuate uteri, lie anterior to the prostate and are very noticeable at necropsy.

Pregnancy

Gestation in the guinea pig is relatively long. Depending upon the litter size, it ranges from 60-70 days, being longer with small litters and shorter with larger ones. Average litter size is about three young, but up to eight have been reported. Litters greater than five are often born dead. Commercial breeders are usually satisfied with 10 to 12 young reared annually per female, but some sows will produce 18 if the postpartum heat is utilized.

Embryos can be palpated easily by four to five weeks or as early as two to three weeks with practice. Because of the sensitive nature of the pregnant sow, the wisdom of transporting her to the clinic for palpation is debatable.

The pubic symphysis will begin to open 10 days prior to delivery and will be ¾ inch wide at parturition. This can be easily palpated from beneath with the forefinger and is indicative of impending birth.

Babies weigh 50 to 100 g at birth; those less than 50 g usually do not survive. A 10% stillbirth and weaning mortality rate is not uncommon under even the best of conditions. The sow is not very motherly; she makes no nest and even remains in the sitting position while nursing. The young are born precocious, i.e., fully haired, with teeth, and with their eyes open. They are thus able to survive without nursing, although they are usually not weaned until they are three weeks old or 150 g. Cannibalism is rare, but fatal trampling is not uncommon in large groups. The mother and young can be removed from the group for awhile if necessary.

Clinical Techniques
Blood Sampling

Routine blood sampling presents a problem in that there are no readily accessible, large, superficial veins. Small amounts of blood for capillary tubes can be obtained from the dorsolateral penile or the saphenous veins with light syringe pressure and a small-gauge needle. Direct capillary tube filling can be done by incising the saphenous vein of a leg previously smeared with petroleum jelly or by incising a toenail, or it can be obtained from the orbital sinus under anesthesia.

Larger volumes of blood can be obtained from the femoral triangle or by direct cardiac puncture while under light anesthesia. The latter procedures for diagnostic purposes may appear radical, but individuals have been so bled repeatedly at weekly intervals without adverse incidence.

Drug Administration

Intramuscular injections may be given into the posterior lateral thigh 0.5 to 1 cm above the stifle or into the lumbar musculature. Subcutaneous injections are easily made into any dorsolateral location from the flank to the nape of the neck. Small amounts of drug can sometimes be injected into the dorsolateral penile veins or the larger ear veins, or one can do a cutdown on the saphenous vein above the hock as it turns inward and upward. Intraperitoneal injections are made slightly to the right of midline about 1 inch anterior to the pubic bone while elevating the rear of the animal. Beware of this procedure in heavily pregnant sows.

The oral route is by far the simplest. Medication can be mixed in food or water, passed through a stomach tube, or dropped into the mouth. A makeshift speculum is helpful when attempting to pass a stomach tube.

REFERENCE
1. Williams CSF: *Practical Guide to Lab Animals.* St. Louis, CV Mosby Co, 1976.

The Guinea Pig: An Overview Part II

Larry J. Peters, DVM
Post Doctoral Fellow
Division of Laboratory Animal
and Wildlife Medicine
College of Veterinary Medicine
University of Florida
Gainesville, Florida

The guinea pig is susceptible to a vast array of diverse organisms, the majority of which are not encountered in the typical pet. The literature on the iatrogenic diseases and research-related problems is voluminous; they will not be discussed here. This article will be limited to those problems that are most likely to be encountered in a pet in a household environment. Even though the guinea pig is physiologically a hardy animal, it is very sensitive to stress associated with temperature, feeding, handling, etc., and many of its health problems are related to primary problems in these areas.

The Anamnesis

A complete history can be the best diagnostic tool available. The anamnesis should cover the following items: source of the pig; clinical signs; onset of signs; previous illnesses; type, source, and age of diet; type of feed and water containers used; bedding type; humidity, temperature, airflow, and light cycle of pet's environment; method and frequency of cage cleaning; new animals introduced to the household; and other pets or local wildlife.

Common Diseases and Health Problems

Cutaneous

Differential diagnoses of some of the more commonly seen cutaneous or externally evident problems in the guinea pig are listed in Table I.

Suppurative cervical lymphadenitis, or *lumps*, is an infection and abscessation usually of the cervical lymph nodes, but involvement of any node is possible. This condition is caused by a Lancefield group C, gram-positive, beta-hemolytic streptococcus normally contracted through mucous membrane abrasions.[1-3] The involved nodes form abscesses containing a thick, yellowish white suppurative exudate. Cellulitis and arthritis may be present, but animals often display no apparent discomfort. Small abscesses are sometimes noted in the visceral organs, and uterine infections have caused abortions. Treatment varies from surgical excision or drainage with lavage in severe cases to conservative therapy utilizing an appropriate antibiotic in less involved situations.

TABLE I

CUTANEOUS OR EXTERNALLY EVIDENT PROBLEMS

Clinical Sign	Differential Diagnosis
Open lesions	Bite wounds Trauma from sharp objects Draining abscesses Thermal or caustic burns Self-trauma
Cutaneous or subcutaneous swelling	Abscesses Aberrant parasite larvae Mastitis Arthritis (Vitamin C deficiency)
Dermatitis	Fungal infection (*Trichophyton* spp.) Bacterial infection Parasites: Mites, *Trixacarus caviae*; lice, *Chirodiscoides caviae*, *Gliricola porcelli*
Alopecia	Nutritional Mites Barbering (nibbling hair from each other) Mechanical (rubbing on feeders or cage parts) Fungal Unknown (diffuse loss over flanks and backs is common during pregnancy)

Another form of *chronic abscessation* of the cervical lymph nodes has been attributed to a gram-negative organism, *Streptobacillus moniliformis*. This condition is usually not lethal, but it causes encapsulated, often unilateral swellings similar to those of suppurative cervical lymphadenitis. It can be acquired through breaks in the oral mucous membrane and is found as a normal respiratory inhabitant in the rat.[2] Treatment of these abscesses is the same as that for suppurative cervical lymphadenitis.

Superficial fungal infections on the guinea pig are frequently encountered. The most common causative agent is *Trichophyton mentagrophytes*. With this condition, scaley, scabby lesions usually begin around the face, and they may later spread to other parts of the body. Diagnosis should be by fungal culture, because this organism does not fluoresce under uv light.[2] Treatment consisting of 25 to 100 mg/kg griseofulvin po for four weeks has been successful.

Septicemia

A fulminating septicemia with or without pneumonia has been associated with a Lancefield group C streptococcus. Hematuria, hemoglobinuria, depression, fever, and death (acutely or within three to four days) often occur with the condition.[2,4,5]

Naturally occurring *pseudotuberculosis* caused by *Yersinia pseudotuberculosis* is not uncommon in the pet cavy. This gram-negative coccoid- to bacillary-shaped organism survives and multiplies in feces, necessitating good sanitation. This condition is generally chronic, manifesting itself as emaciation, diarrhea, nodules in the lymph nodes and viscera, and death in three to four weeks. A more acute death can occur from miliary lesions in the lungs and liver. The primary lesions in chronic cases often begin in the mesenteric nodes, which become palpably enlarged. Necrotic white or yellow nodules containing thick, smooth, caseated pus can also occur in the gastrointestinal tract and mammary tissues. Nonfatal cases exhibiting only enlarged nodes have been reported. Spread is through oral ingestion; it is believed that the organism might be acquired from greens contaminated by the feces of wild birds and rodents.[6] Treatment of this condition is difficult and, except in very early cases, the prognosis is poor. Thorough washing of greens before feeding is important in prevention.

Salmonellosis (paratyphoid) is one of the most lethal infections that can be contracted. It is caused by the bacilli *Salmonella typhimurium* and *Salmonella enteritidis*, and it can remain latent until exacerbated by stress. Salmonellosis often occurs acutely, causing sudden death, but it can also be chronic, with emaciation and diarrhea. Conjunctivitis is common. The more chronic cases show granulomatous lesions in the spleen, liver, and lymph nodes. Acute cases show liquid gut contents composed of purulent exudate in the lumen of the intestines. Lymph nodes will be grossly increased in size within 48 hours postinfection. The route of infection is oral or conjunctival. Salmonellosis closely resembles syndromes caused by *Yersinia pseudotuberculosis* and *Corynebacterium pyogenes*. It can be latent or it can be acquired from feedstuffs and bedding contaminated with rodent excreta.[6] Treatment is usually unsuccessful unless it is begun very early in the case.

Respiratory System

Differential diagnoses of the more commonly seen respiratory syndromes are listed in Table II.

Guinea pigs are susceptible to *pneumonia* caused by a variety of pathogens. The pigs are usually predisposed by stressful situations, i.e., weather change and exposure, shipping, or following purchase from a group colony. Subclinical vitamin C deficiency can also be a predisposing factor.

Streptococcal pneumonia is a devastating disease in the guinea pig that can reach epizootic proportions.[2,4,5] It can be manifested clinically as an acute or chronic condition. The acutely affected animal may be found dead. Any of the following signs may be noted in longer-term illnesses: pleuritis, peritonitis, pericarditis, arthritis, localized abscesses, emaciation, respiratory distress, rise in temperature, coughing, sneezing, blood-stained crusts around the nose, purulent conjunctivitis, hemoglobinuria, and hematuria. Since all

TABLE II

RESPIRATORY SYNDROMES

Clinical Sign	Differential Diagnosis
Conjunctivitis	Bacterial infection
	Chlamydial neonatal conjunctivitis
	Foreign body
	Trauma
Nasal discharge/ dyspnea	Pregnancy toxemia
	Heat stress
	Allergy
	Dry hay as bedding
	Bacterial rhinitis
	Bacteria pneumonia
	Foreign body

TABLE III

REPRODUCTIVE SYNDROMES

Clinical Sign	Differential Diagnosis
Infertility	Nutritional deficiency
	Environmental stress
	Genital infections
	Immature or old age
	Feed toxins or
	hormone contaminations
	Seasonal phenomena
Perinatal mortality	Nutritional deficiency
	Bacterial diseases
	Pregnancy toxemia
	Environmental stress
	Aflatoxin in feed
Dystocias	Large fetuses
	Uterine torsion
	Sick, malnourished, or weakened sow
	Fused pubic symphysis
	Obese female
Litter desertion or cannibalism	Maternal inexperience
	Environmental disturbances
	Mastitis

of these signs except hematuria are manifested in acute salmonellosis, detection of hematuria is valuable in making a differential diagnosis.[4,5] Streptococcal pneumonia is often noted in sows shortly following parturition. Streptococcus is a common surface organism of humans and animals and is contracted via the respiratory system.[2]

Bordetella bronchiseptica, a small, gram-negative bacillus or coccobacillus, often seen in pairs, has been isolated from the respiratory tract of clinically normal animals and is a normal inhabitant of the respiratory tract of rabbits.[2] Disease caused by this organism often occurs secondary to stress, resulting in sudden death or typical bronchopneumonic signs including dyspnea, congestion, consolidation, and purulent bronchial exudate. The source of infection is often other guinea pigs or rabbits, and it is contracted by contact or airborne routes.[4]

A *gram-positive diplococcus* has been implicated in some cases of severe pneumonia, causing hemorrhagic lungs, pulmonary abscesses, purulent otitis, pleuritis, and pericarditis.[2]

There is a *naturally occurring pneumonia* caused by a filterable virus which results in an acute illness approximately one week following inhalation.[2] Congestion and consolidation of the lungs are the primary signs. Treatment entails early diagnosis, use of an appropriate antibiotic, and intense supportive measures.

Reproduction

Differential diagnoses of the common reproductive syndromes are listed in Table III.

Vaginitis of diverse etiologies can occur in guinea pigs. Various bacteria, often secondary to bedding or other foreign bodies, have been isolated from such infections.[2] Treatment of vaginitis consists of thorough examination of the vagina for foreign matter and therapy with appropriate antibiotics. Vaginoscopy is more easily accomplished during estrus, when the vaginal membrane is relaxed.

Mature boars may accumulate a mass of sebaceous material in the folds of skin between the two halves of the scrotum; this is called a *scrotal plug*. It can be up to 1 inch in diameter and is often confused with an external rectal impaction at first glance.[5] Treatment consists of thorough cleaning with soap and water.

Obstetrical problems such as stillbirths and abortions are not uncommon in guinea pigs, and often no cause can be incriminated. Stress of pregnancy can be great upon the sow. Often the total fetal mass may weigh more than the mother, prohibiting her from walking the last few days prior to delivery.[5] If this occurs, food and water should be made easily accessible.

Fusion of the pubic symphysis, excess fat in the pelvic cavity, too large a fetus, and uterine inertia can all contribute to *dystocia*. The only solution for the first three problems is a cesarean section. To overcome uterine inertia, one unit of oxytocin can be injected IM.[4,5] Surgery is indicated if no positive results are achieved within 15 minutes.

Situations such as dual presentation of fetuses, uterine torsion, and dystocia in immature, old, and weak sows can be occasionally corrected via external manipulation.

The pressure of the gravid uterus upon the liver can cause bile blockage and hepatic dysfunction, resulting in a vitamin-K–deficient *hemorrhagic syndrome*. This can cause complications during cesarean sections and even following vaginal deliveries.

Pregnancy toxemia is fairly common in the guinea pig. It is typically seen in stressed, heavily pregnant sows that are 56 or more days into gestation and carrying three or more fetuses. Acute deaths can occur within 24 hours with no history of clinical illness. Treatment is usually too late and ineffective; however, 1 to 2 ml 50% dextrose in 3 to 5 ml saline IV or IP can be tried.[5] The condition can also be chronic, beginning with a ruffled hair coat, lethargy, and anorexia three to five days prior to death and progressing to a reluctance to move, prostration, and coma. The eyes are dull, yellow crusts form along the eyelids, and abortion may occur. A similar syndrome can occur 7 to 11 days postpartum. It is nearly 100% fatal despite treatment. Hyperlipemia and ketone-positive urine with high protein and a pH of 5 or less are consistent findings. The etiology of pregnancy toxemia is unknown, but obesity is an important factor. Stress should be kept to a minimum and the animal should not be transported or fasted during the latter periods of gestation. A genetic predilection may exist.

TABLE IV
CNS AND MUSCULOSKELETAL DISORDERS

Clinical Sign	Differential Diagnosis
Incoordination/convulsions	Guinea pig paralysis Trauma Pregnancy toxemia Toxicity Toxoplasmosis
Paralysis or reluctance to move	Guinea pig paralysis Fractures Luxations Vitamin C deficiency Arthritis Vitamin E deficiency Urinary calculi Prostatitis Late, heavy pregnancy Toxoplasmosis Imbalance of Ca:P
Torticollis	Otitis interna Encephalitis Trauma

CNS and Musculoskeletal Systems

Table IV is a listing of differential diagnoses of some CNS and musculoskeletal disorders found in the guinea pig.

A syndrome called *guinea pig paralysis* is noted occasionally. A filterable agent has been incriminated. Urinary incontinence is the first sign, with gradually increasing hindlimb hypotonia and weakness progressing to complete posterior paralysis. A mild fever and weight loss also occur during the course of the disease. There is no known treatment, and it does not appear to be readily, if at all, transmissible between animals.

Parasites

Endoparasites are not common in the guinea pig. Cysts of the ciliate *Balantidium coli* or *Balantidium caviae* may be noted in direct smears.[2,5] There are usually no clinical signs, and the endoparasites are usually considered nonpathogenic.

The coccidian *Eimeria caviae* is sometimes found in the guinea pig; it also is usually not pathogenic.

Extremely heavy infestations, though, can result in colitis, mucoid diarrhea without blood, loss of appetite, emaciation, and occasionally, death from complications. The sporulation time of this coccidium is 6 to 12 days. Good sanitation will break the cycle of reinfestation—reinfestation is via ingestion. The greatest losses occur in the four- to eight-week-old age groups following stress. Regular cleaning and keeping no open water or feed containers are the best preventive measures. Treatment has been undertaken with sulfamethazine, sulfaquinoxaline, and sulfathiazole added to the drinking water to make a 0.05% solution or with succinyl sulfathiazole in a 0.1% solution for at least two weeks.[5]

Eggs of the *cecal pinworm Paraspidodera uncinata*, an ascarid of the cecum and colon, are occasionally noted on fecal exam. This parasite is normally nonpathogenic and nonzoonotic, but it can cause diarrhea and unthriftiness in heavy infestations. It has a direct life cycle, with eggs infective within one week after passing and mature worms present two weeks postingestion. Treatment with piperazine and proper cleaning of the premises usually alleviate the problem.[2,5]

External parasitic infestations are normally of minor significance in guinea pigs. *Chirodiscoides caviae*, the guinea pig fur mite, generally causes no clinical manifestations. Repeated infestations have been reported to cause skin lesions. The fur mite can usually be treated effectively with any flea powder suitable for use on cats. The cages should be cleaned thoroughly twice weekly for at least three weeks.

Trixacarus caviocoptes caviae, a sarcopticlike mite causing typical mange-type lesions, has only recently been recognized in this country.[8] It can cause alopecia, epidermal scaling, pruritus with self-trauma, and, in extreme cases, anorexia, emaciation, and death (Figures 2 and 3). Details concerning its life cycle are not known. It appears that the mite is capable of existing subclini-

TABLE V
GASTROINTESTINAL PROBLEMS

Clinical Sign	Differential Diagnosis
Diarrhea	Nonspecific Acute cecitis Antibiotic toxicity Salmonellosis Coccidiosis Parasitism Toxicosis
Hypersalivation	Dental malocclusion[7] Vitamin C deficiency Adrenocortical insufficiency Oral foreign body Rectal impaction (Figure 1)
Constipation/vomiting	Calcification of stomach or colon Tumor Impacted cecum Torsion Intussusception

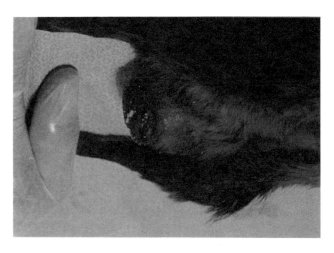

Figure 1—One gastrointestinal problem in the guinea pig is rectal impaction.

cally, becoming active with stresses such as shipping or pregnancy. Young guinea pigs may acquire the mite from the sow before weaning but show no signs until maturity. The mite is sometimes extremely difficult to

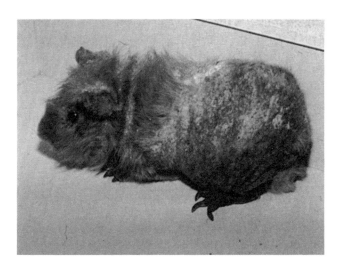

Figure 2—*Trixacarus caviocoptes caviae* mange is commonly seen in the guinea pig.

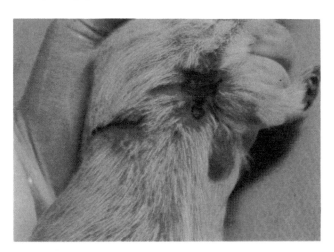

Figure 3—Self-trauma secondary to *Trixacarus caviocoptes caviae* mange.

demonstrate by scrapings. A negative scraping does not rule out the possibility of the condition if clinical signs are consistent with the diagnosis. Treatment with lime sulfur or benzene hexachloride has been reported to be effective if repeated two to three times at three-week intervals.[8,9] No species cross-infestation has been demonstrated.

The guinea pig lice *Gyropus ovalis* and *Gliricola porcelli* are common. There are usually no clinical signs associated with their presence, but the owner may become alarmed by the visible mites on the animal. Treatment with a feline flea powder is usually successful.

Miscellaneous Conditions

Miscellaneous guinea pig problems and their differential diagnoses are listed in Table VI.

Pododermatitis is manifested as a chronic, fibrous granuloma on the ventral surface of the foot (Figure 4). Staphylococci are often isolated from the lesions. The lesions occur more commonly in animals kept on wire flooring. Treatment consists of moving the animal to dry, soft bedding and administering antibiotics if necessary. The feet seldom return to normal following disfigurement.

Overgrowth of nails is another frequent condition in animals kept on wire or smooth flooring (Figure 5). Routine clipping is necessary.

A mild to severe exudative *conjunctivitis* has been attributed to an unnamed viral agent. It appears to be self-limiting, and treatment is symptomatic.[2]

TABLE VI
MISCELLANEOUS GUINEA PIG PROBLEMS

Clinical Sign	Differential Diagnosis
Weight loss	Nutritional deficiencies
	Anorexia
	Metastatic calcification
	Chronic disease
	Malocclusion
	Ectoparasitism
	Endoparasitism
	Tumors
	Inability to reach food
	Aflatoxicosis
Sudden death	Acute enteritis
	Pregnancy toxemia
	Hemorrhagic syndrome
	Starvation/dehydration
	Lymphosarcoma
	Trauma
	Antibiotic toxicity
	Dystocia
	Urinary calculi
	Septicemia
	Toxemia
	Chilling/overheating
	Aflatoxicosis
	Toxoplasmosis

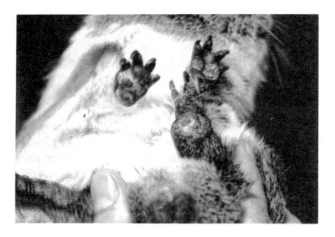

Figure 4—Pododermatitis is one of the miscellaneous conditions seen in the guinea pig.

Vitamin C deficiency is not a common problem in well-cared-for pets, because they normally receive plenty of greens in their diets. It becomes a problem if rabbit food alone or outdated guinea pig chow is fed as the sole diet. An anorexic animal should always receive forced supplementation of some form. A normal animal needs 10 to 20 mg/kg/day. Two weeks on a deficient ration can cause lameness. The first clinical signs of a vitamin C deficiency are a depressed, anorexic animal with ruffled fur. Hemorrhage into joints and muscles subsequently occurs causing lameness and a stiff posture. If treatment at 50 mg/day PO or parenterally is initiated at this stage, the animal can usually be saved. Fast-growing young and pregnant sows die first. Subclinical or marginal deficiencies often predispose animals to many other diverse problems.

Slobbers is really a clinical sign of a condition of unknown etiology. The fur under the jaws and down the neck remains wet from the constant drooling of saliva. The saliva is sometimes green or yellow colored. Overgrowth of teeth due to a selenium excess has been incriminated, but often the teeth are normal. Treatment is symptomatic at best. Teeth should be trimmed if

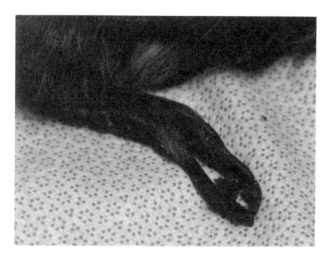

Figure 5—Overgrown toenails in the guinea pig should be clipped.

overgrown and a well-balanced ration should be provided.

Animals in the 12- to 18-month age range have been noted to develop *calcification of* various *soft tissues*, especially of the stomach and colon. This can lead to steady emaciation and death if severe enough; it is usually a postmortem finding.

The guinea pig appears to be particularly susceptible to *anaphylaxis*. This condition is often marked by severe respiratory distress because of a well-developed smooth muscle coat around the bronchial tree and pulmonary vessels.[2] Sensitivity testing is generally impractical, so clients should be made aware of the potential of reactions prior to any injection.

Antibiotics do not usually adversely affect guinea pigs immediately via anaphylaxis, as is often thought. Rather, the animals develop problems later subsequent to the antimicrobial effects of the drugs. The gastrointestinal tract of the guinea pig is populated predominately by gram-positive organisms. Antibiotics that attack principally gram-positive organisms, allowing a secondary increase in gram-negative organisms, may cause diarrhea, enterotoxemia, coliform bacteremia, and, possibly, death in three to five days. Thus, antibiotics specifically affecting gram-positive bacteria are contraindicated. Broad-spectrum antibiotics that affect both gram-positive and gram-negative organisms lessen this risk of harmful bacterial overgrowth.

Neoplasms are rare in guinea pigs less than three years of age. In older animals, neoplasms occur most often in the pulmonary system.

Treatment

Most conditions diagnosed in the pet cavy can be handled similarly to the way the equivalent entity is handled in the more common pet species. Sound medical common sense is used while making special considerations of specific anesthetic, antibiotic, and handling needs. The treatment of any condition should always include alleviating the cause as well as the presenting signs.

Antibiotic Therapy

Antibiotics in the guinea pig, as in many species should be chosen with consideration given to the bacterial sensitivity of the organism, ease of administration, cost, toxicity, and public health implications of the disease. Antibiotics of choice should be broad spectrum. Table VII lists some antibiotics and their doses that have been used effectively in guinea pigs.[4]

Anesthesia

Anesthesia in the guinea pig has long presented a major problem in proper care and treatment. The animal's small size, high metabolic rate, sensitivities, lack of superficial veins, inaccessible glottis, and respiratory system that is very sensitive to anesthetic-induced suppression all combine to complicate anesthesia.

TABLE VII

ANTIBIOTICS COMMONLY USED IN THE GUINEA PIG

Antibiotic	Dose	Route of Administration	Period of Administration
Chloramphenicol palmitate[4,5]	50 mg/kg	PO	Daily for 5 to 7 days
Chloramphenicol sodium succinate[4,5]	30 mg/kg	IM	Daily for 5 to 7 days
Cephaloridine[3,4]	10-30 mg/kg	IM	Daily for 10 days to 2 weeks
Sulfamethazine[4,5]	4 ml of 12.5% stock solution in 500 ml drinking water	PO	1 to 2 weeks
Carbenicillin[12]	200 mg/kg	PO	Divided doses daily for 1 to 2 weeks

Some of the more commonly utilized anesthetic regimes are described below.

Ether has classically been used as an inhalant by dropping the animal into ether vapor in a closed container. Ether gives good analgesia and muscle relaxation, but it is sporadically unsafe. The animals tend to salivate profusely, so they should be given atropine. Also, they hold their breath at first exposure and often succumb thereafter with one fatal gasp.[4]

Halothane has proved to be a satisfactory drug for induction and maintenance of anesthesia when used at 1% concentration. A 35 to 40% decrease in blood pressure has been reported with its use. Chamber induction with face-mask maintenance is a common technique with halothane anesthesia.

Methoxyflurane, at a concentration of 3% for induction and 1% for maintenance, has proved to be an excellent anesthetic. Induction is slow—up to 15 minutes—but relaxation is good and recovery is within 10 minutes. Atropine should be given prior to induction. Methoxyflurane should be administered the same as halothane.[2,4,5]

Sodium pentobarbital is administered at 30 to 40 mg/kg IP. Its effects last 30 minutes but are unpredictable.[5]

Sodium thiopental has been used with success at 55 mg/kg IP.

Innovar-Vet™a is administered at 0.22 to 0.88 ml/kg IM. Its effects range from tranquilization to surgical anesthesia.[10] Anesthesia is very good, but IM injection causes a severe inflammatory reaction in the surrounding tissues, causing nerve, vessel, and muscle necrosis and, sometimes, sloughing of extremities. Self-mutilation of the affected area has been noted.[2,4]

Ketamine hydrochloride is administered at 44 to 100 mg/kg. It produces good sedation but only poor to good anesthesia even at higher dosages.[4] Excellent

results have been obtained by using ketamine for induction and methoxyflurane for maintenance.

A combination of 20 mg *acepromazine* added to 100 mg *ketamine* given at 0.2 to 0.4 ml/kg has produced good results.[11] Xylazine 14 mg plus 100 mg ketamine given at 0.4 ml/kg has also been used successfully.[4]

With any anesthesia, the guinea pig should be fasted for 12 hours prior if possible to prevent vomiting and/or dose miscalculations. The heart beat, respiration, muscle relaxation, mucous membrane color, and reflexes should be monitored to determine depth of anesthesia. The pedal reflex is not a reliable indicator in this species.

In case of respiratory arrest, ventilation is sometimes possible by blowing into a plastic syringe cover or cupped hand held over the nose.[4] Tracheal intubation is difficult to accomplish.

Signs of anesthetic overdose include dilatation of pupils, protrusion of eyeballs, and cyanosis.

Surgery

Surgery in the guinea pig is not unlike that in the more common pet species after adequate anesthesia has been achieved. Aseptic technique should be strictly adhered to because of the stress-sensitive nature of the animal and the desirability of minimal antibiotic usage.

Commonly encountered surgical cases include traumatic lacerations and bite wounds, cesarean sections, fractures, cystotomies, tumor and abscess removals, ovariohysterectomies, and castrations.

Radiology

Radiology is a useful tool in the diagnosis of guinea pig maladies, and there are no normal contraindications for its use. It has been used as an aid in diagnosing such diverse conditions as arthritis, malocclusions, fractures, luxations, otitis media, pyometra, neoplasms, and abscesses.

aPitman-Moore, Inc., Washington Crossing, NJ 08560.

Vaccinations

There are no vaccinations indicated for the pet guinea pig.

Public Health

Some problems of potential importance to humans can exist in guinea pigs. Guinea pigs have long been incriminated as offenders in human allergies. They are very susceptible to both the human and bovine type of tuberculosis and can transmit the disease to humans as well. Owners should thus be directed to consult their physicians should one of these conditions be confirmed in their pets. Other human pathogens rarely harbored

by guinea pigs include bordetella, salmonella, pasteurella, streptococcus, and diplococcus. Rabies virtually never occurs in pet rodents in the United States.

Euthanasia

Placing the guinea pig in a closed container with a supersaturated atmosphere of ether, chloroform, or halothane is an acceptable method for euthanasia. An overdose of pentobarbital, 80 mg/kg, given IP is, however, probably the most acceptable and convenient method.

REFERENCES

1. Henderson JD: Cervical lymphadenitis in the guinea pig. *VM SAC* 71:462-463, 1976.
2. Wagoner JE, Manning PJ: *The Biology of the Guinea Pig.* New York, Academic Press, 1976.
3. Diaz, J, Soave DA: Cephaloridine treatment of cervical lymphadenitis in guinea pigs. *Lab Anim Dig* 8:60, 1973.
4. Wagoner JE, Harkness JE: *The Biology and Medicine of Rabbits and Rodents.* Philadelphia, Lea & Febiger, 1977.
5. Williams CSF: *Practical Guide to Lab Animals.* St. Louis, CV Mosby Co, 1976.
6. Townsend J: The guinea pig: General husbandry and nutrition. *Vet Rec* 96:451-454, 1975.
7. Olson GA: Malocclusion of the cheek teeth of a guinea pig. *Lab Anim Dig* 7:12-14, 1971.
8. McDonald SE, Lavvipierre MJ: *Trixacarus caviae* infestation in two guinea pigs. *Lab Anim Sci* 30(1):67-70, 1980.
9. Henderson JD: Treatment of cutaneous acariasis in the guinea pig. *JAVMA* 163:591-592, 1973.
10. Rubright WC, Thayer CB: Innovar-Vet, a surgical anesthetic for the guinea pig. *Pract Vet* 43(3):15-25, 1971.
11. Mulder JB, Johnson HB: Anesthesia with ketaset plus in guinea pigs and hamsters. *VM SAC* 74:1807-1808, 1979.
12. Jacobson E: Personal communication, University of Florida, 1980.

UPDATE

ANESTHESIA

Newer, popular anesthetics for use in guinea pigs are as follows:

Isoflurane—Induction is quick and effective at 2.5% to 3.0% and maintenance is usually adequate at 1.5% to 2.0%. An accurate vaporizer is required.

Tiletamine/zolazepam—When adminstered at a dose of 10 to 30 mg/kg, IM, anesthesia will result in two to three minutes with a duration of over 30 minutes.

Ketamine/xylazine—Lower dose ranges such as 40 mg of ketamine and 5 mg of xylazine per kg body weight, given IM, have proven effective and safe for repeated use.

ANTIPARASITIC DOSAGES

An effective new treatment for mange is the use of ivermectin. The Cambridge Cavy Trust recommends the following dosages using the Ivomec® injection formulation for

cattle (Merck, Sharp & Dohme).
—age three weeks to three months; 0.1 ml (1000 g) by subcutaneous injection
—age three months to adult; 0.2 ml by subcutaneous injection or one drop given orally
(Treatment may be repeated in 10 to 14 days.)

ANTIBIOTIC DOSAGES

Antibiotic	Dose	Route	Period
Enrofloxacin	5–10 mg/kg	IM/SQ	Daily for 5–7 days
Cephalexin	50 mg/kg	IM	Daily for 5–7 days
Metronidazole	20 mg/kg	PO	In drinking water for 7–10 days

BIBLIOGRAPHY

Richardson VC: *Diseases of Domestic Guinea Pigs.* Oxford, Blackwell Science Ltd, 1992.

The Pet Guinea Pig

Margi Sirois, MS, RVT
Gaston College
Veterinary Technology Program
Dallas, North Carolina

Guinea pigs (*Cavia porcellus*) are docile rodents that are popular as pets. They are more closely related to porcupines and chinchillas than to mice and rats. Their tranquil nature, relatively low cost, and ease of maintenance make guinea pigs excellent pets. They seldom bite or scratch, respond pleasantly to regular handling, and can be conditioned to squeal before such reward situations as the owner approaching the cage.

Although guinea pigs are generally hardy, poor husbandry practices will lead to immediate deterioration in health. A good husbandry program provides a system of housing and care that permits animals to grow, mature, and maintain good health. A thriving guinea pig has a higher resistance to disease than an unhealthy one does. Part of an owner's responsibility is to prevent the occurrence of disease and injury.[1]

The average life span of domesticated guinea pigs is three to four years. The most common pet variety is the English, or short-haired, guinea pig. Other varieties are the Abyssinian (with short, rough hair arranged in a rosette pattern) and the long-haired Peruvian. Because the varieties are often interbred, an abundance of colors and hair lengths is available[2] (Figure 1).

Handling and Restraint

Guinea pigs are easily frightened, make energetic attempts to escape being caught, and often struggle and squeal when handled. They can be lifted by grasping the trunk with one hand while supporting the hindquarters with the other hand (Figure 2). A pig must be handled gently because the lungs can be injured if the animal is grasped too firmly on the back. Support of the hindquarters is especially important when pregnant animals are being handled because it prevents struggling.[3]

Factors Predisposing to Disease

Housing and nutrition must be emphasized in the client education program, as these factors play important roles in disease predisposition. Guinea pigs are ordinarily quite vigorous but are extremely susceptible to environmental factors that reduce resistance to infection. These factors include poor sanitation, overcrowding, improper temperature and humidity control, and inadequate diet (particularly insufficient vitamin C).[1] Even a simple change in the location of a cage can cause some weight loss.

Illness might not be immediately obvious to an untrained observer. In general, healthy guinea pigs are tense, anxious, and alert. On the other hand, listlessness and leanness are unfavorable signs.[4]

Housing

Guinea pigs are not apt to climb and thus can be kept in open-top cages with sides at least 10 inches high.[1] A full-grown guinea pig requires approximately 101 square inches of floor space. A large aquarium is usually suitable. Solid floors with approximately two inches of bedding are difficult to clean but are preferred, especially for breeding animals. The bedding can be wood shavings or shredded paper. A box with a grid or mesh floor is easier to clean, but limbs are often broken if pigs that have not been raised on wire are then placed in housing with this type of floor.

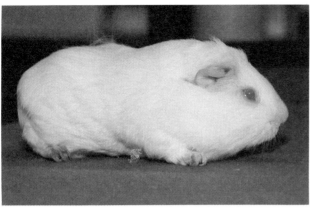
Figure 1A

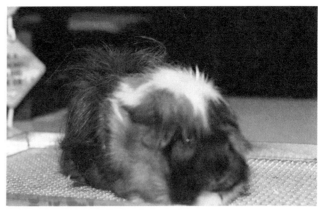
Figure 1B

Figure 1—The wide variety of hair color and length among guinea pigs includes (**A**) white short-haired guinea pigs and (**B**) tricolored Abyssinian guinea pigs.

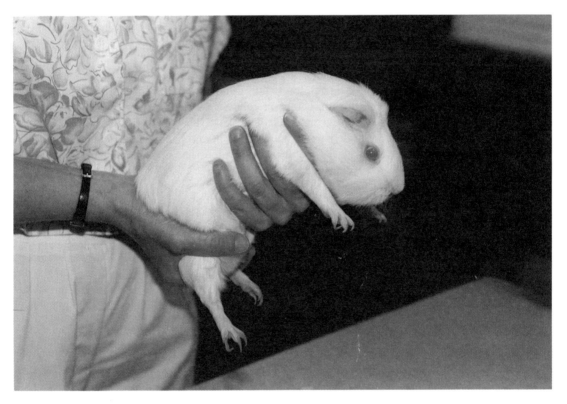

Figure 2—Guinea pigs must be carefully lifted and well supported with two hands.

If a young guinea pig must be put on mesh flooring, a piece of cardboard placed on the floor will ease the transition from a solid floor. By the time the animal has chewed up the cardboard and grown larger, it will have learned to walk safely on wire.[4]

Room temperature should be maintained between 65° and 75°F, and the cage should not be placed in direct sunlight. Guinea pigs kept singly in cages with wire floors require a higher room temperature than those kept in groups or in cages with solid sides and floors.[5] Ideal environmental humidity is between 45% and 55%. Temperature and humidity should be kept constant because guinea pigs are sensitive to extremes.

Adequate ventilation without excessive drafts should be provided. A simple method of air exchange is the use of a cage that has one or more wire-mesh sides. High temperature without adequate airflow predisposes to heat stress; low temperature and wet bedding predispose to pneumonia.[2]

Feeding and Nutrition

Feed is usually supplied ad libitum in a hanging feeder.

Porcelain bowls placed inside cages have been used, but this method allows feed to be contaminated with excreta. The preferred feed is pelleted and specifically labeled for guinea pigs. Like humans and monkeys, guinea pigs require a dietary source of vitamin C.[2] Rabbit feed looks like guinea pig chow but is lower in protein and lacks vitamin C. A guinea pig fed rabbit feed will demonstrate signs of vitamin C deficiency (scurvy) within two weeks.[1] It is important that the chow be no more than three months old (from time of manufacture) because vitamin C quickly loses its potency. The feed bag will normally be stamped with the date of manufacture[5]; feed should be purchased in small amounts to ensure its use within the three-month period.[6]

If there is doubt about the freshness of the feed, vitamin C should be supplemented directly. The preferred method of supplementation is mixing a small amount of L-ascorbic acid powder in the pet's water daily. Vitamin C can also be supplied in the form of such fresh vegetables as cabbage, kale, and carrots. These are relatively expensive sources of vitamin C. Some guinea pigs, however, will refuse to eat pelleted food if offered fresh vegetables. Lettuce in large amounts produces diarrhea and should be avoided.[7]

Like feed bowls, open water bowls usually become contaminated with excreta. An inverted bottle with a small sipper tube can be attached to the inside of the cage and suspended just above the bedding. Guinea pigs often play with the sipper tube, causing excessively wet bedding and wasted water; to alleviate this problem, a ball-bearing rather than a valveless sipper tube can be used.[6]

Guinea pigs often mix food and water in their mouths and then pass the mixture back into the sipper tube, causing a green discoloration of the water that resembles the color of algae.[2] The bottle and sipper tube should therefore be cleansed with each daily water change to avoid bacterial overgrowth in the bottle.

Reproduction

Guinea pigs are normally bred at three to five months of age. Females bred later often experience dystocia caused by fusion of the pubic symphysis.[2]

Sexing

In guinea pigs, unlike other rodents, anogenital distance is not an accurate method of determining sex. Instead, the guinea pig should be restrained and the shape of the external genitalia examined. The female's genital area appears Y shaped; the male's looks more like a straight slit. Gender can also be verified by exerting slight digital pressure cranial and caudal to the genital region; this pressure causes extrusion of the penis in males.[2]

Pregnancy and Parturition

The gestation period ranges from 63 to 70 days; average litter size is three to four (Table I). Most females come into estrus 2 to 15 hours postpartum; another mating is likely if the male remains in the cage. The young are born fully

TABLE I
Normal Physiologic Data for Guinea Pigs[7-9]

Parameter	Value
Gestation	63 to 70 days
Weaning age	21 to 28 days
Puberty	45 to 70 days
Breeding age	12 to 14 weeks
Life span	2 to 5 years
Water consumption	10 ml/100 g body weight/day
Food consumption	5 g/100 g body weight/day
Rectal temperature	100° to 104°F
Respiratory rate	110 to 150/min
Heart rate	150 to 160/min
Average adult body weight	
Male	900 to 1000 g
Female	700 to 900 g
Urine	Creamy white or yellow; thick, turbid
Feces	Dark green or brown; hard, cylindric pellets

haired and with eyes open. They can walk immediately after birth and will eat solid food within a few hours. Guinea pigs are usually weaned at 14 to 21 days by simply removing them from the mother. The young can reach puberty as early as four weeks of age. They should not be housed together after weaning because it is preferable that they not be bred for several months.[1]

Diseases Related to Poor Husbandry
Scurvy

As mentioned, when not provided sufficient amounts of vitamin C, guinea pigs quickly demonstrate deficiency. Clinical signs include prolonged periods of immobility, unthrifty appearance, distention around the joints, diarrhea, cutaneous sores, and anorexia. Patients often succumb to secondary infection before profound evidence of scurvy is apparent.[1]

Patients with signs of vitamin C deficiency should be given large amounts (20 to 50 mg/day) of ascorbic acid until recovery is evident. Vitamin C therapy should be considered in all guinea pigs that become anorectic from any cause. Guinea pigs usually enjoy the taste of ascorbic acid solution and will readily drink it from the end of a syringe or a glass dropper.[1]

Salmonellosis

Salmonellosis is a rare but highly fatal disease in guinea pigs. The most common source of infection is ingestion of contaminated feed, particularly green and leafy vegetables that have not been properly washed.

Clinical signs usually include anorexia; weight loss; light-colored, soft feces; conjunctivitis; and dyspnea. Positive diagnosis is subject to recovery of the organism from

172 *The Compendium Collection*

blood or feces. Because of its zoonotic potential and the difficulty of eliminating the organism, salmonellosis is usually not treated.[1]

Ulcerative Pododermatitis

Staphylococcus aureus is the primary causative agent of ulcerative pododermatitis in guinea pigs. A granuloma is present on the ventral surface of one or more of the patient's feet. The condition is also called bumblefoot and is comparable to that in poultry. Bumblefoot occurs most frequently in guinea pigs housed in cages with wire-mesh floors, particularly if the floors are rusted or soiled. Treatment involves removing the pigs to cages with clean, dry, soft bedding and giving antibiotics. Results are often discouraging because the inflammation is chronic and diffuse.[1,4]

Coccidiosis

Eimeria caviae is the usual causative agent of coccidiosis. The condition is normally nonpathogenic but rarely can cause colitis, diarrhea, and death. Because the sporulation time is 6 to 12 days, good sanitation disrupts the life cycle; prevention is thus uncomplicated. Clinical disease is rare. Diagnosis depends on isolation of the organism in feces. Sulfonamides given in the drinking water are effective if treatment is required.[4]

Trauma

In pet guinea pigs, the most common traumatic injury is fracture of the rear leg. The tibia is usually the bone involved. As mentioned, such fracture can occur when the pig catches a leg in wire flooring material. In addition, the fracture might result from the animal being dropped by a child. A simple, lightweight splint can be applied to provide support for the fractured bone.[7]

Ketosis

Ketosis is usually seen in well-nourished sows in late pregnancy, but it can occur in males or virgin females. The exact cause of ketosis is unknown, but a history of change in diet or housing is often noted.

Onset is acute. Patients demonstrate signs of lassitude and severe depression. Treatment consists of intravenous or intraperitoneal lactated Ringer's solution, calcium gluconate, or dextrose in conjunction with corticosteroids. The prognosis is poor.[1]

Alopecia

Diffuse alopecia over the flanks and back develops in all sows in late pregnancy. Thinning of hair occurs near the time of weaning during the transition from baby fur to adult hair.[7] Although the exact cause is unknown, alopecia is also apparently associated with stress conditions. Alopecia with a distinctive pattern or patch distribution can result from hair chewing, or so-called barbering. Animals can chew their own hair or that of a cage mate. The location of hair loss can provide a clue as to whether the loss is self-

inflicted or has resulted from barbering by a cage mate. Because pigs that barber themselves cannot reach the head or neck, these areas will not show evidence of hair loss.[3]

There is no specific treatment for alopecia other than the removal of an offending animal if hair loss resulted from barbering. When separation of the animals is impossible, providing good-quality hay might be a beneficial treatment for barbering problems by allowing the offending pig to chew and tug at something else as well as smaller pigs to escape by burrowing and hiding in the hay. Other measures to lower stress should also be taken.[1]

Preputial Infection and Vaginitis

Male guinea pigs sometimes develop preputial infections as a result of foreign material (e.g., bedding) becoming lodged in the preputial folds. Treatment consists of removing the particles and cleansing the area. Vaginitis in female guinea pigs is usually caused by entrapment of bedding in the vagina; a foreign-body reaction results. The problem is corrected by washing the area carefully and swabbing away the chips. It is usually helpful to place the patient on a different type of bedding until the area heals.[1]

Water Deprivation

Guinea pigs occasionally experience water deprivation even though an apparently adequate supply of water is present. Such deprivation occurs when (1) the pet is unfamiliar with or does not know how to manipulate the water-supplying device, (2) water devices are positioned too high or otherwise out of reach, (3) water is undrinkable because of impurities or odors in the device or in the water itself, (4) water devices or sipper tubes become unworkable because of air locks or lodged foreign material, or (5) territorialism on the part of dominant animals prevents less-aggressive individuals from drinking.[1]

Socialization

Because guinea pigs live in clans in the wild, domesticated pigs are generally more content when kept in pairs, especially if the owner is away for long periods. A single guinea pig, however, will thrive and develop a strong attachment to its owner if given an adequate amount of attention and affection. If two animals are kept, it is preferable that they be females, which are less likely to fight.[8]

Allergenicity

The guinea pig is among the worst animals for provoking allergic reactions in people. Children who are asthmatic or develop severe allergies should not keep guinea pigs as pets.[1]

Conclusion

Many practical reasons account for the popularity of guinea pigs as pets. They are inexpensive to purchase and maintain, have little odor, and are quiet and pleasant. The owner's attention to proper husbandry practices will lead to a rewarding relationship with the pet and assure it a long, healthy life.

REFERENCES

1. Holmes D: The guinea pig, in *Clinical Laboratory Animal Medicine*. Ames, IA, Iowa State University Press, 1984, pp 34–44.
2. Harkness JE, Wagner JE: *The Biology and Medicine of Rabbits and Rodents*. Philadelphia, Lea & Febiger, 1977, pp 14–16.
3. Arrington LR: *Introductory Laboratory Animal Medicine*, ed 2. Danville, IL, Interstate Printers and Publishers, 1978, pp 13–151.
4. Williams CSF: The guinea pig, in *Practical Guide to Laboratory Animals*. St. Louis, CV Mosby Co, 1976, pp 12–25.
5. Clifford DR: What the practicing veterinarian should know about guinea pigs. *VM SAC* 68:678–685, 1973.
6. Herrlein HG: *A Practical Guide on the Care and Use of Small Animals in Medical Research*. New City, NY, Rockland Farms, 1949, pp 49–54.
7. Wagner JE, Manning PJ: *The Biology of the Guinea Pig*. New York, Academic Press, 1976, pp 6–23.
8. Bielfeld H: *Guinea Pigs*. Woodbury, NY, Barron's Educational Series, 1983, pp 23–34.
9. Manning PJ, Wagner JE, Harkness JE: Biology and diseases of the guinea pig, in Fox JG (ed): *Laboratory Animal Medicine*. New York, Academic Press, 1984, pp 149–155.

Dermatology of Rabbits, Rodents, and Ferrets

Diplomate, ABVP (Avian Practice)
Petra Burgmann, BSc, DVM

It has been said that diseases in exotics are basically no different than those in any other species, and that the same principles of diagnosis apply equally well to these species as they do to any other. This is in fact true, but it is important not to extrapolate too far from one species to another. Just as there is no canine version of feline "endocrine" alopecia, one must recognize that certain species-specific peculiarities do exist.

The purpose of this chapter is to describe not only those skin diseases most frequently seen in the commonly kept exotics—rabbits, rodents, and ferrets—but to present them in such a way that the species-specific differences can be easily identified.

The Parasite Diagnostic Key (Table I) lists the most commonly encountered skin parasites, while the Therapeutic Key (Table II) lists the most common treatments. Certain parasitic skin diseases and some treatments are described more fully in the text because of their importance in that species.

Therapeutics in exotics is a controversial issue because practically none of the drugs commonly used are approved for use in these species. Because most treatments have evolved through a "hit and miss" type of system, there are great discrepancies in the literature concerning not only which drugs to use, but at what dose to administer them. The treatments listed are those that I have used myself, or that have had at least two references in the literature. A special caution must be given with reference to the use of antibiotics. Fatal reactions to antibiotics are common, as either a direct toxic effect or indirectly because of an alteration of the normal bacterial flora. If a certain drug is not listed for a particular species, try to choose one that has been listed.

MICE

Although they are one of the less frequently encountered exotic pets in private practice, mice are prone to a variety of unique dermatologic conditions.

Bacterial Conditions

Bacterial dermatitis and abscesses are most commonly caused by *Staphylococcus aureus* and *Streptococcus* spp. These infections are often secondary to a pri-

TABLE I
Parasite Diagnostic Key

Parasite	Description	Distinguishing Features	Host	Usual Habitat	Life Cycle	Pathologic Effects	Other Health Significance
Ornithonyssus bacoti	Blood-sucking mite, rare	750 μm long	Wild rodents, mice, rats, hamsters	Crevices, bedding, wild rodent burrows	13 days; female survives off host up to 70 days	Anemia, debilitation	Can harbour eastern equine encephalitis (EEE) virus, typhus, Q fever, plague, natural vector for tularemia, dermatitis in humans
Trombicula alfreddugesi	Chigger mite, rare	200–400 μm long; red to yellow, 6-legged larvae	Rodents, rabbits	Only larval stage is parasitic; other stages free-living in soil	On host only a few hours or days	Intense pruritus, swelling, lasting days to weeks	Painful bite, pruritus in humans
Fleas, various spp.	Common	1–3 mm long	Rabbits, ferrets, rodents	Pelage, bedding, environment	16–21 days; can survive off host for months	Pruritus, allergic dermatitis, anemia, debilitation	Vector for sylvatic plague, tularemia, intermediate host for tapeworms
Cuterebra spp.	Fly larvae, common	20–42 mm long	Rabbits, rodents, ferrets	Eggs at entrance to burrows	Enter via nose or mouth; migrate to subcutaneous location	Subcutaneous mass, weight loss, debilitation	None
Myobia musculi	Fur mite, common	300–500 μm long; single empodial claw or tarsi of second pair of legs	Mice	Pelage, especially head, ears, back	23 days; eggs hatch in 8 days	Inapparent to severe allergic dermatitis with pruritus, alopecia, ulceration	None known
Myocoptes musculinis	Fur mite, common	200–300 μm long; dark brown; 3rd and 4th leg pairs	Mice	Pelage, especially inguinal region, abdomen, and back	Probably 8–14 days; eggs hatch in 5 days	Inapparent to erythematous dermatitis, patchy alopecia	None known
Radfordia affinis	Fur mite, common	300–500 μm long; pair of subequal terminal claws on tarsi of second pair of legs	Mice	Pelage, especially head, back	Unknown, probably 21–23 days	Dermatitis, pruritus, alopecia	None known
Psorergates simplex	Follicle mite, rare	90–150 μm, rounded body	Mice	Fur follicles	Unknown	Dermal pouches on visceral skin surface, occasionally scabby dermatitis of ears	None
Polyplax serrata	Sucking louse, rare	0.6–1.5 mm long; eggs fastened near skin	Mice	Pelage, especially shoulders	13 days; eggs hatch in 5–6 days	Pruritus, dermatitis, restlessness, debilitation, anemia	Vector of murine haemobartonellosis, eperythrozoonosis, possible vector of tularemia

TABLE I (continued)

Parasite	Description	Distinguishing Features	Host	Usual Habitat	Life Cycle	Pathologic Effects	Other Health Significance
Notoedres spp.	Burrowing mite, rare	200–400 µm long; anus located dorsally	Hamsters	Ears, especially nose, feet, genitalia, tail	6–10 days	Papilloma-like yellow crusts, hyperkeratosis	None
Demodex criceti	Follicle mite, common	80–100 µm long; short stubby body	Hamsters	Skin follicles	Unkown; probably 10–15 days	Unknown	None
Demodex aurati	Follicle mite, common	150–200 µm long; cigar-shaped	Hamsters	Skin follicles	Unknown; probably 10–15 days	Moderate to severe dry, scaly alopecia usually nonpruritic	None
Demodex spp.	Follicle mite, uncommon	100–400 µm long	Gerbils	Skin follicles	Unknown; probably 10–15 days	Alopecia, dermatitis	None
Radfordia ensifera	Fur mite, common	300–500 µm long; pair of equal terminal claws on tarsi of second pair of legs	Rats	Pelage, especially head, back	Unknown	Dermatitis, pruritus, self-inflicted trauma	None known
Notoedres muris	Burrowing mite, rare	200–400 µm long; anus located dorsally	Rats	Especially ears, nose, tail; occasionally genitalia, limbs	19–21 days; eggs hatch in 4–5 days	Papilloma-like, yellow crusts on ears, nose; papular dermatitis; hyperkeratosis	None
Polyplax spinulosa	Sucking louse, rare	0.6–1.5 mm long; eggs fastened near skin	Rats	Pelage, especially back	26 days; eggs hatch in 5–6 days	Pruritus, dermatitis, restlessness, debilitation, anemia	Vector of murine haemobartonellosis, typhus between rodents
Chirodiscoides caviae	Fur mite, common	350–500 µm long; often joined in pairs	Guinea pigs	Deep in pelage, especially back	Unknown	Inapparent to pruritus, alopecia	None
Trixacarus caviae	Burrowing mite, common	200–400 µm long; anus located terminally	Guinea pigs	Especially neck, shoulders, lower abdomen	Probably 10–14 days	Intense pruritus, hyperkeratosis, alopecia, self-inflicted trauma, debilitation	Dermatitis in humans
Gliricola porcelli	Biting louse, common	1–1.5 mm long; narrow head and body; eggs fastened to fur	Guinea pigs	Pelage, especially around ears	Unknown	Pruritus, unthriftiness, alopecia	None known

TABLE I (continued)

Parasite	Description	Distinguishing Features	Host	Usual Habitat	Life Cycle	Pathologic Effects	Other Health Significance
Gyropus ovalis	Biting louse, common	1–1.2 mm long; wide head, oval body; eggs fastened to fur	Guinea pigs	Pelage, especially around ears	Unknown	Pruritus, unthriftiness, alopecia	None known
Cheyletiella parasitovorax	Fur mite, common	350–500 μm long	Rabbits	Pelage, especially between shoulders, ears, back	14–21 days; female can survive off host 10–14 days	Mild alopecia, scaling to erythematous, oily dermatitis with pruritus	Transient dermatitis in humans
Listrophorus gibbus	Fur mite	300–500 μm long	Rabbits	Back, abdomen	Unknown	None	None known
Sarcoptes scabei cuniculi	Burrowing mite, rare	200–400 μm long; anus located terminally	Rabbits	Especially head, neck, ears, then generalized	17–23 days; eggs hatch in 3–8 days	Intense pruritus, alopecia	Dermatitis in humans
Notoedres cati var. *cuniculi*	Burrowing mite, rare	200–400 μm long	Rabbits	Skin of head, ears, neck, forelegs	21 days	Crusts, hyperkeratosis, pruritus, alopecia, self-inflicted trauma	Transient dermatitis in humans
Psoroptes cuniculi	Ear mite, common	400–800 μm long	Rabbits	Ear canals, occasionally face, neck, legs, inguinal region	21 days; eggs hatch in 4 days	Dry tan crusty exudate; when removed reveals moist, red painful otitis; pruritic dermatitis	None known
Haemodipsus ventricosis	Sucking louse, rare	1.2–2.5 mm long; eggs oval with operculum	Rabbits	Pelage, especially back and sides	30 days; eggs hatch in 7 days	Extreme pruritus, alopecia, anemia debilitation	Vector of *Francisella tularensis* in rabbits (cause of tularemia)
Sarcoptes scabei spp.	Burrowing mite, uncommon	200–400 μm long; anus located terminally	Ferrets	Feet, or generalized	17–23 days	Erythematous, swollen feet, or generalized alopecia, intense pruritus	Dermatitis in humans
Otodectes cynotis	Ear mite, common	450 μm long	Ferrets	Ear canals, skin	21–28 days	Otitis, occasionally pruritus	Zoonotic to cats, dogs

TABLE II
Therapeutic Key

	Mice	Hamsters	Gerbils	Rats	Guinea Pigs	Chinchillas	Rabbits	Ferrets
Antibiotics								
Amikacin*	10 mg/kg IM/SC sid	10 mg/kg IM/SC sid	10 mg/kg IM/SC sid	10 mg/kg IM/SC sid	10–15 mg/kg IM/SC sid	8–16 mg/kg IM, IV, SC sid	8–16 mg/kg IM, IV, SC sid	8–16 mg/kg IM, IV, SC sid
Ampicillin†	20–100 mg/kg divided dose PO/SC tid	DO NOT USE	20–100 mg/kg divided dose PO/SC tid	20–100 mg/kg divided dose PO/SC tid	DO NOT USE	DO NOT USE	DO NOT USE	5–10 mg/kg IM/SC bid
Chloramphenicol succinate	30 mg/kg IM/SC sid 5–7 days	30 mg/kg IM/SC sid 5–7 days	30 mg/kg IM/SC sid 5–7 days	30 mg/kg IM/SC sid 5–7 days	30 mg/kg IM/SC sid 5–7 days	30 mg/kg IM/SC sid 5–7 days	30 mg/kg IM/SC sid 5–7 days	30 mg/kg IM/SC sid 5–7 days
Chloramphenicol palmitate	50 mg/kg PO bid 5–7 days	50 mg/kg PO bid 5–7 days	50 mg/kg PO bid 5–7 days	50 mg/kg PO bid 5–7 days	50 mg/kg PO bid 5–7 days	50 mg/kg PO bid 5–7 days	50 mg/kg PO bid 5–7 days	50 mg/kg PO bid 5–7 days
Doxycycline	2.5 mg/kg PO bid	2.5 mg/kg PO bid	2.5 mg/kg PO bid	2.5 mg/kg PO bid	2.5 mg/kg PO bid	2.5 mg/kg PO bid	2.5 mg/kg PO bid	2.5 mg/kg PO bid
Enrofloxacin‡	2.5–10 mg/kg PO bid	2.5–10 mg/kg PO bid	2.5–10 mg/kg PO bid	2.5–10 mg/kg PO bid	2.5–10 mg/kg PO bid	2.5–10 mg/kg PO/IM/SC bid	2.5–10 mg/kg PO/IM/SC bid	2.5–10 mg/kg PO/IM/SC bid
Gentamicin*	2.5–5 mg/kg IM/SC sid 5 days	2.5–5 mg/kg IM/SC sid 5 days	2.5–5 mg/kg IM/SC sid 5 days	2.5–5 mg/kg IM/SC sid 5 days	2.5–5 mg/kg IM/SC sid 5 days	2.5–5 mg/kg IM/SC sid 5 days	2.5–5 mg/kg IM/SC sid 5 days	4–8 mg/kg IM/SC sid 5 days
Tetracycline hydrochloride	10–20 mg/kg SC/PO bid	10–20 mg/kg SC/PO bid	10–20 mg/kg SC/PO bid	10–20 mg/kg SC/PO bid	10–20 mg/kg SC/PO bid	25 mg/kg SC/PO bid	25 mg/kg SC/PO bid	25 mg/kg SC/PO bid
Trimethoprim/ sulfadiazine	30 mg/kg SC sid	30 mg/kg SC sid	30 mg/kg SC sid	30 mg/kg SC sid	30 mg/kg SC sid	30 mg/kg SC sid	30 mg/kg SC sid	30 mg/kg SC sid
Trimethoprim/ sulfamethoxazole	15 mg/kg PO bid	15 mg/kg PO bid	15 mg/kg PO bid	15 mg/kg PO bid	15 mg/kg PO bid	15 mg/kg PO bid	15 mg/kg PO bid	15 mg/kg PO bid
Tylosin	10 mg/kg IM sid 5 days	10 mg/kg IM sid 5 days	10 mg/kg IM sid 5 days	10 mg/kg IM/PO sid 5–7 days				10 mg/kg PO sid 5–7 days
Antifungals								
Griseofulvin	25 mg/kg PO sid 14 days	25 mg/kg PO sid 14–28 days	25 mg/kg PO sid 14–28 days	25 mg/kg PO sid 14–28 days	25 mg/kg PO sid 14–28 days	25 mg/kg PO sid 4–6 weeks	25 mg/kg PO sid 4–6 weeks	25 mg/kg PO sid 4–6 weeks

*Nephrotoxic; concurrent fluid therapy advised; total daily dose may also be divided bid-tid.
†Prolonged use may result in changes in microbial flora and diarrhea.
‡Parenteral use may cause skin slough; not for use in young animals.

TABLE II (continued)

	Indications	Dosage (for all of the above species)	Route
Antiparasitics[1]			
Amitraz (Mitaban® — Upjohn)	*Demodex, Sarcoptes*	3–6 treatments 14 days apart	Topical
5% Carbaryl powder	Fur mites, fleas, lice	Dust lightly once weekly for 3–6 treatments	Topical
Ivermectin (Ivomec® — MSD AGVET)	*Sarcoptes, Psoroptes, Otodectes,* fur mites, lice	200–400 µg/kg 7–14 days apart	Per os or subcutaneously
Lime sulfur	*Sarcoptes,* fur mites	Dilute 1:40 with water; apply once weekly for 6 weeks	Topical
Lindane (Rogar® — STB)	Fur mites	0.03% dip once weekly for 3 weeks	Topical
Malathion	Fur mites, lice	2% dip every 10 days for 3 treatments	Topical
Pyrethrin .05% shampoo	Mites, lice, fleas	Shampoo once weekly for 3–6 treatments	Topical
Tresaderm® (MSD AGVET)	*Otodectes, Psoroptes*	2–5 drops in each ear bid for 7 days; repeat in 2 weeks	Topical

[1]The applications for antiparasitics are appropriate for all animals mentioned in previous page.

(continued from page 174)

mary wound caused by fighting amongst males, or by self-trauma because of acariasis. Treatment consists of eliminating the inciting cause, lancing the wound if necessary, cleansing the wound with 3% hydrogen peroxide, and treating with an appropriate antibiotic. Topical preparations are often unrewarding in this species because of their fastidious grooming habits.

Corynebacterium kutscheri and *Pasteurella pneumotropica* have also been identified as infrequent, opportunistic pathogens of mice. *C. kutscheri* can produce septic emboli, causing infarction of dermal vessels that results in skin necrosis and ulceration. *P. pneumotropica* can cause superficial lesions and subcutaneous abscesses. Culture and sensitivity will aid in diagnosis and choice of an appropriate antibiotic.

Furunculosis in genetically nude mice has also been reported, but is obviously rarely encountered in private practice.

Viral Conditions
Mousepox (Ectromelia)

Although not uncommon in breeding stocks of mice in China, Japan, England, and Europe, mousepox is rare in North America and is unlikely to be encountered in private practice. It has been imported into laboratory facilities in the United States on several occasions via live mice, mouse tissues, or tumors, causing severe epizootics. Caused by an orthopoxvirus, the usual route of infection is via skin abrasions on the face, feet, or abdomen from virus-contaminated bedding or cage surfaces. Most susceptible mice die shortly after the primary eruption, but those that survive the acute infection often develop a dermatitis. The severity of the eruption is determined by the extent of secondary viremia. The lesion can be solitary or generalized. The eruption goes through a macular, vesicular, and pustular stage, and will recede within a few weeks. Necrosis of the dermal epithelium can produce a surface scab that heals as a hairless scar, but severe infection of the feet or tail can cause them to become gangrenous and drop off, hence the name *infectious ectromelia*.

Diagnosis is by microscopic examination of tissues revealing eosinophilic cytoplasmic inclusion bodies, or by electron microscopy revealing the orthopoxvirus. Treatment consists of eradication and disinfection, or vaccination with the vaccinia virus by scarification of the base of the tail.

Fungal Conditions

Several dermatomycoses have been reported to occur in mice, but these infections, commonly known as *ringworm*, are caused most often by *Trichophyton mentagrophytes*. Mice are often asymptomatic, but stressed or debilitated animals may exhibit clinical signs of a sparse haircoat or a well-demarcated crusty lesion with focal hair loss, erythema, and scaling. Lesions on the tail are common.

Diagnosis is by microscopic examination of skin scrapings macerated in 10% potassium hydroxide (KOH) for 30 to 60 minutes and identification of mycelia or arthrospores, or by growth of the fungus on dermatophyte test medium (for example, Fungassay®-Pitman-Moore). Because the organism grows slowly, cultures should be held for 3 weeks for a definitive diagnosis.

Treatment includes disinfecting the environment, clipping the hair around the lesions, and treating orally with griseofulvin. Griseofulvin should not be used in pregnant animals because of possible teratogenic effects. Topical creams are of little use in this species because of their fastidious grooming habits. It is always important to remember the zoonotic potential of dermatophytes, particularly because many of these "pocket pets" are carried around inside their owners' clothing, and *T. mentagrophytes* is highly infectious for humans. It is not unusual for lesions to be noticed first on an owner, while the rodent remains an asymptomatic carrier.

Parasitic Conditions

Mites are very common in mice and infestations are frequently encountered in private practice. *Myocoptes musculinis* is the most common ectoparasite, although it frequently is found in conjunction with *Myobia musculi*. When both mites are present on the same host, *Myocoptes* tends to crowd out populations of *Myobia*. *Radfordia affinis* is also frequently encountered.

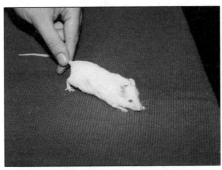

Figure 1—Clinical lesions of *Myobia musculi* infestation on the head and flank.

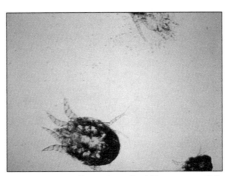

Figure 2—*Myobia musculi*. (Courtesy of S. W. Barthold, Yale University, New Haven, Connecticut)

Lesions consist of varying degrees of alopecia and ulceration, usually involving the neck, lateral thorax, and flank regions (Figure 1). The scabby to ulcerative dermatitis of *Myobia* is actually caused by self-trauma, induced as a pruritic response to the mite allergen. It has been found that certain genetic strains of mice are more susceptible to an allergic response to the mites than other strains. In these mice even a very low parasite burden can cause extensive skin lesions. The mite is spread by direct contact, usually from parents to offspring, but lesions usually do not develop until the mouse reaches maturity, indicating that a period of sensitization is required even in susceptible strains. Once the hypersensitivity has developed, however, exposure to even a few mites will result in an anamnestic response, with lesions developing within 1 to 2 days of exposure. The lesions of *Myocoptes* are also pruritic, but tend not to be as ulcerative as those of *Myobia*. It has been said that the mites are difficult to eliminate, but I suspect that in those cases treatment likely was not intensive enough.

Diagnosis is by skin scrapings and mite identification (Figure 2). The main differences between the three mites are described in the Parasite Diagnostic Key (Table I).

Treatment consists of a weekly light dusting with a 5% carbaryl powder, thorough cage disinfection, and the use of a dichlorvos-impregnated resin strip hung in the pet's room for 24 hours once a week for 6 weeks. Certainly this approach is not applicable in a laboratory setting, but it can be quite efficacious for treatment of an individual pet. Because of the 23-day life cycle of the mite *Myobia* and the resistance of the egg to insecticides, treatment in a laboratory setting must consist of at least two treatments, with the second treatment occurring between 8 and 10 days after the first. A 1 x 2-inch piece of a dichlorvos-impregnated resin strip placed on the cage for 24 hours for two treatments is the most widely advocated treatment for the laboratory setting. An alternative treatment consists of two subcutaneous injections of ivermectin given at 200 µg/kg 8 days apart. Concurrent treatment of the environment is still advisable.

Polyplax serrata, the mouse louse, is rare, but when encountered is significant because of its zoonotic importance as a possible vector of tularemia. It is spread by direct contact. Treatment is the same as that described for mites.

Nutritional Conditions

Recognition of nutritional deficiencies in rodent species encountered in private practice is rare. Most of the deficiencies described in the literature have been experimentally induced; the most important of these experimental findings have been included for the sake of completeness. Mice have an absolute requirement for linoleic and arachidonic acids. Chronic essential fatty acid deficiency can lead to hair loss and dermatitis with scaling and crusting of the skin. Zinc deficiency can cause hair loss on shoulders and neck.

Several varieties of rodent chow are commercially available and are nutritionally complete; however, owners must be reminded that freshness and quality should be considered when purchasing these foods.

Neoplastic Conditions

Spontaneous skin tumors are rare in mice, although many have been experimentally induced. Of those encountered naturally, squamous cell carcinoma appears to be the most prevalent. Spontaneous tumors of the Harderian gland occur frequently. These tumors appear late in life and grow slowly, but may cause proptosis of the eye.

Miscellaneous Conditions
Facial Hair Loss

Facial hair loss resulting from friction on cage bars or feeders, or barbering of the vibrissae or head by a dominant mouse or cage-mates during crowding or stress, is common in mice (Figure 3). A thorough history and examination of the cage will often provide a simple solution, such as separating cage-mates or removing offending objects from the environment. In most cases hair regrowth will be complete in 30 days, although some small patches of alopecia can remain for up to 90 days depending on the phase of the hair cycle.

Dry Gangrene

Dry gangrene of the ear tips in mice was reported in one instance, and appeared to be associated with cold environmental temperatures as well as self-trauma caused by parasite infestation. An area of hyperemia was first noted in the distal third of the ear, followed by a distinct line of demarcation and a gray ear tip that would slough within a few days. The lesions were self-limiting once the inciting causes had been eliminated.

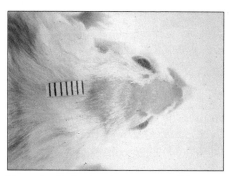

Figure 3—Barbering in a mouse. (Courtesy of D.H. Percy, Ontario Veterinary College, Guelph, Ontario, Canada)

RATS
Chromodacryorrhea

Of all the rodents, rats are the species most frequently presented because of chromodacryorrhea. Chromodacryorrhea refers to the ability of various rodents to secrete a porphyrin-containing pigment from the eyes. The red pigments are produced in the Harderian gland and are secreted in response to parasympathetic stimulation under stress or as a result of certain diseases. Discharge from the eyes can be profuse and can also stain the forepaws, and is often mistaken for blood by the owner. Treatment consists of identifying and removing the underlying cause of stress, or identifying and treating the disease state. Sialodacryoadenitis virus can also cause marked Harderian gland secretion and is described below.

Bacterial Conditions

An ulcerative dermatitis caused by *Staphylococcus aureus* is common in rats, particularly in young males. Lesions begin on the neck and shoulders and appear as irregularities in the haircoat with small focal areas of alopecia or ulceration, and can progress to involve the entire anterior trunk with extensive ulcerations. Some lesions scab and regress spontaneously, while others are pruritic and stimulate scratching and self-mutilation. Treatment includes cleaning the wounds with hydrogen peroxide, choosing an appropriate oral antibiotic, and clipping the toenails to reduce self-mutilation. Underlying acariasis may be a contributing factor and should be considered in the etiology of the lesions.

Pasteurella pneumotropica has also been implicated as a cause of skin abscessation, although it often occurs as a secondary opportunist. Treatment is the same as that described above.

Ulcerative pododermatitis is also encountered from time to time in private practice. The cause is unknown, but wire-bottomed cages or rough cage surfaces may be contributing factors. One report implicated exercise wheels used in their experiments as a contributing factor. The lesions are often difficult to treat; bandaging to allow healing may be of use in severe cases as well as eliminating the inciting cause and treating with an appropriate antibiotic.

Viral Conditions

Sialodacryoadenitis, a very common disease in research facilities, is caused by a coronavirus. Transmission occurs by direct exposure to virus-laden nasal secretions or fomites. Clinical signs include profuse chromodacryorrhea, cervical lymphadenitis, sneezing, keratoconjunctivitis, and corneal lesions. Clinical signs develop within 8 to 10 days of exposure to virus-infected rats. Complete recovery usually occurs within 30 days, and no latent carrier state is known. Diagnosis is by the characteristic clinical signs, virus isolation, or acute and convalescent antibody titers. Immunity is conferred for one year after exposure. No vaccine exists, and prevention is best accomplished by preventing exposure.

Pox infection in rats has been reported but is extremely rare. Lesions are similar to those described for mousepox.

Fungal Conditions

Dermatophyte (ringworm) infections are rare in rats. If present, *Trichophyton mentagrophytes* is the most commonly encountered fungus. Rats usually are asymptomatic, but a patchy alopecia with scale, papules, and pustules is sometimes seen, primarily over the back. Diagnosis and treatment are the same as that described for mice.

Parasitic Conditions

Radfordia ensifera is a commonly encountered fur mite of rats. Small scabby lesions around the head and shoulders are caused by self-inflicted trauma as a result of the pruritus caused by the mite allergen. Diagnosis and treatment are the same as that described for mice.

Polyplax spinulosa, the blood-sucking louse of rats, is rarely encountered in private practice, as is the mite *Notoedres*. Both are described in the Parasite Diagnostic Key (Table I). Treatment for lice is the same as that described for fur mites in mice. Treatment of *Notoedres* consists of bathing the affected area with a 0.05% pyrethrin shampoo and applying lime sulfur topically to the affected areas with a cotton swab. Two oral doses of ivermectin given at 200 μg/kg a week apart will also be beneficial in treating this condition.

Nutritional Conditions

Of all the species maintained under laboratory conditions, the most is known about the dietary requirements of rats. Again, dietary deficiencies are seldom reported in private practice, but are included here for completeness. Deficiencies in linoleic, linolenic, or arachidonic acids have been reported to result in reduced hair growth, alopecia, scaly skin, and cutaneous ulceration in rats. As is reported for hamsters, vitamin A deficiency may result in a thin, coarse haircoat and keratinizing squamous metaplasia. Deficiency in vitamin B₂ (ri-

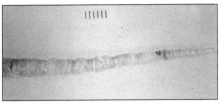

Figure 4—Ringtail in a rat. (Courtesy of D.H. Percy, Ontario Veterinary College, Guelph, Ontario, Canada)

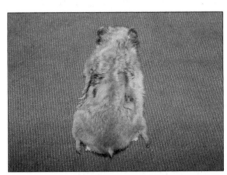

Figure 5—Normal pigmented "hip" or "flank" gland in a male hamster.

boflavin) can cause dermatitis and alopecia, whereas deficiency in vitamin B₆ (pyridoxine) can cause hair loss and achromotrichia (loss of hair pigmentation). Achromotrichia is also reported in copper deficiency in rats. Biotin deficiency can cause dermatitis, alopecia, and achromotrichia.

Neoplastic Conditions

Spontaneous tumors of the skin and subcutis are uncommon in rats; when they do occur, they usually are found around the head, tail, or paws. Papillomas, basal cell carcinomas, and squamous cell carcinomas are the most frequent types. Basal cell tumors may be locally invasive, but tend not to metastasize. Squamous cell carcinomas are locally invasive and may metastasize to other areas. Squamous cell carcinomas of the face and head are highly invasive but seldom metastatic and often start as a sebaceosquamous tumor from the glands of Zymbal in the ear.

Subcutaneous mesenchymal tumors, such as fibromas, fibrosarcomas, lipomas and undifferentiated sarcomas, are more common than epithelial tumors. Benign mammary fibroadenomas are the most frequently encountered tumors in rats in private practice, and can occur in both males and females.

Treatment of all tumor types is surgical excision where applicable. A subcuticular line of closure will prevent the rat from chewing out the stitches.

Miscellaneous Conditions

Ringtail describes a condition in which there are one or more annular constrictions of the tail (Figure 4). Distal to the constrictions the tail can become edematous, then necrotic, and, if sloughed, usually heals without complications. The condition occurs most often in unweaned rats 7 to 15 days of age and is caused by housing the animals in less than 20% humidity. Seen most frequently in winter as a result of the use of heating systems, treatment consists of raising the humidity level to 50%, reducing air turnover in laboratory facilities, and providing solid-bottomed cages with nesting material for nursing dams. Ringtail is rarely encountered in private practice.

HAMSTERS

Hamsters have two well-developed dark-pigmented "hip glands" located on either side of the midline in the flank region (Figure 5). Poorly developed and scarcely visible in the female, the glands are more prominent in the male. Thought to be used for olfactory identification of territory, when the male becomes sexually excited the fur around the gland becomes wet and he scratches and rubs at the gland. This activity often is incorrectly interpreted as pruritus of a skin lesion by the owner, who is often unaware that these glands exist.

Bacterial Conditions

Skin and cheek pouch abscesses caused by *Staphylococcus aureus* and *Streptococcus* spp. are fairly common in hamsters (Figure 6). Treatment is the same as that described for mice.

Viral Conditions

A papovavirus has been identified as a cause of cutaneous epitheliomas in hamsters. The lesions usually are wart-like, and occur most often around the eyes, mouth, or perianal area. The condition is rare but the virus is highly contagious, has a long incubation period, and is very resistant. It has also been implicated in several other disease processes in infected colonies. No individual treatment for this condition has been described, but its presence in a laboratory setting could have serious consequences; therefore, depopulation and strict sanitation is advised.

Fungal Conditions

Dermatophytosis (ringworm) is rarely reported in hamsters but it can occur. As in other rodents, *T. mentagrophytes* is the most likely cause. Treatment is the same as that described for mice.

Parasitic Conditions

Demodex is particularly common in hamsters older than 1.5 years of age and is frequently secondary to immunosuppression malnutrition, or concurrent systemic disease. Two types of demodectic mange mites are recognized in hamsters. *Demodex criceti* is a short stubby-bodied mite that generally is considered to be non-pathogenic. *D. aurati* is a cigar-shaped mite that burrows in the pilosebaceous component of the skin, causing a moderate to severe, dry, scaly alopecia which starts over the back and can extend to involve the entire body (Figure 7). Transmission occurs from mother to young during the time of suckling. Diagnosis is by recovering mites from skin scrapings, although examination of clinically normal hamsters has revealed mild to

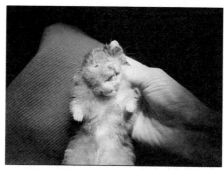

Figure 6—Jaw abscess in a hamster.

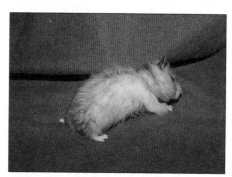

Figure 7—Demodicosis in a hamster.

moderate infestations with *D. aurati* and in other cases the mites have been difficult to demonstrate on skin scrapings.

A variety of different miticidal preparations have been used with varying success, but in my experience it is important to recognize that the mange is more likely indicative of an underlying problem that has predisposed the hamster to the condition than a serious disease entity in its own right. Weekly bathing of the hamster with a benzoyl peroxide shampoo will stimulate follicular flushing and reduce the mite load, followed by topical application of a miticidal preparation, such as amitraz, by cotton swab to the most severely affected areas. Lime sulfur is an additional option.

Nutritional Conditions

As with most of the commonly kept small rodents, dietary deficiencies are seldom seen if the animal is maintained on a fresh, good quality, commercially available rodent chow. Several nutritional deficiencies have been produced experimentally, however, and are included here for the sake of completeness. Essential fatty acid deficiency causes hair loss, tight skin, and increased ear wax production in hamsters. Vitamin A deficiency results in a thin, coarse haircoat and keratinizing squamous metaplasia. Deficiency in vitamin B_2 (riboflavin) results in dermatitis and alopecia, whereas deficiency in vitamin B_6 (pyridoxine) results in hair loss and achromotrichia. Achromotrichia is also recorded in copper deficiency. Niacin deficiency has also been reported as a cause of alopecia and rough haircoat.

Neoplastic Conditions

Adenomas and carcinomas of the adrenal cortex and thyroid gland are common in hamsters, and it is reasonable to assume that they may present with some of the same cutaneous manifestations as do other species. Melanomas are also common, with a much higher incidence in males than females. Several other neoplasms have been described, although their incidence is sporadic. Diagnosis of these tumors can be made by skin biopsy. Treatment consists of surgical removal of the tumor where applicable.

One interesting report of cutaneous lymphoma resembling mycosis fungoides in humans was described in three pet hamsters. Clinical signs included erythema, alopecia, pruritus, and flaking skin, progressing to plaques or tumors (Figure 8). Anorexia, lethargy, and weight loss were also noted. No treatment was described.

Miscellaneous Conditions

Allergic dermatitis attributable to cedar or pine shavings has been seen by the author. Lesions consist of swelling of the face and feet with associated pruritus. In one instance several cases occurred in the course of one month. All the owners had recently purchased a fresh bag of shavings produced by a leading pet company. When the animals were housed on plain newspaper the lesions regressed spontaneously. Since then I have seen several more cases in which people have purchased bulk shavings from landscaping or nursery outlets. Presumably the shavings have been chemically treated in some way that causes a contact allergy.

One report described another lesion caused by wood shavings. In this case the footpads became thickened and developed granulomata. Histologic examination revealed a foreign body, giant cell reaction with wood shavings and sawdust seen within the lesions. When shredded paper was substituted for the shavings, no more lesions developed. A similar case recently presented to the author resolved with removal of the shavings.

GERBILS

Gerbils have an ovoid hairless ventral midline sebaceous gland which is especially pronounced in the male and is used for scent marking (Figure 9). The area is normally a tan color and has a clearly defined smooth border. This area is frequently involved in bacterial infections and tumors. Other than the conditions described below, skin conditions are less frequent in gerbils than in other species.

Bacterial Conditions

Nasal dermatitis in gerbils is a common problem af-

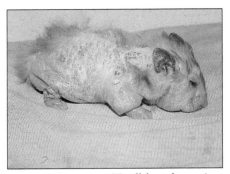

Figure 8—Cutaneous T-cell lymphoma in a hamster. (Courtesy of L.J. Ackerman, Mesa, Arizona)

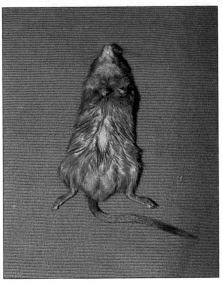

Figure 9—Normal sebaceous "scent" gland in a gerbil.

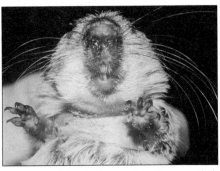

Figure 10—Nasal dermatitis in a gerbil. (Courtesy of R.D. Axelson, Willowdale, Ontario, Canada)

fecting 5% of the gerbil population. The lesions, which begin as erythemic, small crusts, or alopecia, surround the external nares, but often go on to involve the entire face, forepaws, and sometimes the abdomen with extensive moist dermatitis and alopecia (Figure 10). If not resolved, gerbils may become unthrifty and anoretic and die. Various theories have been presented to explain this phenomenon, including abrasion on rough cage surfaces, or staphylococcal or streptococcal infections. A recent theory postulates that hypersecretion of the Harderian gland or failure to spread the material by grooming leads to the dermatitis. The worst damage appears to be self-inflicted, as scratching with the forepaws leads to bleeding, scabbing, and alopecia. Treatment involves (1) cleaning the lesions of moist dermatitis with 3% hydrogen peroxide; (2) oral antibiotics to treat the secondary bacterial infection if present; and (3) permitting sandbathing to decrease the amount of Harderian gland lipids on the pelage.

The midventral sebaceous glands can become infected and abscessed, most often with staphylococci or streptococci. Because of the fastidious grooming habits of gerbils, topical ointments are not advised. Cleaning the lesions with 3% hydrogen peroxide and administering an appropriate oral antibiotic are more efficacious.

Fungal Conditions

Dermatophytosis (ringworm) is extremely rare in gerbils, although it can occur. Diagnosis and treatment is the same as that described for mice.

Parasitic Conditions

Apart from one reported case of demodicosis, external parasites are extremely rare in gerbils. In the one case of demodicosis reported, alopecia and focal ulcerative dermatitis was seen, but, as with hamsters, debility of aging appeared to be the predisposing factor in this case.

Nutritional Conditions

Information on the nutritional needs of gerbils is sparse; presumably they would exhibit clinical signs of deficiency similar to those of other rodents.

Neoplastic Conditions

Tumors have been reported in various sites in gerbils; the most frequent site of tumor development is the scent gland area. Sebaceous gland adenomas are most common, but basal cell and squamous cell carcinomas also occur. Treatment is by wide surgical excision of the tumor.

Miscellaneous Conditions

Gerbils are known for their sleek, smooth haircoat; however, when relative humidity is greater than 50%, the hair will often appear greasy and stand out instead of lying smoothly. Pine shavings can also cause this appearance.

Biting near the base of the tail causing denuded spots is common in overcrowded conditions. Tail chewing can occur because of boredom.

GUINEA PIGS

Skin diseases in guinea pigs are frequently encountered in private practice, particularly in recently purchased pets or in older males. A complete physical examination will often reveal at least one of the conditions listed below.

Bacterial Conditions
Ulcerative Pododermatitis

Ulcerative pododermatitis is caused by the organism *Staphylococcus aureus*. It is most frequently seen in obese animals housed on rough or soiled wire mesh floors, and presents as firm, ulcerated masses on the plantar surfaces, most commonly on the forefeet. If not treated, it can progress to osteoarthritis as the infection penetrates the tendon sheaths and joints. Amyloidosis of many organs has also been reported as a common sequel to severe infection.

Treatment consists of moving the animal to a smooth, clean cage surface, or in severe cases, housing the animal on 2 to 3 inches of clean, soft bedding. The nails should be trimmed and the feet treated topically. In cases of osteoarthritis, systemic antibiotics and bandaging may be of benefit.

Cervical Lymphadenitis

Cervical lymphadenitis is caused most frequently by the organism *Streptococcus zooepidemicus*. Soft, fluctuant subcutaneous masses appear in the ventral cervical region. These abscessed cervical lymph nodes can rupture spontaneously, exuding a thick, cream-colored pus. Diagnosis can be easily made by examination of a Gram stain of the material, which will reveal chains of gram-positive cocci. The organism is believed to be transmitted by a variety of routes, through small abrasions in the oral cavity caused by coarse plant feeds, such as hay or oats; through cutaneous bite wounds; or via the respiratory tract or conjunctiva. Septicemia is not an uncommon sequel, and in young animals may cause a fatal, generalized disease. The mortality rate is lower in older animals, although generalized lymphadenitis, pleuritis, pericarditis, arthritis, and nephritis have been described. Treatment consists of surgical drainage and debridement of the wound where required. Culture and sensitivity of the organism is warranted; chloramphenicol palmitate given at 50 mg/kg orally for 5 to 7 days is often the first drug of choice because it is one of the few antibiotics that is relatively safe in guinea pigs. Affected animals should be isolated to prevent the spread of infection.

Slobbers

Slobbers describes a condition in which excessive drooling, dysphagia, and weight loss are the predominant signs. The excessive drooling leads to matting of fur under the chin which may lead to a secondary bacterial dermatitis. Several causes have been suggested, the most likely of which is malocclusion because of the lower molars bridging over the tongue, or some other dental condition. Treatment consists of a thorough examination of the oral cavity under general anesthesia to determine the underlying cause, and cleaning the skin lesions with hydrogen peroxide and topical ointments.

Fungal Conditions

Spontaneous dermatophytosis has been reported to occur frequently in young guinea pigs, but any age group can be affected. Most often caused by *Trichophyton mentagrophytes*, the lesions usually involve the nose, face, and ears with a scaly alopecia. More generalized infection with moist, raised, hairless lesions called *kerions* can occur. Tufts of hair lifted from these lesions provide excellent specimens for examination. Fungal by-products diffused into the vascular tissue can be deposited as antigens in other parts of the skin. These lesions, usually found on the dorsal trunk or underside of the limbs, contain a sterile, clear liquid and represent an immune-mediated hypersensitivity reaction. Diagnosis and treatment is the same as that described for mice. An alternative treatment consists of using a 1.5% solution of griseofulvin in dimethyl sulfoxide (DMSO) applied daily to the lesions for 5 to 7 days. Topical antifungal preparations-such as miconazole nitrate (Conofite®—Pitman-Moore), are useful in guinea pigs.

Parasitic Conditions

The lice *Gyropus ovalis* and *Gliricola porcelli* are both very common in guinea pigs. Distinguishing features are listed in the Parasite Diagnostic Key (Table I). Mild infestations can be asymptomatic, although the nit eggs are readily visible attached to the shafts of the hairs around the ear and eye region (Figure 11). Severe infestations may cause alopecia and pruritus.

The fur mite *Chirodiscoides caviae* is also considered common, but infestations usually are asymptomatic. The small, nonburrowing mites can be found deep in the fur, usually over the dorsum. Pruritus and alopecia have been observed in heavy infestations.

Both of these parasite types can be treated with weekly insecticide baths, followed by a light dusting with a 5% carbaryl powder for six treatments. Disinfecting the environment and once weekly 24-hour exposure to a dichlorvos-impregnated resin strip hung in the pet's room for 6 weeks is also advisable.

The sarcoptic mange mite *Trixacarus caviae* causes a severe dermatitis with alopecia, epidermal scaling, hyperkeratosis, and intense pruritus (Figure 12). Lesions are first seen on the neck, shoulders, lower abdomen, and inner thighs, but can progress to a generalized, debilitating dermatitis. Diagnosis is best accomplished by deep skin scrapings cleared with 10% potassium hydroxide to reveal the sarcoptic mite. Weekly bathing with an antiparasitic shampoo, followed by 1:40 lime sulfur dips for 6 weeks or three weekly applications of 1% lindane, is usually effective. Ivermectin given at 200 μg/kg orally is also effective. This disease is also important because of its zoonotic potential.

Nutritional Conditions

As is well known, scurvy is an important condition in guinea pigs, and may first present as a roughened haircoat, anorexia, and a mild white crusty discharge from the eyes. A complete description of this condition is available in other reference texts.

Metastatic soft tissue calcification has often been reported over the years, but to date no clear cause has been identified. An imbalance in the relationship between calcium, phosphorus, and magnesium is suspected as the cause. Clinical signs include mineral deposits in soft tissue near the elbows and ribs, in the spinal column, gastrointestinal tract, and skeletal muscle. Stiff and sore carpi and small white foci of calcium phosphate crystals in the footpads also occur. No treatment is known.

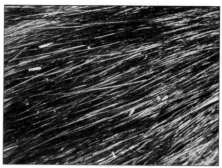

Figure 11—*Gliricola porcelli* in a guinea pig. (Courtesy of P. Lautenslauger, Ontario Veterinary College, Guelph, Ontario, Canada)

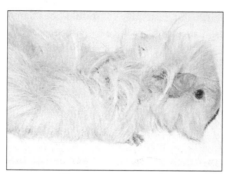

Figure 12—*Trixacarus caviae* infestation in a guinea pig. (Courtesy of L.J. Ackerman, Mesa, Arizona)

Fatty acid deficiency has been known to cause dermatitis, fur loss, and skin ulceration. Rough haircoat and skin atrophy have been seen with riboflavin deficiency.

Endocrine Conditions

Diffuse hair loss over the flanks and back in sows in late pregnancy is quite common, as is thinning of the haircoat in weanlings during the time of transition from baby fur to adult fur.

Marked shedding during stress is also very common. When a guinea pig is frightened or very ill, it is easy to epilate an entire spot of hair when tenting the skin for an injection.

Neoplastic Conditions

Neoplasms of the skin and subcutis occur infrequently in guinea pigs. Of these, benign trichofolliculomas occurring over the lumbar area appear to be the most common. They are described as unencapsulated multiloculated cysts lined by stratified squamous epithelium with abortive hair follicles. They are confined to the hypodermis and often contain hair, keratin, and sebum. Fibrosarcomas, sebaceous adenomas, and fibrolipomas have also been reported.

Miscellaneous Conditions

Overcrowding or stress often leads to barbering, either self-inflicted or by a cage-mate. Inadequate roughage can also cause this condition. Separating incompatible animals and adding alfalfa hay to the diet may help.

Mature males can produce a sebaceous secretion around the circumanal region that can almost occlude the anus. The plug can be softened with soap and water and removed. Washing the area periodically will prevent recurrence.

Mature males can also develop preputial infections when foreign materials, such as bedding, become entrapped in the preputial folds after mating. Bedding is drawn into the preputial fornix by adhering to the moistened prepuce. Once there it can cause a severe foreign body reaction. Removing the foreign body and treating the area locally with an antiinflammatory cream is usually sufficient to resolve the lesions. Preputial dermatitis can also be caused by physical irritation from rough cage flooring and subsequent fecal contamination or urine scalding. Cleaning the wounds and treating locally with zinc oxide ointment is usually sufficient.

Guinea pigs also have a tendency to develop small horny growths on the lateral aspects of the front footpads. Keeping the toenails trimmed and occasionally trimming back the nonvascular portions of the growths will keep these lesions under control.

CHINCHILLAS

Chinchillas are known for their soft, thick haircoats and are mentioned here briefly because of several common skin conditions.

Fungal Conditions

Dermatophytosis (ringworm) is relatively common. Most often caused by *Trichophyton mentagrophytes*, lesions tend to start around the face, axilla, groin, and base of the tail. Erythema, white flaky dermatitis, and easy fur epilation are the predominant clinical signs. Diagnosis is the same as that described for mice. Treatment consists of removing all the affected fur at the periphery of the lesions, bathing the chinchilla with an iodine-based shampoo, such as Welladol® (Pitman-Moore), and using oral griseofulvin and topical antifungal preparations. As with other species, environmental sanitation by thorough vacuuming and disinfection will prevent recurrence and minimize the zoonotic potential.

Miscellaneous Conditions
Fur Chewing

Fur chewing is a common vice in chinchillas. The cause is unknown, but environmental stress, overcrowding, heredity, dietary deficiencies, a low-roughage diet, boredom, and nesting activity have all been implicated as possible causes. Treatments described have been varied, but providing fresh alfalfa hay, proper chinchilla pellets, and reducing stress should help.

Fur-Slip

Fur-slip is the term used to describe the chinchillas' ability to shed large tufts of fur suddenly when frightened or attacked. The loss of fur causes no pain to the animal, although large patches of bare skin may be exposed. It can take 3 to 5 months for the fur to regrow, however, so it is a situation best avoided. Quiet surroundings and calm, gentle handling will minimize the chances of occurrence.

Fur Ring

Fur ring describes a condition in which a ring of fur becomes entrapped within the prepuce, causing paraphimosis. Treatment consists of lubricating the penis to free up the ring of fur and trimming the fur away.

Chinchillas tend to have fewer coat problems if sand-bathing with chinchilla dust, which is available commercially, or Fuller's earth. The dust should be poured 2 inches deep in a tray large enough to accommodate the chinchilla and allow rolling. Bathing should be allowed for half an hour two to three times a week. To prevent the possibility of fungal spores contaminating the dust, regularly placing the dust bath in an oven for 20 minutes at 300°F (148.8°C) has been suggested.

RABBITS

Rabbits are prone to a number of dermatologic conditions. One of the most significant effects of these conditions, however, is the tendency of rabbits to develop gastric trichobezoars. Because of the rabbit's inability to vomit and its narrow pyloric antrum, these trichobezoars do not always respond well medically, and surgical intervention is almost invariably fatal. For this reason, any dermatologic condition in which ingestion of hair is a component must be treated and resolved swiftly to prevent this secondary condition.

Bacterial Conditions

Ulcerative pododermatitis, also known as "hock sores," actually involves the ventral metatarsal region. It is often encountered in heavy rabbits kept on wire mesh or rough or dirty flooring, or in any rabbit in which the plantar fur pad is too thin. For this reason, it is often encountered in Angora rabbits after they have been groomed or trimmed because the desire to trim the matted, soiled fur from this region is natural. The lesions appear as well-circumscribed, ulcerated areas covered by a dry scab. Abscess formation under the scab occurs frequently, and infection can spread to nearby joints causing a septic arthritis. Treatment consists of providing a clean, smooth environment, and treating topically with an appropriate antibiotic and bandaging the wounds. If an abscess or arthritis is present, culture and sensitivity and systemic antibiotics are required.

Sore dewlap refers to a localized submandibular dermatitis, caused by drooling from malocclusion or by drinking from an open pan or crock. Treatment consists of removing the inciting cause by trimming the affected teeth, or by replacing the crock with a sipper tube waterer, and treating the dermatitis topically with hydrogen peroxide and an appropriate cream.

Staphylococcus aureus, *Pasteurella*, *Salmonella*, and *Streptococcus* have all been implicated as causes of dermatitis or abscessation (Figure 13). Self-trauma can be an important cause of progression of these lesions. Treatment consists of cleaning or debriding the wounds and treating with an appropriate antibiotic.

Venereal spirochetosis is caused by the spirochete *Treponema cuniculi*. It is transmitted by direct contact, especially during mating or by infection of the offspring at birth or during nursing. The rabbit is the only known natural host for the organism. The most common clinical signs are hyperemia and edema of the vulva or prepuce, followed by macules, papules, erosions, ulcers, and crusts on the external genitalia, perineal areas, eyelids, nose, and lips. Affected rabbits remain alert, and the disease regresses after several weeks. Lesions may heal with minimal scarring or persist as proliferative areas suggestive of papillomas. Diagnosis is by finding fine spiral-shaped bacterium 10 to 30 μm long on dark field examination of skin scrapings; or by the use of serologic tests, although a positive titer might not occur until 5 to 6 weeks after lesions have already appeared. Treatment success has been reported using three subcutaneous injections at 7-day intervals of 42,000 IU/kg penicillin G benzathine-penicillin G procaine.

Necrobacillosis, or Schmorl's disease, is caused by the organism *Fusobacterium necrophorum*. Clinical signs include ulceration and abscessation of the skin and subcutaneous swellings about the face, neck, and oral cavity. The lesions have a foul odor and may be present for weeks or months. Affected animals are usually pyrexic and anorectic as a result of the lesions in and around the mouth. The organism is a gram-negative, non-spore-forming, pleomorphic anaerobe present in the digestive tract of rabbits and other animals. Infection occurs under filthy conditions in which continuous fecal contamination of feet or wounds is possible. Diagnosis is by anaerobic culture of the organism. Treatment consists of cleaning and debriding the wounds and treating with an appropriate antibiotic. Prevention is easily accomplished by practicing proper husbandry; thus, this condition is rarely encountered in commercial facilities or in private practice.

Pseudomonas aeruginosa has also been identified as a cause of a dermatitis that has been referred to as "blue fur" because of the blue-green pigment produced by the organism. *Pseudomonas* is a ubiquitous gram-negative bacillus readily found in water and soil. Most infections are opportunistic, and are associated with immunosuppression or prolonged broad-spectrum antibiotic administration. Chronic wetting of the fur, usually caused by pan waterers or dripping water bottles, appears to be the major contributing factor. Skin lesions are often edematous, hemorrhagic, and necrotic. Pseudomonas is resistant to a number of different an-

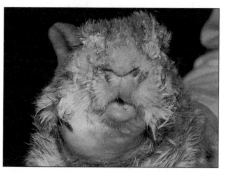

Figure 13—Dermatitis and jaw abscess caused by *Pasteurella multocida* infection in a rabbit. (Courtesy of R.D. Axelson, Willowdale, Ontario, Canada)

tibiotics; therefore, culture and sensitivity is imperative in establishing a proper therapeutic approach. Clipping the hair, debriding the wounds, and treating locally with 3% hydrogen peroxide may slow the spread until proper antibiotic therapy is instigated.

Viral Conditions

Myxomatosis is primarily an arthropod-transmitted poxvirus endemic in wild rabbits but is of great importance to domestic rabbit owners in Europe, Australia, and the western United States. Because the disease is transmitted by arthropod vectors, the incidence varies greatly from year to year based on the number of arthropods parasitizing the species. Birds, plants, and fomites can also act as mechanical vectors in the transmission.

Natural attenuation of the virus has led to the development of various strains, ranging from a mild avirulent fibroma-causing strain to an almost uniformly lethal strain. Clinical signs associated with the California strain most often include erythema, palpebral edema, purulent conjunctivitis, and gelatinous subcutaneous swellings of undifferentiated mesenchymal cells, especially of the face, ears, and external genitalia. Death usually occurs 8 to 12 days after exposure, but in those that survive, the lesions usually regress in 1 to 3 months. Diagnosis is based on the clinical signs and characteristic histopathologic lesions. Virus isolation and identification by fluorescent antibody technique is required in those cases in which lesions do not provide a definitive diagnosis. No treatment is known, and prevention is best accomplished by keeping pets in insect-proof enclosures and eliminating exposure to wild rabbits. Vaccinating with an attenuated vaccine prepared in the face of an outbreak may be helpful in rabbitry situations.

The Shope fibroma virus is a poxvirus antigenically related to the myxomatosis virus. Usually regarded as a cause of benign, localized fibromas in cottontail rabbits throughout North America, the virus has caused severe epizootics in commercial rabbitries in the United States. The disease is transmitted primarily by arthropod vectors, although mechanical transmission can occur. Tumors usually occur on the legs and feet, but may be seen on the muzzle or eyes of infected rabbits. The tumors are subcutaneous, localized, benign fibromas, and may persist for months without causing any other clinical signs. Diagnosis is by the characteristic clinical signs and histopathology of the lesions, or by virus isolation and identification. No treatment is known, but because arthropod vectors are important in the transmission, eliminating exposure to wild rabbits and insect-proof enclosures will aid in prevention.

The Shope papillomavirus causes wart-like lesions most frequently found on the neck, shoulders, or abdomen of cottontail rabbits. The virus causes a benign disease of cottontail rabbits in the midwestern United States, but has also been seen in domestic rabbits in that area. The warts begin as red, raised areas at the site of infection, then grow to become papillomas with rough, rounded surfaces, or large keratinized horny growths. These lesions usually regress spontaneously within 6 months, but occasionally go on to form malignant squamous cell carcinomas. Diagnosis is by the characteristic clinical signs, or by histopathology of the affected tissue. Because the infection appears to be transmitted by arthropod vectors, eliminating exposure is the best prevention.

Rabbit pox is caused by a poxvirus only distantly related to the other poxviruses of rabbits. Only six outbreaks have been recorded since the 1930s, so it is unlikely that disease would be encountered in private practice. Skin lesions begin as erythematous or macular eruptions which progress to form papules all over the body. Extensive edema of the face and oral cavity and purulent conjunctivitis are also seen frequently. Death usually occurs 7 to 10 days after infection. Diagnosis is by clinical signs, histopathology, and virus isolation and identification. Depopulation and strict sanitation is advised.

Fungal Conditions

Dermatophytosis occurs more frequently in pet rabbits than in the laboratory setting. *Microsporum canis, M. gypseum, M. audouinii,* and *Trichophyton shoenleini* infections do occur, but *T. mentagrophytes* is the most common cause of ringworm in domestic rabbits. Often appearing first on the head, face, or forelimbs, lesions on the back are also common (Figure 14). The lesions appear as an irregularly coin-shaped alopecic area, with a ridge of acute inflammation and mild to moderate crusting around the periphery. An area of central heal-

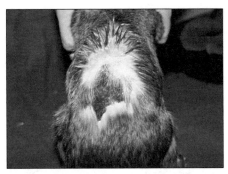

Figure 14—*Trichophyton mentagrophytes* infection in a rabbit.

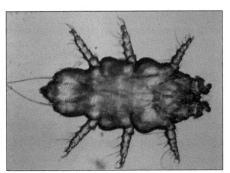

Figure 15—*Psoroptes cuniculi.* (Courtesy of D.H. Percy, Ontario Veterinary College, Guelph, Ontario, Canada)

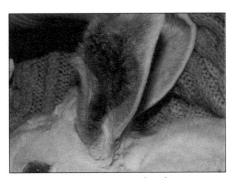

Figure 16—*Psoroptes cuniculi* infestation in a rabbit. (Courtesy of R.D. Axelson, Willowdale, Ontario, Canada)

ing and hair regrowth is characteristic. The lesions are often pruritic. Secondary bacterial infection of hair follicles is common. Diagnosis and treatment is the same as that described for chinchillas.

Parasitic Conditions

Psoroptes cuniculi is an obligate, nonburrowing ear mite that is extremely common in domestic rabbits (Figure 15). The lesions first appear inside the ears at the bottom of the ear canal, then gradually extend higher up as a dry, tan, crusty exudate which, when removed, exposes a moist, red, very painful skin surface (Figure 16). Head shaking, intense pruritus, self-mutilation, and secondary bacterial infections are common. The ear mite's life cycle is 3 weeks under favorable conditions, and owners may insist that the lesions were not there a week ago despite the fact that the ear canal is full of debris. Although usually confined to the ears, lesions can also be found on the external genitalia or on the face, neck, and limbs in conjunction with the ear lesions. Many authors maintain that simply instilling a few milliliters of mineral oil/miticide in the canal, repeating the process in 7 to 10 days, and allowing the rabbit to shake out the crusts itself is sufficient. Because the condition is extremely painful, I feel that anesthetizing the rabbit, flushing the ear canal with a dilute chlorhexidine solution, and then using an antibiotic-antiparasitic-corticosteroid otic preparation, such as Tresaderm® (MSD AGVET), is the preferred method of treatment in private practice. Ivermectin given orally at 400 µg/kg is also effective, but secondary bacterial infection of the canal should still be treated if present. The mite can exist off the host for a short period and is very contagious between rabbits; therefore, it is also advisable to treat the environment with an insecticide for 4 weeks to reduce the chance of spread.

Cheyletiella parasitovorax is a nonburrowing fur mite found very commonly in private practice in certain geographic regions. Clinical signs include thinning of the fur and scaling between the shoulder blades, progressing to reddened, oily, hairless patches over the back and head if not treated. Lesions are mildly to moderately pruritic in rabbits and can cause a transient dermatitis in humans. Treatment is the same as that described for fur mites in guinea pigs. Because the female *Cheyletiella* can exist for 2 weeks off the host, treating the environment with an insecticide for several weeks is also advised.

Listrophorus gibbus is an obligate, nonpathogenic fur mite of the rabbit found throughout the world. It is considered to be nonpathogenic and thus is often not mentioned in the literature. It is included here for the sake of completeness. Treatment would be the same as that described for *Cheyletiella.*

Haemodipus ventricosis, Notoedres cati, and *Sarcoptes scabiei* can occur in rabbits but are rare and are described in the Parasite Diagnostic Key (Table I). Treatment is the same as that described for lice and mange in guinea pigs.

Cuterebra larvae are common, particularly in rabbits housed outdoors. In northern climates there is a marked seasonality to myiasis. Flies usually emerge in June or July, and mating and egg laying follow within 7 to 8 days. Eggs are laid at the openings of rabbit burrows or around the rabbit hutch. The ova hatch in response to rapid increases in environmental temperature and moisture, likely caused by the immediate presence of the host. Larvae enter the host through nasal or oral openings, and larval development and migration occur in about one month. When the larvae are mature they exit the host, fall to the ground, and burrow in the soil to pupate and overwinter. Development resumes in the spring. The peak incidence of myiasis thus occurs in the late summer and early fall. No such periodicity is seen in southern climates, where myiasis can occur year round. The lesions consist of painful, 2- to 3-cm masses with fistulae in the center surrounded by moist matted fur. Treatment consists of anesthetizing the rabbit and lancing the lesion or enlarging the fistula to facilitate removal of the larvae. It is very important not to rupture the cystic cavity containing the larvae during this process because an anaphylactic reaction could ensue. After removal, the wound should be thoroughly cleansed and treated with an appropriate topical antibiotic.

Fleas are common in rabbits housed outdoors. Of the 1500 or so known species of fleas, approximately 25 have been identified as attacking wild or domestic rabbits. Of these, however, only *Cediopsylla simplex* (the common eastern rabbit flea) and *Odontopsyllus multispinosis* (the giant eastern rabbit flea) have been reported frequently in domestic rabbits. *C. simplex* is found most commonly around the head and neck region, while *O. multispinosis* is most common on the hind end. Infestation leads to pruritus and self-inflicted trauma, and severe infestations can be debilitating. Treat-

ment consists of bathing with an insecticidal shampoo, and treating the rabbit and environment with insecticidal preparations suitable for cats. It is important to remember that fleas found on rabbits can serve as vectors of tularemia, myxomatosis, plague, and Rocky Mountain spotted fever as well as other diseases of zoonotic potential.

A number of ticks have been known to affect rabbits, but of these, only *Haemaphysalis leporis-palustris* (the continental rabbit tick) has been reported with any frequency in North America. Ticks are voracious blood suckers and are most important as vectors of disease, including Q fever, tularemia, and Rocky Mountain spotted fever. Treat with any commercially available tick spray suitable for cats.

Nutritional Conditions

A lack of roughage in the diet is an important cause of fur chewing in domestic rabbits. Rabbit pellets supplemented with fresh timothy hay must form the basis of the diet, with fresh fruits and greens, oats, and other treats added only in small amounts as supplements. Most diets contain 16 to 20% fiber, but diets with 25% fiber are required in some cases.

Several dietary deficiencies have been produced experimentally in rabbits. Pyridoxine deficiency resulted in scaling and thickening of the skin around the ears, and encrustations of the nose and paws. Biotin deficiency resulted in dermatitis; hair loss on the back, lips, eyelids, and tail; and scaliness and flaking of skin. Magnesium deficiency has been reported to cause alopecia and changes in fur texture and luster. Zinc deficiency resulted in achromotrichia and patchy alopecia 6 to 9 weeks after being on a zinc-deficient diet. Copper deficiency can cause achromotrichia, alopecia, and dermatosis.

Endocrine Conditions

Fur plucking for nest building by preparturient does is very common and usually begins several days before kindling. Hair is most often plucked from the dewlap, underbelly, or sides. Diagnosis is made by eliminating any other cause of the lesions. No treatment is required.

Neoplastic Conditions

Other than those tumors already described under Viral Conditions, spontaneous tumors of skin in rabbits are relatively rare, although both squamous cell carcinoma and basal cell adenoma do occur. Treatment of these two tumor types is by surgical excision where applicable.

Miscellaneous Conditions

Both male and female rabbits possess two sebaceous

scent glands on either side of the vulvar/testicular region that secrete a brown waxy debris. This secretory substance can build up from time to time, and can be easily removed by gentle traction or soap and water. Hutch-burn is caused by urine scalding of the perineal region because of an unclean environment or inability of the rabbit to void without soiling itself, such as after a fractured limb or a spinal injury

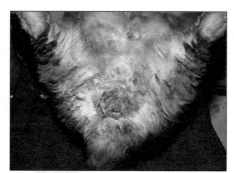

Figure 17—Hutchburn in a rabbit.

(Figure 17). Washing the wounds with an antiseptic and applying zinc oxide cream has been remarkably successful in mild cases. In severe cases in which a limb or spinal injury is involved, baby diapers to absorb the urine, zinc oxide, and an Elizabethan collar to prevent the rabbit from pulling off the diaper are very effective until the inciting cause has healed, but owner compliance is essential.

FERRETS

Of all the species described in this chapter, the pet ferret is the most similar to dogs and cats. Because ferrets have become popular only in recent years, information on dermatologic conditions seen in this species is relatively sparse. Nonetheless, several conditions are seen regularly in private practice and are described below.

Bacterial Conditions

Bite wounds to the neck by cage-mates during play or during mating are common. Mild lesions often appear as a thinning of hair or a scabby, erythematous area around the neck and shoulders that can be mistaken for self-trauma resulting from pruritus if the history of contact with another ferret is unknown. Separating the ferrets will usually result in complete resolution of the lesions without medical intervention. Severe bite wounds may result in subcutaneous abscesses, most often caused by *Streptococcus* spp. or *Staphylococcus aureus*. Diagnosis is by cytology or culture and sensitivity of the organism. Treatment consists of lancing and flushing the wound and treating with an appropriate antibiotic.

Viral Conditions

Canine distemper is a highly infectious disease in domestic ferrets that has several very distinctive skin lesions. Caused by a paramyxovirus, it is spread via aerosolization of viral particles from nasal secretions or saliva from infected dogs or other ferrets. The incubation period ranges from 4 to 10 days, with clinical signs appearing 7 to 9 days after exposure. A mucopurulent conjunctivitis is usually one of the first signs, progress-

ing to erythematous eruptions on the chin, footpads, and inguinal region over the next few days. Vesicle formation and secondary pyoderma are common, as is pruritus. Hyperkeratosis of the footpads is highly suggestive of canine distemper, but should not be confused with sarcoptic mange (described under Parasitic Conditions). Anorexia, fever, and respiratory and gastrointestinal signs are common, and animals surviving the acute phase may develop central nervous system signs before death. Death occurs anywhere from 2 days to a month after exposure. Infection with distemper offers a poor prognosis, as mortality approaches 100%. Prevention is best accomplished by annual vaccination with a modified live chick embryo origin vaccine. Canine cell origin vaccines should not be used, as they have been implicated as causing the disease in ferrets.

Fungal Conditions

Dermatophytosis (ringworm) in ferrets is most frequently caused by *Microsporum canis* or *Trichophyton mentagrophytes*. Clinical signs include circumscribed areas of alopecia and a scaly dermatitis most frequently seen around the eyes, nose, or limbs. *Microsporum canis* will sometimes display positive green fluorescence under a Wood's lamp, but diagnosis is best accomplished by microscopic examination of skin scrapings macerated in 10% potassium hydroxide (KOH) for 30 to 60 minutes and identification of mycelia or arthrospores, or by growth of the fungus on dermatophyte test medium. Because the organism grows slowly, cultures should be held for 3 weeks for a definitive diagnosis. Treatment includes disinfecting the environment, clipping the hair around the lesions, bathing with an iodine-based shampoo, and using topical creams and oral griseofulvin. Griseofulvin should not be used in pregnant animals because of possible teratogenic effects.

Parasitic Conditions

The mite *Otodectes cynotis* is very common in pet ferrets. It is transmitted by direct contact with infected ferrets, dogs, or cats. Clinical signs of head shaking and scratching may or may not be present, but waxy brown sebum and demonstration of the mites or eggs on an otic smear is diagnostic. The mites can exist on other areas of the body or off the host for short periods of time; therefore, whole body treatment with an insecticide is recommended as well as an otic preparation suitable for use in cats. Ivermectin given at 200 µg/kg twice at 14-day intervals is also effective.

Fleas are found on ferrets, and are often associated

with homes that are infested with fleas as a result of the other pets in the household. Pruritus is the most common clinical sign, and lesions are consistent with self-trauma. Heavy flea burdens can cause severe anemia and debilitation. Treatment with a 0.05% pyrethrin or 0.5% carbaryl shampoo followed by a weekly light dusting with 5% carbaryl powder is effective, as long as the environment is also treated. The environment may be treated with any of the commercially available premise insecticides, but ferrets should only be treated with products considered safe for use in kittens.

Sarcoptes scabiei is an uncommon parasite of domestic ferrets. Infection is more common in areas where ferrets are used for hunting rabbits and may be exposed to the parasite in rabbit burrows. Transmission is by direct contact with an infected animal or by exposure to a contaminated environment. Two forms of infestation have been described. The most frequently encountered form involves the feet and toes, which are swollen, erythematous, and may become ulcerated as a result of self-trauma. If left untreated the ferret can lose its claws. In the more generalized form, skin lesions predominate, with focal to generalized alopecia, hyperkeratosis, and intense pruritus. Diagnosis is best accomplished by deep skin scrapings cleared with 10% potassium hydroxide to reveal the sarcoptic mite. Treatment consists of weekly insecticide shampoos followed by lime sulfur dips for at least six treatments. Soaking the feet before removing the affected portion of the claw and debriding the foot lesions is helpful. Ivermectin given at a dose of 200 μg/kg is also useful in treating this condition. Because of the zoonotic potential, thorough disinfection of the environment and use of dichlorvos-impregnated resin strips is also advised.

Cuterebra spp. infestation can occur in ferrets housed outdoors or used for hunting, but is rare in house pets. Treatment is the same as that described for rabbits.

Nutritional Conditions

The most common cause for alopecia and dull, dry haircoat in ferrets is poor dietary practices. Many misconceptions exist in the general population concerning what constitutes an adequate diet for ferrets. Ferrets are no different than dogs and cats in their need for good quality protein and essential fatty acids for maintenance of a healthy haircoat. They are different in that their very short digestive tract provides them with only a limited ability to digest fiber. Food passage averages 3 to 4 hours in ferrets; therefore, diets high in protein

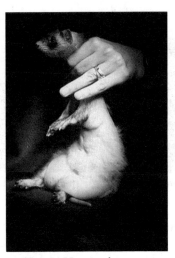

Figure 18—Hyperadrenocorticism caused by an adrenal adenoma in a ferret.

and fat but low in fiber are important. I believe that most of the commercially available cat foods are not adequate for ferrets, and that top quality nutrition, such as commercial ferret food, Hill's Science Diet Feline Maintenance®, or IAMS Cat Food, is required as well as a fatty acid supplement containing both linoleic and α-linolenic acids. No data are available concerning specific vitamin and mineral deficiencies in ferrets, but it is reasonable to assume that they may exhibit clinical signs similar to those seen in dogs and cats. Biotin deficiency has been seen in practice resulting from the feeding of raw eggs in the diet. Clinical signs include alopecia, hyperkeratosis, and achromotrichia.

Endocrine Conditions

Bilaterally symmetric alopecia of the ventral abdomen and tail area, enlarged vulva, and possible superficial perivulvar dermatitis are all part of the estrogen-induced aplastic anemia syndrome of unspayed female ferrets. Diagnosis is easily made by the obvious clinical signs. Treatment consists of spaying the ferret and improving the level of nutrition to aid in the recovery. Another treatment consists of the use of 50 to 100 IU of human chorionic gonadotropin (HCG) given subcutaneously to take the female out of heat as a temporary measure until she can be spayed, or bred on a subsequent heat.

A heavy shed can be seen in female ferrets after the first heat of the season, and in males during October and November. Hair regrowth occurs spontaneously provided that the diet is adequate.

Hyperadrenocorticism caused by a functional adrenal adenoma, carcinoma, or a pituitary tumor causing bilateral adrenocortical hyperplasia occurs infrequently in domestic ferrets. Clinical signs include progressive hair loss, muscle atrophy, and a thin skin with prominent blood vessels (Figure 18). Muscle weakness, polydipsia, and polyuria are infrequent findings. Skin biopsy reveals sparse hair follicles with irregularly arranged collagen. Dexamethasone suppression tests or resting cortisol levels are not always rewarding in trying to make a diagnosis, although they can be attempted. The disease seems to progress slowly, and currently there is no well-recognized method of treatment. Surgical removal of the tumor should be attempted but can be difficult because of the large fat pad surrounding the kidney and adrenal gland in the ferret. Chemotherapy with the antineoplastic drug o,p'-DDD may be attempted. Little data are available concerning dosages used or success rates. A dose of 50 mg/kg given once daily for 7 days and then twice weekly until signs resolve has been suggested.

Neoplastic Conditions

Skin tumors are the third most common tumor type reported in ferrets. Of these, squamous cell carcinoma is the most common, followed by poorly differentiated sebaceous gland adenocarcinoma. Mast cell tumors, myxosarcoma of the subcutis, basal cell carcinoma, neurofibroma/sarcoma, histiocytoma, sebaceous gland adenoma, and hemangioma have all been reported. Diagnosis is by cytology, or biopsy and histopathology. Treatment consists of surgical excision when applicable.

Miscellaneous Conditions

An unusual condition that I have seen in practice but not reported in the literature is a condition I refer to as "blue ferret syndrome." Male or female ferrets, neutered or unneutered, present with a history of "bruising" on the abdomen. Though the skin has a bluish discoloration, no obvious hematomas are evident. The lesion is bilaterally symmetric, and usually progresses over several weeks to involve most of the abdomen. There is no pain or pruritus associated with the lesion, the ferret's behavior does not change in any way, and the lesions regress spontaneously over the course of a few weeks. To date no hematologic or histologic abnormality has been identified. The cause of the condition is unknown, though rupture of subcutaneous blood vessels has been suggested. No treatment is necessary.

SELECTED READINGS

Ackerman LJ: *Trixacarus caviae* infestation in a guinea pig. *Can Vet J* 28:313, 1987.

Anderson LC: Guinea pig husbandry and medicine. *Vet Clin North Am [Small Anim Pract]* 17(5):1045–1060, 1987.

Barthold SW, Bhatt PN, Johnson EA: Further evidence for papovavirus as the probable etiology of transmissible lymphoma of Syrian hamsters. *Lab Anim Sci* 37(3):283–288, 1987.

Battles A.: The biology, care, and diseases of the Syrian hamster. *Compend Contin Educ Pract Vet* 7(10):815–825, 1985.

Besch-Williford CL: Biology and medicine of the ferret. *Vet Clin North Am [Small Anim Pract]* 17(5):1155–1183, 1987.

Besch-Williford CL, Wagner JE: Bacterial and mycotic diseases of the integumentary system. In: Foster HL, Small JD, Fox JG (eds): *The Mouse in Biomedical Research. Volume II: Diseases.* New York, Academic Press, 1982, pp 55–74.

Burke TJ: Rats, mice, hamsters, and gerbils. *Vet Clin North Am [Small Anim Pract]* 9(3):473–486, 1979.

Collins BR: Dermatologic disorders of common nondomestic animals.In: Nesbitt GH (ed): *Dermatology. Contemporary Issues in Small Animal Practice,* vol 8. New York, Churchill Livingstone, 1987, pp 235–294.

Cunliffe-Beamer TL, Fox RR: Venereal spirochetosis of rabbits: Description and diagnosis. *Lab Anim Sci* 31(4):366–371, 1981.

Davidson M: Canine distemper virus infection in the domestic ferret. *Compend Contin Educ Pract Vet* 8(7):448–453, 1986.

Estes PC, Richter CB, Franklin JA: Demodectic mange in the Golden hamster. *Lab Anim Sci* 21(6):825–828, 1971.

Flynn RJ: *Parasites of Laboratory Animals.* Ames, IA, Iowa State University Press, 1973.

Fox JG: *Biology and Diseases of the Ferret.* Philadelphia, Lea & Febiger, 1988.

Fox JG, Goad MEP, Garibaldi BA, Wiest LM: Hyperadrenocorticism in a ferret. *JAVMA* 191(3):343–344, 1987.

Fox JG. Cohen BJ, Loew FM (eds): *Laboratory Animal Medicine.* Orlando, Academic Press, 1984.

Frisk CS: Bacterial and mycotic diseases. In: Van Hoosier GL, McPherson CW (eds): *Laboratory Hamsters.* Orlando, Academic Press, 1987, pp 112–133.

Harkness JE, Wagner JE: *The Biology and Medicine of Rabbits and Rodents,* ed 3. Philadelphia, Lea & Febiger, 1989.

Harkness JE: Rabbit husbandry and medicine. *Vet Clin North Am [Small Anim Pract]* 17(5):1019–1044, 1987.

Harris IE: Rabbits: Medicine and other veterinary aspects. *Austr Vet Pract* 18(1):6–11, 1988.

Jacobson E, Kollias GV, Peters LJ: Dosages for antibiotics and parasiticides used in exotic animals. *Compend Contin Educ Pract Vet* 5(4):315–325, 1983.

Olsen GH, Turk MAM, Foil CS: Disseminated cutaneous squamous-cell carcinoma in a ferret. *JAVMA* 186(7):702–703, 1985.

Ryland LM, Bernard SL, Gorham JR: A clinical guide to the pet ferret. *Compend Contin Educ Pract Vet* 5(1):25–32, 1983.

Saunders GK, Scott DW: Cutaneous lymphoma resembling mycosis fungoides in the Syrian hamster. *Lab Anim Sci* 38(5):616–617, 1988.

Small JD: Drugs used in hamsters. In: Van Hoosier GL, McPherson CW (eds): *Laboratory Hamsters.* Orlando, Academic Press, 1987, pp 179–199.

Wagner JE, Farrar PL: Husbandry and medicine of small rodents. *Vet Clin North Am [Small Anim Pract]* 17(5):1061–1087, 1987.

UPDATE

Since this material was first published, a number of advances in small exotic animal medicine have occurred as more veterinarians have begun to view these species as pets rather than as laboratory animals. For example, there has been a dramatic decrease in the incidence of hyperestrogenism since most ferrets are now spayed early; however, reports of alopecia and swollen vulvas in spayed females have increased. Differential diagnoses include remnants of ovarian tissue or hyperactive or neoplastic adrenal glands.

Whereas hyperadrenocorticism was previously believed to be infrequent, it is now recognized as a common disorder in ferrets, most frequently involving the left adrenal gland, although both glands can be diseased. Adrenalectomy is currently considered the treatment of choice, although mitotane therapy as described is still being used in some cases. Ketoconazole has not been effective in treating ferrets with adrenal gland disease.

Mast cell tumors in ferrets also have been recognized with increasing frequency and can cause pruritus and alopecia. They are most often described as small, slightly raised, tan to erythematous circumscribed skin lesions found along the neck or dorsum. As the lesions often have a black crusty exudate, they may be mistaken for a wound that doesn't heal.

Several other points mentioned in the text also warrant some minor revision. Ivermectin has proven to be a very useful insecticide, and may be considered the treatment of choice for many of the parasitic conditions listed. Nasal dermatitis in gerbils has since been shown conclusively to be caused by secretions of the Harderian gland, often with secondary bacterial infection with *Staphylococcus*. Treatment remains the same. A recent report of dermatophytosis in rabbits involved fur loss on the footpads and toes and resulted in a progressive pododermatitis with infective fungus in nail beds. Dipping the infected toes in an iodine solution several times daily for weeks was suggested, although in another article ketoconazole, given at 10 to 40 mg/kg/day per os for 14 days, was reported as an effective treatment for dermatophytosis, and, I expect, should be efficacious for mycotic pododermatitis as well.

An oversight in the text was a failure to mention myiasis (fly strike) in exposed, untreated wounds or sores in rabbits housed outdoors. It is not uncommon in cases of marginal husbandry for an owner not to notice even a severe infestation with maggots in a rabbit with hutchburn until they pick the rabbit up and examine its underside. Prognosis in these cases can be grave, as an overwhelming number of maggots can lead to terminal toxic shock.

Although I had underplayed the importance of nutrition somewhat when this text first appeared, I have since become increasingly aware that, unlike their laboratory counterparts, most pet rodents and rabbits are kept on woefully inadequate diets. Rodent mixes available in pet stores are neither balanced nor fresh, and likely lack sufficient protein, unlike the lab chows most often used in a laboratory setting. Drinking water in water bottles is often not changed for days, and fresh fruits and vegetables are seldom offered. I suspect a predisposition to many illnesses is due to these inadequate diets, resulting in depressed immune system function and a delayed or impaired healing response. In these species, a thorough assessment of the diet is an essential part of any treatment plan, regardless of the cause of the illness.

REFERENCES

Allen DG, Pringle JK, et al: *Handbook of Veterinary Drugs*. Philadelphia, PA, JB Lippincott, 1993.

Burgmann PM, Percy DH: Antimicrobial drug use in rodents and rabbits, in Prescott JF, Baggot JD (eds): *Antimicrobial Therapy in Veterinary Medicine*, ed 2. Ames, Iowa, Iowa State University Press, 1993 pp 524-541.

Harkness JE, Wagner JE: *The Biology and Medicine of Rabbits and Rodents, ed 4*. Media, PA, Williams and Wilkins, 1995.

Hawk LT, Leary SL: *Formulary for Laboratory Animals*. Ames, Iowa, Iowa State University Press, 1995.

Hillyer EV: Ferret endocrinology, in Kirk RW (ed): *Current Veterinary Therapy XI*. Philadelphia, PA, WB Saunders, 1992, pp 1185-1188.

Smith DA, Burgmann PM: Formulary, in Hillyer EV, Quesenbury K (eds): *Clinical Medicine and Surgery of Ferrets, Rabbits and Rodents*. Philadelphia, PA, WB Saunders, 1996 (in press).

Diseases of the Integumentary System of Reptiles

Elliott R. Jacobson, DVM, PhD

A great variety of infectious and noninfectious integumentary diseases have been reported for reptiles. Many of these diseases primarily affect the integumentary system while others are generalized infections with both systemic and cutaneous involvement.

To appreciate abnormalities of the reptilian integument, an understanding of the normal structure is imperative. The first part of this chapter includes a brief review of the anatomy and histology of the reptilian integument. Infectious and noninfectious diseases of the integument are reviewed next, followed by a discussion of diagnostic techniques.

ANATOMY AND HISTOLOGY

Reptiles are the first truly terrestrial group of vertebrates. To avoid excessive water loss in a dehydrating environment, one of the major modifications that evolved over the ancestral amphibian plan included the integumentary system. For the most part, amphibians have a thinly keratinized skin containing an elaborate array of mucus and poison glands. In some amphibian species, the skin acts as a respiratory structure. The thin moist skin of amphibians restricts these animals to living in macro- or microenvironments that are moist or humid. With the evolution of reptiles, the integument went through some significant modifications to prevent dehydration and allowed the ancestral reptiles to radiate out into many untouched habitats. Invasion of aquatic systems resulted in further modifications. While crocodilians, lizards, and snakes all have a structurally similar integument, chelonians (turtles and tortoises) have developed a biologically unique integumentary structure, the shell. The chelonian shell evolved early in the evolutionary history and had a great selective value because it has changed minimally over millions of years.

From the standpoint of diagnostic work, the chelonian shell is extremely difficult to biopsy and evaluate histologically compared with the soft integument of other reptiles. The chelonian shell consists of outer epidermal scutes overlying a series of dermal plates. In most species, the epidermis is quite hard and is covered by a keratin-like material. In tortoises, new areas of growth are seen at the suture lines equidistant between the embryonic shields.[1] These growth lines may be more obvious in the plastron than the carapace (Figure 1). The dermal bone is metabolically active[2] and in calculating dosages of medicaments to be

Updated from original publication in *Dermatology for the Small Animal Practitioner*, Trenton, NJ, VLS Books, 1991 administered, the weight of the shell must be considered in the calculation. The dermal bone of the chelonian shell integrates with the ribs and the vertebral column. In green turtles, Rathke's glands exit through small openings in the axillary and inguinal portions of the infra-marginal scutes.[3] While terrestrial chelonians shed the outer portions of their shell as small, often imperceptible, flakes, many aquatic turtles shed the outer portions of entire scutes (Figure 2).

The soft tissue of the integument shows similarities between the various orders of reptiles. The skin is composed of several layers of epidermal cells overlying a dermis composed of loose and dense connective tissue (Figure 3). Many species of crocodilians have bony plates within the dermis called *osteoderms*; the best developed osteoderms are in the cervical region. Overlying the epidermal cells is a thin layer of keratin. In turtles the skin is covered by a keratin-like substance and is unique among vertebrates in composition.[4] A multitude of chromatophores are located within the dermis immediately below the basement membrane and consist of melanophores, erythrophores, xanthophores, and iridophores (Figure 4). The reptile integument has relatively few glandular structures and typically is dry. The scent glands that do exist in reptiles probably function to ward off predators or function in sex discrimination and species recognition during the breeding season.

Lizards and snakes have a unique method of periodic epidermal ecdysis (skin shedding).[4a] In snakes and some lizards (night lizards, some geckos) the cornea is covered by a spectacle, which is also involved in the shedding process. In this process only the superficial portion of the skin is lost. In snakes ecdysis is characterized by six stages of epidermal development.[5] Clinically, as a snake enters a cycle of ecdysis the skin and spectacle take on a bluish tinge. During this time a new epidermal generation is laid down and matures. Approximately 4 to 7 days after

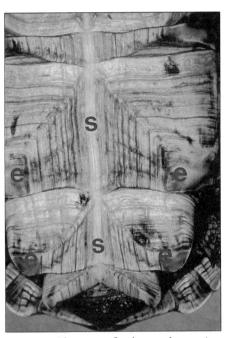

Figure 1—Plastron of a leopard tortoise. Lightly pigmented areas of new growth are seen at suture line *(s)*, equidistant between embryonic shields *(e)*.

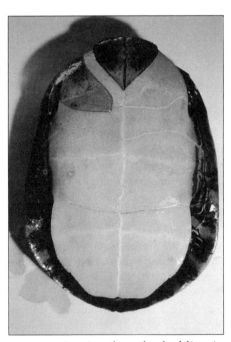

Figure 2—A painted turtle shedding its scutes.

the height of development of this dullness to the skin, the snake's color rapidly brightens and the spectacle of the eye clears completely and shedding occurs. After shedding, the epidermis enters a resting phase composed of the following three subdivisions: (1) postshedding resting phase, (2) perfect resting phase, and (3) late resting phase.[6] Subsequently, a renewal phase (lasting approximately 14 days) begins and the cycle repeats itself. If the snake goes one day beyond the normal time of shedding, the skin becomes roughened and somewhat dehydrated in appearance.

INFECTIOUS DISEASES
Viral Skin Diseases
Gray Patch Disease of Green Sea Turtles

A virus with the morphologic appearance of herpesvirus has been shown to be the causative agent of epizootics of skin lesions termed *gray patch disease* in young green turtles (*Chelonia mydas*) between 56 and 90 days after hatching in aquaculture.[7] Skin lesions commenced as small circular papular lesions which coalesced into spreading patches (Figure 5) containing epidermal cells with basophilic intranuclear inclusions. Electron microscopy revealed inclusions to consist of viral particles having an electron-dense core. Particles were found enveloping from nuclear membranes and mature enveloped particles found in the cytoplasm measured 160 to 180 nm. The most severe epizootics occurred in the summer under stressful environmental conditions of high water temperature (>39°C [102°F]), crowding, and organic pollution. In controlled experiments turtles that were subjected to a gradual temperature increase from 25 to 30°C (77 to 86°F) with subsequent maintenance at 30°C and those that were abruptly shifted from water temperatures of 25 to 30°C showed a significantly shorter period before the onset of clinical signs and an increase in the severity of the lesions compared with control turtles.[8]

Poxvirus Skin Disease of Caimans and Nile Crocodiles

The first report of a virus-associated disease in a crocodilian is that of a poxvirus skin disease of captive caimans (*Caiman sclerops*).[9] Infected caimans were found to have gray-white circular skin lesions scattered over the body surface (Figure 6). Oral proliferative lesions also were seen on the tongue and hard palate. While in some caimans severe lesions resulted in digital sloughing, other individuals only had focal lesions often involving only the palpebrae. By light microscopy large eosinophilic intracytoplasmic inclusions were seen within hypertrophied epithelial cells. Numerous inclusions were present in an extremely thickened keratin layer. By electron microscopy inclusions were found to consist of myriads of viral particles that were morphologically typical of poxvirus. The size of 200 x 100 nm was smaller than previously reported poxviruses of vertebrates and insects. A similar poxvirus disease was identified in juvenile farm-reared Nile crocodiles (*Crocodylus niloticus*) in Zimbabwe[10] and South Africa.[11]

Desert Tortoise Poxvirus

An amelanotic California desert tortoise (*Xerobates agassizi*) with multiple raised papular-to-vesicular lesions on the skin of the head, neck, and legs was found by light microscopy to have ballooning of the epidermal cells in the stratum granulosum.[12] Large intracytoplasmic inclusions were seen in many of these cells with hematoxylin and eosin (H&E) staining. Although the author of that report considered these inclusions to be consistent with those of poxvirus infection, there was no confirmation of this interpretation because no supportive electron photomicrographs were provided. Accumulations of protein and/or keratin within the cytoplasm of a dysplastic epidermal cell can be confused with intracytoplasmic viral inclusions.

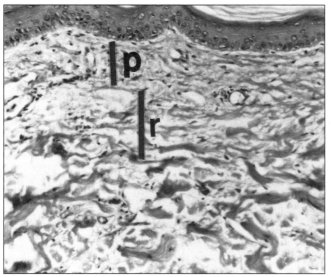

Figure 3—Histologic section of skin of a green turtle. The epidermis is approximately four to seven cells thick and is covered by a thin keratin-like substance corresponding to the stratum corneum. Immediately below the papillary layer *(p)* is the reticular layer *(r)*, which is composed of large collagenous bundles. (H&E stain, ×160) (From Jacobson ER, Mansell JL, Sundberg JP, et al: Cutaneous fibropapillomas of green turtles (*Chelonia mydas*). *J Comp Pathol* 101:34–52, 1989, with permission).

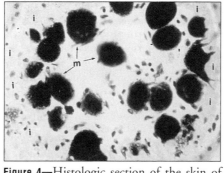

Figure 4—Histologic section of the skin of an American anole. Melanophores *(m)* and iridophores *(i)* are seen in the dermis. (H&E, ×160)

Papillomavirus of Bolivian Side-Neck Turtles

Papilloma-like viral crystalline arrays were observed in skin lesions of recently imported Bolivian side-neck turtles (*Platemys platycephala*).[13] The turtles were submitted for examination with circular papular skin lesions that in some animals coalesced into patches (Figure 7). The gross appearance of this disease was similar to that seen with herpesvirus infection of green turtles and poxvirus of caimans. Light microscopic evaluation of skin lesions, however, revealed hyperkeratosis and hyperplasia with acanthosis; no inclusions were noted. Electron microscopic examination of skin biopsies revealed intranuclear crystalline arrays of hexagonal particles measuring approximately 42 nm. These aggregates were morphologically consistent with those of papillomavirus. The lesions were more benign in appearance than papillomavirus-induced wart lesions of mammals.

Lacertid Lizard Papillomas

Cutaneous papillomas are commonly seen in lacertid lizards (Figure 8). Raynaud and Adrian presented a detailed report on the distribution of papillomas in European green lizards (*Lacerta viridis*) maintained as a breeding colony.[14] The papillomas ranged in diameter from 2 to 20 mm and numbered 2 to 25 per individual. In females the papillomas were most commonly found in the caudal lumbar area of the body, in the vicinity of the tail base; papillomas were rarely found around the head. In males the papillomas had a dorsocranial distribution around the base of the head. Neither sex had papillomas associated with ventral scales. The authors associated the distribution to the reproductive behavior whereby males inflict bite wounds on females at the base of the tail and combative behavior between males during which males inflict bites at the base of the neck of other males. Histopathologic examination of papillomas showed hyperkeratosis and hyperplasia of epidermal cells. The nucleus of epidermal cells was often hypertrophied with margination of chromatin material and intranuclear inclusions. Papillomas submitted for electron microscopy revealed three morphologically distinct virus particles resembling papovavirus, herpesvirus, and reovirus.

Treatment/Management of Viral Skin Diseases

There are no vaccines available for any of the viral diseases of reptiles. In most cases the lesions are colonized by bacteria and fungi that often contribute to the severity of the lesions. Biopsies and microbial culture of these lesions allow selection of the most appropriate chemotherapeutic agent for treatment of these secondary invaders. Ill reptiles should be removed from healthy cage-mates and maintained under ideal environmental conditions. For aquatic species water quality control is imperative; water should be changed at least daily.[14a]

Bacterial Skin Diseases
Bacterial Shell Diseases of Chelonians

Septicemic cutaneous ulcerative disease of turtles was first described by Jackson and Fulton[15] and is commonly seen in freshwater turtles of the genera *Pseudemys* and *Chrysemys* that have been recently purchased from biologic supply companies. Often these turtles are kept under suboptimal environmental conditions and have not been fed adequately. Clinically the disease is seen as necrotizing ulcerative cutaneous lesions with both shell and skin involvement. Typically there is a septicemia with lesions in the liver, heart, kidney, and spleen. Although the organism *Citrobacter freundii* has been incriminated as the etiologic agent, *Serratia* may be necessary to initiate the infection.[15] Unfiltered aquatic systems with excess accumulations of fecal ma-

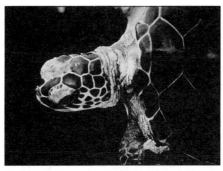

Figure 5—Gray patch disease in a juvenile green turtle. Note the prominent lesions on the head and cervical region. (From Jacobson ER: Diseases of reptiles. Part I. Noninfectious diseases. *Compend Contin Educ Pract Vet* 3:122–126, 1981, with permission)

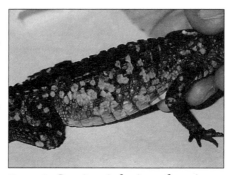

Figure 6—Poxvirus infection of a caiman. Multiple white patches are seen on the body surface.

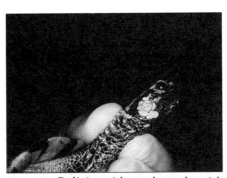

Figure 7—Bolivian side-neck turtle with confluent white skin lesions caudal to the right eye. (From Jacobson ER, Gaskin JM, Clubb SL: Papilloma-like virus infection in Bolivian side-neck turtles. *JAVMA* 181: 1325–1328, 1982, with permission)

terial will exacerbate the disease. Good water quality and a good feeding schedule are necessary for controlling this problem. Chloramphenicol was recommended as the antibiotic of choice. Wallach subsequently described an ulcerative shell disease of several species of aquatic turtles, with softshell turtles (*Trionyx* spp.) being most severely affected.[16] The gram-negative bacillus *Beneckea chitinovora* was cultured from these lesions on blood agar at 24°C (75.2°F) but not at 37°C (98.6°F). The disease was experimentally produced in softshell turtles and painted turtles (*Chrysemys picta*), and it was demonstrated that a prior injury to the shell was necessary for the bacteria to cause the disease. *B. chitinovora* is commonly isolated from shrimp and crayfish fed to turtles and the author recommended that these food items be avoided.

Middle Ear Infections of Chelonians

This disease is seen as a bulging of the skin (tympanic scale) overlying the middle ear.[17] It has been seen in free-ranging eastern box turtles (*Terrapene carolina*), either unilaterally or bilaterally (Figure 9). I have also seen this disease in freshwater turtles and the green sea turtle. The lesion consists of caseous laminated material surrounded by mixed inflammatory cells. In advanced cases osteomyelitis may occur. *Citrobacter, Enterobacter, Morganella morgani, Providencia rettgeri, Pseudomonas,* and *Pasteurella* have all been cultured from these lesions. Treatment consists of removing the caseated material and flushing the area with a dilute organic iodine solution. In severe cases use of an injectable broad spectrum antibiotic is recommended.

Subcutaneous Abscesses

Subcutaneous abscesses of bacterial origin are commonly encountered in lizards and snakes (Figure 10). In snakes, subcutaneous abscesses are most often secondary to trauma from prey items biting the snake, bite wounds from cage-mates, or penetration of foreign bodies. An adult mangrove snake (*Boiga dendrophila*) with a large sub-cutaneous abscess was found to have a tooth from another snake within the center of the abscess. A mixture of gram-negative organisms, includ-ing *Pseudomonas, Providencia, Es-cherichia coli,* and *Proteus,* have been cultured from these lesions. In the Cuban anole (*Anolis equestris*), *Ser-ratia anolium* has been isolated from subcutaneous abscesses.[18] Subcuta-neous abscesses associated with *Ser-ratia marcescens* have been seen in a green iguana (*Iguana iguana*) and spiny-tailed iguana (*Ctenosaura acanthura*).[19] In the same report, *Salmonella marina* and *Micrococcus* were also cultured from subcuta-neous abscesses in a green iguana and spiny-tailed iguana. Recently a *Neisseria* species was isolated from tail abscesses in green iguanas and from the oral cavity of healthy igua-nas.[20] Bite wounds inflicted by oral carriers were believed to be the source of the infection. The abscess-es could not be effectively managed with either systemic antimicrobial therapy or localized treatment; thus, the *Neisseria* was considered a high-ly pathogenic organism. I have also isolated *Corynebacterium pyogenes* from an iguana with a subcutaneous abscess (Figure 11) and a variety of anaerobes have also been isolated from abscesses of reptiles.[21]

Whatever their origin, subcuta-neous abscesses should be surgically removed. In some situations the ab-scess may be a single large focal le-sion surrounded by a fibrous cap-sule, while in other cases abscesses may be miliary and diffusely found in surrounding tissues. After removal, it is not uncommon for abscesses to recur at the same site, especially if they are in the miliary form. Antibiot-ic therapy includes use of a broad spectrum antibiotic and, if an anaerobe is present, an appropriate drug such as metronidazole.[21]

Necrotizing Bacterial Dermatitis

Necrotizing skin lesions colonized by *Pseudomonas*

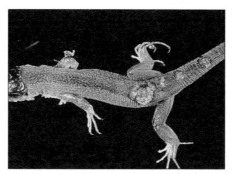

Figure 8—Papillomas on a European emer-ald lizard are seen as darkly pigmented pro-liferative lesions.

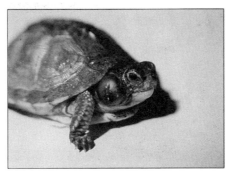

Figure 9—Middle ear infection in a juvenile eastern box turtle. (From Jacobson ER: Diseases of reptiles. Part I. Noninfectious diseases. *Compend Contin Educ Pract Vet* 3:122–126, 1981, with permission)

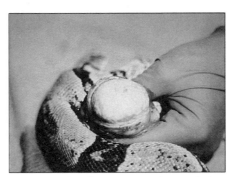

Figure 10—A subcutaneous abscess being surgically removed from a boa constrictor. The abscess was the result of a bite wound from a rodent.

have been seen secondary to burn wounds in several snakes (Figure 12). In humans *P. aeruginosa* colo-nizes 60% of burn patients by the fifth day after the burn.[22] Snakes are commonly burned from electrical heating pads used within their cages. The lesions consist of hemor-rhagic body scales with edema and necrosis. The lesions most often in-volve ventral scales in areas of direct contact with heating devices. Large areas of skin may slough, exposing subcutaneous tissue. Severe cases of *Pseudomonas* skin disease can result in a pneumonic condition after in-halation of microorganisms being shed into the surrounding atmo-sphere from the lesion site. Snakes with extensive skin lesions need to be soaked in a dilute iodine solu-tion followed by application of a burn ointment, such as mafenide acetate (Sulfamylon® Cream-Winthrop Pharmaceuticals). Sys-temic antibiotics, such as amikacin, should also be used.

Pseudomonas aeruginosa, as well as *Corynebacterium xerosis, Staphy-lococcus* spp., *Streptococcus* spp., and *Citrobacter freundii*, were isolated from a necrotizing skin lesion in a rattlesnake, *Crotalus mitchelli pyrrhus.*[23] A recently imported adult Indonesian blue tongue skink, *Tili-qua gigas*, which arrived with a multifocal *P. aeruginosa* dermatitis, died despite treatment with appro-priate broad spectrum antibiotics and was found to have a large intra-coelomic perihepatic abscess con-nected to the overlying skin lesion by a thin stalk.[24] A pure growth of *P. aeruginosa* was cultured from this lesion. I have seen similar lesions in turtles in which shell ulcerations were continuous with coelomic abscesses via fistulous tracts.

Pseudomonas, one of the most common bacterial or-ganisms associated with oral and respiratory disease in snakes, in advanced cases may enter the vascular com-partment and ultimately produce necrotizing lesions at multiple sites, including the skin. Coagulation necrosis of the dermis results in sloughing of the overlying epi-dermal layer.

A condition has been seen in boa constrictors,

pythons, and other snakes in which obstipation, necrosis of the gastrointestinal tract, or infection of the reproductive tract in females results in loss of the stratum corneum of the epidermis.[25] The outer portions of each scale are seen to "flake off" (Figure 13). At first only a few scales may be seen in the cage, but as the disease progresses almost the entire body can be involved. If the primary cause of the problem can be identified and corrected, the outer portions of the skin will be replaced at the next cycle of ecdysis.

Aeromonas hydrophila is a significant opportunistic pathogen of crocodilians. Die-offs of American alligators, *Alligator mississippiensis*, caused by *A. hydrophila* have been reported in the wild.[26] Deaths have also been seen in farm-reared alligators that have suffered from heat stress. Organisms from the intestinal tract enter the vascular compartment and invade multiple visceral structures. Peripherally, necrotizing hemorrhagic skin lesions are commonly seen. Because *Aeromonas* often cannot be cultured from skin lesions, it is thought that the lesions result from bacterial toxins released into the vascular compartment or thrombosis of subjacent vessels in the dermis.

Mycobacteriosis

Cutaneous disease caused by mycobacteria has been described in reptiles, either as a primary skin disease or secondary to systemic involvement.[27] The lesions appear as subcutaneous swellings and must be distinguished from other causes, such as bacterial abscesses, mycotic granulomas, and neoplasia. The skin over the granuloma may ulcerate. Organisms from the subcutaneous lesions can spread elsewhere. In a boa constrictor with primary subcutaneous mycobacteriosis, a proliferative ulcerating oral lesion developed from which a mycobacterium was isolated.[28]

Several species of atypical mycobacteria have been isolated from reptiles and include *Mycobacterium marinum*, *M. chelonei*, and *M. thamnopheos*. Acid-fast staining of granulomas is often diagnostic for the presence of mycobacteria. In many situations an abundance of

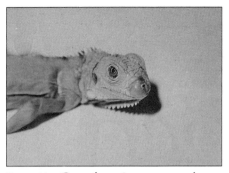

Figure 11—*Corynebacterium pyogenes* abscess in a green iguana.

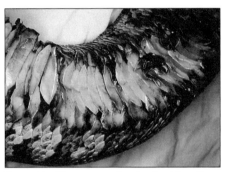

Figure 12—Burn wound colonized by *Pseudomonas aeruginosa* in a Burmese python.

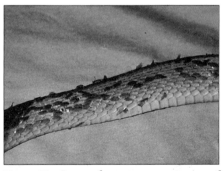

Figure 13—Loss of stratum corneum of body scales in a taipan that had a severe enteritis.

organisms in tissue section makes identification easy. *M. thamnopheos*, however, is minimally acid-fast and may be difficult to demonstrate in tissue section.

There are no reports of treating reptiles with mycobacteriosis. Many of the reptile isolates are resistant to drugs used in mammals. Epizootics are seldom a problem in reptile collections; therefore, control should involve removal of infected animals and decontamination of the cage.

Dermatophilosis

Dermatophilus congolensis is one of two species within the family *Dermatophilaceae*. Members of this family are unique in forming filamentous structures that segment transversely as well as longitudinally to form coccoid cells that become motile spores. *D. congolensis* is gram-positive and is not acid-fast. It is the etiologic agent of dermatophilosis (formerly called streptothricosis), a disease that has been seen in a variety of mammals including ruminants, horses, primates, and carnivores. In reptiles it has been reported in Australian bearded lizards (*Amphibolurus barbatus*)[29] and marble lizards (*Calotes mystaceous*)[30] imported into the United States. It has also been seen in a captive bearded lizard in Australia.[31] I have seen an organism with microscopic characteristics of *D. congolensis* in skin lesions of six recently imported Senegal chameleons (*Chameleo senegalensis*), one

green iguana (*Iguana iguana*), one collared lizard (*Crotophytus collaris*), and one boa constrictor; an organism consistent with *Dermatophilus* was cultured from the chameleons and iguana. In the lizards the lesions were seen as raised brown multifocal encrustations, scattered over the integument (Figure 14). The boa constrictor was found to have multiple subcutaneous nodules that bulged the overlying skin. In those reptiles with epidermal involvement, the encrustations were found to consist of necrotic cellular debris, accumulations of keratin, and inflammatory cells; the underlying epidermis was necrotic. In hematoxylin and eosin-stained tissue sections, numerous basophilic coccoid structures were seen on the surface of the lesions; in sections stained by the

Giemsa method, numerous branching filamentous structures with longitudinal and transverse divisions were observed in the encrusted material (Figure 15). In the boa constrictor, similar-appearing organisms were seen within the caseated center of a subcutaneous nodule. Rough, dry, white-gray colonies developed from skin lesions of a chameleon and iguana cultured on trypticase soy agar. Gram-stained smears of these colonies demonstrated gram-positive filamentous rods consistent with *D. congolensis.*

Treatment for dermatophilosis includes removal of skin encrustations and topical application of a dilute iodine solution. Antibiotics of choice are amikacin and penicillin.

Drug Therapy for Bacterial Skin Disease

Bacterial disease problems in captive reptiles are caused most commonly by aerobic gram-negative microorganisms. Many of these organisms are secondary invaders, requiring predisposing problems before an infection begins. When treating these animals, one must not only isolate and identify the pathogen(s) but identify correct the factors responsible for allowing the organism(s) to become established. For instance, reptiles kept at suboptimal environmental conditions are immunocompromised and are at risk for bacterial (and other pathogen) infections. In these cases treatment includes exposure to an appropriate ambient temperature regime.

The use of chemotherapeutics in reptile medicine been discussed elsewhere[32] and is briefly reviewed here. In selecting the most appropriate antibiotic, ideally the causative agent needs to be identified and sensitivity patterns determined. Next, minimum inhibitory concentrations (MICs) of antibiotics should be determined. Because pharmacokinetic information is only available on a handful of antibiotics (in relatively few species of reptiles), scientifically treating these animals with appropri-

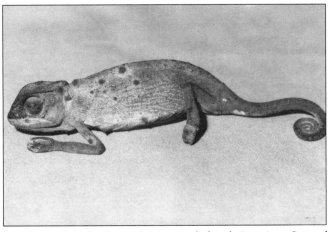

Figure 14—Multifocal raised, encrusted skin lesions in a Senegal chameleon. An organism resembling *Dermatophilus* was isolated from these lesions.

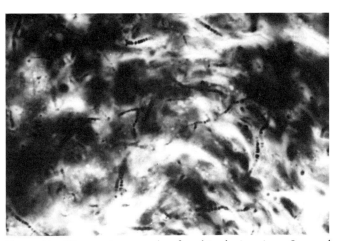

Figure 15—Photomicrograph of a skin lesion in a Senegal chameleon revealing a beaded filamentous organism resembling *Dermatophilus.* (Giemsa stain, ×1000)

ate antibiotics often narrows the range of drugs from which one can select. Pharmacokinetic data are available for chloromycetin, carbenicillin, ceftazadime, gentamicin, and amikacin. Dosages of antibiotics routinely used in treating reptiles with bacterial disease(s) are listed in Table I.

Many of the reptiles submitted with gram-negative sepsis are immunocompromised and thus bactericidal antibiotics would be more efficacious than bacteriostatic drugs. The health status of the reptile patient, the size of the patient, and the potential side effects of the drug should also be considered in selecting the most appropriate drug. In reptiles that are extremely dehydrated, the aminoglycosides should be avoided, at least until the animal is rehydrated. Ideally, reptiles that are being placed on a regimen of aminoglycoside administration (such as gentamicin and amikacin) should have a complete blood count (CBC) and serum chemical profile (including uric acid) performed before the initiation of therapy. For most reptiles normal uric acid levels should be below 14 mg/dl. If the reptile is administered an aminoglycoside, serum uric acid levels ideally should be monitored throughout the course of treatment and after treatment has ended. Isotonic saline at 20 ml/kg body weight should be administered subcutaneously, intraperitoneally, or orally on the days of treatment.

In general, oral administration of antibiotics to reptiles should be avoided. Few pharmacokinetic studies have been done on antibiotics administered orally in reptiles and uptake appears to be extremely variable and unpredictable. Many small species of lizards, however, have relatively small muscle masses and are extremely stressed when handled and injected. In such cases the medicament will have to be offered in the animal's food (if it is still feeding).

TABLE I
Antibiotic Dosages for Reptiles

Antibiotic	Trade Name	Dose (mg/kg)	Frequency	Duration	Route
Chloramphenicol sodium succinate	Chloromycetin® sodium succinate (Parke-Davis)	40	Every 24 hours	5–14 days	SC
Chloramphenicol	Mychel-Vet Tevocin®	50	Every 12–72 hours depending on species	2 weeks	SC
Carbenicillin	Pyopen® (Beecham)	400	Every 48 hours in turtles Every 24 hours in snakes	2 weeks	IM IM
Ceftazadime	Fortz®	20	Every 72 hours in snakes	2–3 weeks	IM
Gentamicin	Gentocin® (Schering-Plough Animal Health)	6 2.5 1.75	Every 72–96 hours in turtles Every 72 hours in snakes Every 96 hours in alligators	7–9 treatments 7–9 treatments 7–9 treatments	IM forelegs IM IM forelegs
Enrofloxacin[32a]	Baytril®	10 5 15	Every 24 hours for resistant infections Every 24 hours for routine infections Every 72 hours for URI in tortoises	3 weeks 3 weeks 3 weeks	IM IM IM
Amikacin	Amiglyde® (Fort Dodge Laboratories)	5, 2.5 2.25	First dose; thereafter, every 72 hours in snakes Every 96 hours in alligators	7–9 treatments 7–9 treatments	IM forelegs IM
Trimethoprim/ sulfadiazine	Tribrissen® (Coopers Animal Health)	30	First two doses 24 hours apart, then every other day	7–14 treatments	IM

(From Jacobson ER: Reptiles. *Vet Clin North Am [Small Anim Pract]* 17:1203–1225, 1987; with permission.)

As a rule hind-leg muscles in quadrupedal reptiles and hind-body muscles in snakes should be avoided as injection sites because of the anatomy of the renal portal system. Such drugs as gentamicin and amikacin, if injected into the hind-leg musculature of a lizard, could go directly to the kidney, which, because these drugs are nephrotoxic, could be disastrous.

Ambient temperature has a marked effect on the uptake, distribution, and elimination of antibiotics in reptiles. As mentioned earlier, when ill reptiles are treated, they should be maintained at their preferred optimum temperature range. For many species a temperature range of 26 to 33°C (78.8 to 91.4°F) is ideal. At high temperatures small species can dehydrate rapidly, and the clinician must constantly be aware of the hydration status of the patient.

Mycotic Diseases

Although at one time considered rare, mycotic diseases of the integumentary system are not uncommon in captive reptiles.[32b] I have also seen several cases of mycotic skin disease in free-ranging reptiles. The common dermatophytes, such as *Microsporum* and *Tri-*

chophyton, are rarely recovered; instead, a variety of fungi, such as *Mucor, Fusarium, Trichosporon,* and *Geotrichum,* have been isolated from these lesions. While fungi are relatively easy to identify in tissue section, isolating the causative agent and making an accurate identification is extremely difficult. For ultimate identification the agent must be sent to an expert familiar with the genus of fungus isolated. Many new species of mycotic agents have been described in reptiles. In this section, mycotic diseases are reviewed by reptile group.

Mycotic Dermatitis of Chelonians

There are relatively few reports of cutaneous mycotic disease in chelonians. Mycotic dermatitis has been described in a radiated tortoise[33] and several other chelonians in a zoologic collection.[34] In the latter report, shell necrosis was associated with invasion of fungi in the order Mucorales with the plastron affected more often than the carapace. Six hatchling Florida softshell turtles (*Trionyx ferox*), representative of a group of approximately 400 with circular gray ulcerating lesions of the shell and skin (Figure 16), were found on histopathology to have bacterial colonies and large numbers of branching nonseptate hyphae (Figure 17).[35] *Mucor* spp., *Proteus* spp., *Escherichia coli*, and *Pseudomonas* were recovered from the lesions. The surviving turtles were immersed for 15 minutes in a solution of malachite green (0.15 mg/L) three times daily for one week. Turtles were thoroughly rinsed with fresh water after the immersion to reduce eye irritation. After one week of treatment, surviving turtles responded with regression of lesions. I have also seen fungal organisms in hatchling Ridley sea turtles (*Lepidochelys kempi*) with necrotizing palpebritis, in subcutaneous granulomas in the cervical region of an adult leopard tortoise (*Geochelone pardalis*), and in pitted shell lesions of hatchling Australian sideneck turtles (*Chelodina longicollis*).

Mycotic Skin Disease of Crocodilians

Relatively few cases of mycotic skin disease have been reported for this group of reptiles. In captivity crocodilians are often kept in cement pools and as a consequence, abrasions of the ventral integument are not uncommon. A bumblefoot-like condition of the footpads occurs and fungal organisms have been seen in these lesions. A *Trichophyton* sp. was isolated from one of these cases.[36]

Mycotic Skin Disease of Squamates (Lizards and Snakes)

Numerous cases of mycotic skin disease have been reported for this group of reptiles. The disease generally is seen as hyperkeratotic skin lesions, necrotizing skin lesions, or subcutaneous granulomas. I have seen numerous cases of mycotic skin disease in imported geckos. Recently a Madagascan day gecko (*Phelsuma madagascariensis*), representative of several species of recently imported *Phelsuma* that developed proliferative skin lesions, was examined. It was found to have raised circular proliferative lesions that became white in color as the lesions progressed. Ultimately there was a complete sloughing of the affected skin with de-

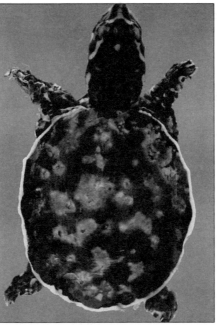

Figure 16—Necrotizing shell and skin lesions in a juvenile Florida softshell turtle. (From Jacobson ER, Calderwood MB, Clubb SL: Mucormycosis in hatching Florida softshell turtles. *JAVMA* 177:835–837, 1980, with permission)

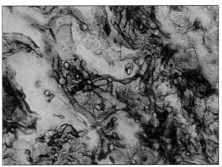

Figure 17—Histologic section of a shell lesion in a juvenile Florida softshell turtle showing a branching nonseptate fungus. (GMS stain, ×1000) (From Jacobson ER, Calderwood MB, Clubb SL: Mucormycosis in hatchling Florida softshell turtles. *JAVMA* 177:835–837, 1980, with permission)

velopment of a moist dermatitis. Examination of skin biopsy specimens revealed numerous branching septate hyphae throughout the tissue. I have also seen similar lesions in several species of recently imported West African ground geckos.

Trichosporonosis, caused by *Trichosporon beigelii* (*cutaneum*), has been isolated from a variety of lesions in reptiles including skin lesions of lizards.[36] I have isolated this fungus from subcutaneous hematomas in the American anole, *Anolis carolinensis* (Figure 18). These lesions are a result of combat and biting by cagemates.

In snakes mycotic diseases of the integument include phycomycosis, penicillinosis, geotrichosis, fusariomycosis, and chromomycosis. In some cases the lesions are extremely necrotizing, as seen in a Burmese python (*Python molurus bivittatus*) with a *Fusarium* infection.[37] In other cases the lesions are proliferative and hyperkeratotic, such as in a *Trichoderma* infection in a ball python (*Python regius*) and *Penicillium* and *Oospora* infections in eastern king snakes (*Lampropeltis getulus*).[37] In a rosy rat snake (*Elaphe guttata rosacea*) with mycotic skin disease in addition to epidermal necrosis, there were well-developed dermal granulomas containing hyphae.[37] A case of dermal fibrosarcoma and chromomycosis was seen in a Mangrove snake (*Boiga dendrophila*), with the skin overlying the mass having several small deeply pigmented fistulous tracts extending into the fungal portion of the mass.[38]

In most cases epidermal skin lesions result in discoloration of the normal pigmentation of the skin. In snakes the scales appear thickened and have a yellow-orange-brown discoloration (Figure 19). Once familiar with the gross appearance of these lesions the clinician will have little problem recognizing them. These are relatively common lesions in snakes that often are misdiagnosed.

Management/Treatment of Fungal Skin Disease

As in higher vertebrates, fungi in reptiles can be either primary or secondary invaders.[36] In my experience, they are more often secondary invaders with a multitude of predisposing factors being involved. In aquatic turtles, poor water quality is contributory. Lower environmental temperature results in immunosuppression in reptiles and may allow secondary agents to become invasive. In one study skin lesions in carpet pythons were associated with high humidity in the cage that may have reduced the capacity of the skin to resist infection.[39] Cages that are not kept clean promote the growth of numerous fungal organisms. In additional, fungal disease may follow a primary viral and/or bacterial skin infection.

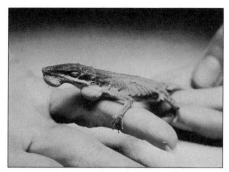

Figure 18—Subcutaneous hematomas in an American anole. *Trichosporon beigelii* was cultured from this lesion.

Relatively few reports discuss treatment of reptiles with fungal skin disease. Localized mycotic infections of scales and subcutaneous mycotic granulomas are best treated by surgical removal. Several cases of mycotic skin disease have been

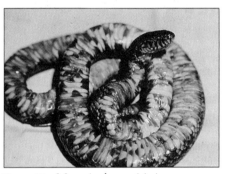

Figure 19—Mycotic dermatitis in an eastern king snake.

treated successfully by soaking in a dilute organic iodine solution twice daily followed by the topical application of an antifungal ointment such as tolnaftate (Tinactin®—Schering-Plough) or miconazole nitrate (Monistat-Derm™—Ortho Pharmaceutical Corp.). As mentioned earlier, malachite green has been used for treating aquatic turtles with mycotic shell disease. Two cage-mate ball pythons (*P. regius*) diagnosed with a *Trichoderma* spp. dermatitis were unsuccessfully treated with oral griseofulvin at 20 and 40 mg/kg body weight, respectively, every 3 days for five treatments. Ketoconazole (Nizoral®—Janssen Pharmaceutica) has also been administered to reptiles with fungal skin disease. In a pharmacokinetic study in the gopher tortoise (*Gopherus polyphemus*), oral administration of 30 mg/kg body weight resulted in therapeutic plasma concentrations (>1 µg/ml) from 4 to 32 hours after dosing.[40]

Parasitic Diseases
Pseudophyllidean Cestodes

Spirometra is a pseudophyllidean cestode that is widely distributed in different species of snakes, which serve as intermediate or paratenic hosts. Each egg releases a larva (coracidium) which, when ingested by a copepod, develops into a procercoid. Upon ingestion of the latter stage by a second intermediate host (reptile), procercoids develop into plerocercoids, which are known as sparganum when they are present in skeletal muscle. When present

subcutaneously, sparganum can cause soft swellings of the overlying skin. Edema and hemorrhage of soft tissues may be found associated with this stage. The definitive host is generally a mammalian carnivore (most often a felid), although reptiles and birds can also serve as final hosts. In some parts of the world, human sparganosis is a common disease, and some cases result from the consumption of raw snake meat.

Mesocercariae Infections

Trematode mesocercariae of the genera *Alaria* and *Fibricola* have been identified in subcutaneous locations in a Texas indigo snake (*Drymarchon corais erebennus*) and red-sided garter snakes (*Thamnophis sirtalis parietalis*).[41] In the indigo snake, the trematodes were found within gelatinous subcutaneous masses in the intermandibular region and tail.

Spirorchidiasis

Adult members of the family Spirorchidae inhabit the circulatory system of susceptible reptiles. Turtles appear to be the most commonly infected reptilian host. Adult parasites generally are found within the great vessels leaving the heart or within the heart chambers, where focal endothelial hyperplasia has been seen. These lesions generally range in intensity from minimal to mild and show no clinical signs of illness that can be attributed directly to their presence.

The most significant lesions resulting from these parasites are a consequence of eggs released within the vascular compartment. Eggs ultimately become trapped within terminal vessels almost anywhere in the animal's body; at these places a severe granulomatous response often is elicited. Infected turtles have been seen with shell lesions ranging from focal to coalescing and ulcerative on the plastron and carapace. Edema of the limbs can also be seen and results from vascular occlusion.

Control of these parasites involves identification and elimination of the snail intermediate host. Transmission should be self-limiting in captivity, provided that no snails are present. Praziquantel (Droncit®—Mobay Corp.) at 8 mg/kg body weight given intramuscularly has been used in treating spirorchid infections of green turtles.

Filariasis

Filarial nematodes have been described for all major

groups of reptiles. Some of the more important genera include *Oswaldofilaria, Foleyella,* and *Macdonaldius.* Limited studies have shown that there seems to be a low degree of host specificity for these genera. As adults all members of this group are found at extraintestinal sites (lungs, circulatory system, subcutaneous areas); these nematodes are either ovoviviparous or viviparous. Microfilariae are released into the circulatory system and transmission is achieved through blood-sucking arthropods, usually ticks and mosquitos.

Most reptilian filarial infections are diagnosed at necropsy. There are relatively few reports documenting clinical signs and gross lesions associated with infection. Several reticulated pythons in a zoologic collection developed cutaneous lesions; the transmission was presumably from boa constrictors kept in the same exhibit.[42] An argasid tick served as the vector. Lesions consisted of a necrotizing dermatitis; numerous parasites were found in the mesenteric arteries and obstruction of peripheral capillaries by microfilariae resulted in ischemic necrosis of the skin. The death of a bull snake (*Pituophis catenifer*) was attributed to the obstruction of the portal vein with *Macdonaldius seetae.*[43] In this case no signs of illness were seen before death.

Diagnosis depends on demonstration of adult parasites (most commonly found in the portal vein) at necropsy or identification of microfilariae in a blood sample. There are no reports describing the use of chemotherapeutic drugs. Telford found that an ambient temperature regime of 35 to 37°C (95 to 98.6°F) for 24 to 48 hours resulted in the death of adult parasites.[44] Care must be taken to carefully monitor snakes at this temperature regime and to ensure that the critical thermal maximum for the species is not exceeded.

Dracunculiasis

Several species of snakes with multifocal raised pustular lesions scattered over the body surface were found to contain myriads of nematode larvae within these lesions.[45] Larger slender nematodes in various stages of degeneration were associated with these lesions and were identified as a member of the superfamily Dracunculoidea. Dracunculoidea larvae develop in *Cyclops* sp. (a copepod) and tadpoles have been used as experimental transfer hosts. The intermediate host(s) is unknown.

Spiruridiasis

Larvae of the spirurid *Eustrongylides* have been reported to cause dermal lesions in red-sided garter snakes (*Thamnophis sirtalis parietalis*).[46] In addition to subcutaneous sites, larvae also were encountered in the lungs and free within the coelomic cavity. Intermediate hosts include fish and frogs. Adult parasites are located in the mucosa of the esophagus or the proventriculus or in the intestine of fish-eating birds.

Pentastomiasis

These primitive-appearing parasites are now placed in their own phylum. The adults are worm-like and superficially segmented; they range in size from 0.5 to 12 cm. All require intermediate hosts for completion of their life cycle. The most important genera infecting reptiles include *Sebekia* (in crocodilians), *Raillietiella* (in lizards and snakes), and *Kiricephalus, Porocephalus,* and *Armillifer* (in snakes). Mammals serve as intermediate hosts and several species within the genus *Armillifer* can infect humans. Most of the reports on human infection involve cases in Africa and Southeast Asia.

Ingested larvae migrate through the intestinal tract and may undergo extensive visceral migration before they reach maturity either in the lung and air sac or in subcutaneous tissues. Parasites distributed in subcutaneous sites may cause bulging of the overlying skin. Pentastomes are known to exit through lesions in the skin of newly captured wild reptiles.

Acarids

Mites. Most free-ranging reptiles are infested with mites. Some species of mites show a high degree of host specificity, whereas others are rather nonspecific in their predilection for a particular host. Because of their small size, mites may be overlooked in the recently acquired reptile.

The most commonly reported mite of reptiles is the snake mite (*Ophionyssus natricis*). This mite has a worldwide distribution and although it is only occasionally found on wild snakes, severe burdens are commonly encountered in recently imported snakes maintained under crowded, filthy conditions. The entire life cycle requires approximately 10 to 32 days, and a single female can lay up to 80 eggs. Eggs are deposited off the host in the immediate environment of the snake.

Severe infestations of *Ophionyssus* can result in a debilitated, anemic snake. Mites are often found in the axes between scales and in the sulcus formed between the spectacle and the periocular scales. The conjunctiva may become swollen and edematous. In addition, *Ophionyssus* is capable of transmitting the gram-negative bacteria *Aeromonas hydrophila.* Some strains of this bacteria are extremely pathogenic and can result in fatal septicemia. Under unusual conditions mites are capable of infesting humans, who may develop focal skin lesions.

Although mites are easy to overlook in light infestations, they appear almost to consume the host in severe cases. Mites generally are first noticed at the bottom of water bowls, where they fall off while the snake is drinking.

Ticks. Reptiles, including several marine species, are commonly infested by ticks. The more important hard-bodied genera infesting reptiles include *Amblyomma,*

Aponomma, and *Hyalomma*. The most common soft-bodied tick is *Ornithidoros*. Even under captive conditions ticks rarely reach the burdens achieved by mites; still, they are significant potential pathogens causing anemia, producing focal ulcerating skin lesions, or acting as vectors for the transmission of other pathogens, such as *Macdonaldius* and rickettsiae.

Diptera. Numerous species of the order Diptera are known to feed upon reptiles and many are responsible for transmitting infectious agents. Several species of flies are known to parasitize reptiles directly in the larval (maggot) stages. Most cases of myiasis involve terrestrial chelonians; a few examples have been seen in debilitated crocodilians. Of turtles, box turtles (*Terrapene carolina*) and gopher tortoises (*Gopherus polyphemus*) in the southeastern United States appear particularly prone to infestation with *Cistudinamyia cistudinis*. In severe infestations maggots can be found at almost any subcutaneous site. Gopher tortoises have been found with focal lesions adjacent to the cloaca containing up to three dozen maggots. These fly larvae are incapable of penetrating intact skin but can utilize small openings, such as those caused by tick bites.

NONINFECTIOUS DISEASES
Environmentally Associated Skin Diseases
Trauma

Various traumatic injuries have been identified in captive reptiles, including abrasions, bite wounds, crushing injuries to turtle shells, damaged mouthparts (especially in turtles), and thermal burns.

Because reptiles are ectotherms, ultimately dependent upon environmental infrared radiation as a heat source, high wattage infrared and incandescent light bulbs are often used as heat sources in captivity. Often the bulb is placed within the cage where the animal can make direct contact, or too "hot" a bulb is used resulting in thermal burns to the animal. Captive reptiles ideally should be exposed to a gradient of temperature that spans the preferred optimum range for the species. Heat sources should originate outside the cage or at a distance where contact cannot be made. Reptiles receiving thermal burns will develop epidermal vesicles followed by necrosis.

Electric heating pads used to provide heat for captive reptiles often develop hot spots and result in ventral burning of the reptile's integument. As discussed earlier, severe necrotizing burn lesions often become invaded with *Pseudomonas* spp. and further add to the problems. Such animals require intensive chronic treatment with broad spectrum injectable antibiotics in addition to organic iodine soaks and topical application of organic iodine ointments.

Trauma in captive reptiles can result from direct aggression between cage-mates or indirectly when reptiles come together at feeding time. With snakes, when an animal is fed a prey species, a feeding frenzy often is elicited whereby anything smelling of the prey species will be attacked. Two snakes feeding upon the same rodent or fish may result in the larger snake inflicting cutaneous lacerations on the smaller snake. Depending upon the temperament of the animals, separation of cage-mates at feeding time may be necessary.

It is recommended that prey items be killed before feeding them to carnivorous reptiles, especially when food items are rodents. Live mice and rats can inflict serious bites upon their reptile predator. Snakes have been seen that have had large areas of skin and underlying musculature removed by prey rodent species left in the cage overnight. As discussed earlier, subcutaneous abscesses can develop several weeks or months after a rodent bite.

Dysecydysis

Humidity is an important environmental consideration when keeping reptiles in captivity. A relative humidity of 50 to 60% is used for many reptile species; however, some species will do better at lower relative humidities while others will thrive at higher relative humidities. In snakes and lizards, if the relative humidity is too low for the species, it may not be able to shed its old skin normally. If a snake's skin is retained for one day beyond the normal time of shedding, the integument will have the appearance of being dehydrated because of the drying of the retained skin. Spectacles also can be retained. If a snake has not molted properly, it should be soaked in a container having just enough water to cover the body. Retained spectacles can be gently removed with forceps or rubbed free with moistened cotton.

Blister Disease

For some species of lizards and snakes excess humidity can cause problems. Some of the fungal skin diseases have been seen in reptiles kept in cages with excess humidity. Another disease that has been described in snakes, although its pathogenesis is not understood, is blister disease. This disease is seen commonly in water snakes, garter snakes, and king snakes that are maintained under excessively moist conditions (Figure 20). It is perplexing as to why this disease develops in water snakes, a species spending most of its time in or around water. Air exchange in the cage may be important in the development of the disease as many of the snakes developing this disease are in cages that have poor air circulation. Stagnant air of high relative humidity in some way may initiate pathologic changes in the skin resulting in cleft formation and accumulation of fluid in the epidermis. The pathogenesis of this disease needs to be elucidated.

Nutritional Deficiency-Associated Skin Diseases
Vitamin A Deficiency

Vitamin A is essential for the maintenance of epithelial integrity. Many cases of vitamin A deficiency in reptiles are epithelial-related problems, particularly disease of the adnexal structures of the eye in aquatic turtles. Turtles often are presented with palpebral edema, anasarca, hyperkeratosis of the skin, and overgrowth of the mandibular and maxillary horny mouthparts. Classic histopathologic changes seen are squamous metaplasia and hyperkeratosis of lacrimal and Harderian gland tubules.

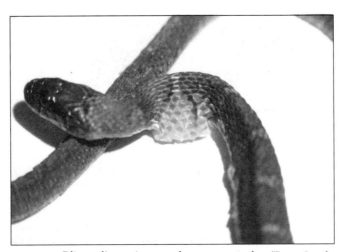

Figure 20—Blister disease in a northern water snake. (From Jacobson ER: Diseases of reptiles, Part I. Noninfectious diseases. *Compend Contin Educ Pract Vet* 3:122–126, 1981, with permission.)

Therapy should include treatment of the immediate problem and improvement of the deficient diet. In severe cases in which the animal's palpebrae are swollen and closed, injectable vitamin A can be administered intramuscularly at 2000 units/kg body weight every 3 days for 2 weeks. The commercial diet ReptoMin® (Tetra-Werke—West Germany), which is available in most pet stores selling reptiles, appears to be nutritionally complete and is readily accepted by most aquatic chelonians.

Collagen Disorders

A very interesting disease of collagen has been seen by the author in several recently imported reticulated pythons (*Python reticulatus*). The snakes were submitted with the epidermis detached from the dermis. The skin would tear after minimal abrasions or manual restraint. Fluid accumulated between the epidermis and dermis and in one snake moved as a column from the head to tail after tilting. One snake also regurgitated after feeding and after euthanasia, necropsy revealed that the gastric mucosa had separated from the submucosa and formed a balloon-like structure over the pylorus. Histologically, collagen in the dermis and submucosa was poorly organized and poorly developed. Chronic malnutrition (that is, protein deficiency) may have been instrumental in initiating this problem. Further because some species of snakes are known to synthesize vitamin C in their kidney,[47] malnourished snakes may not produce enough vitamin C for adequate formation of collagen.

Neoplastic Skin Diseases

Neoplastic diseases are common in older captive reptiles whereas relatively uncommon in young reptiles. Several populations of free-ranging green turtles have been identified with cutaneous fibropapillomas, with both juvenile and adult green turtles equally represented. In crocodilians few neoplasms have been reported for any age group. This is especially surprising because crocodilians are long-lived reptiles (many live for 100 years) and are commonly kept in zoologic collections. The major neoplasms of the integument are discussed below.

Squamous Cell Carcinoma

Squamous cell carcinomas have been reported from the foot of a Ceylonese terrapin (*Geoemyda trijuga*)[48] and from the foot of a common tegu (*Tupinambis teguixin*).[49] In the latter report, the tumor measured 3 cm in diameter and almost destroyed the metacarpus as well as the proximal two phalanges of the fifth right digit. The tumor consisted of neoplastic epithelial cells and pearl formation with large areas of necrosis. Although squamous cell carcinoma has been described for the oral cavity and cloaca of snakes, few cases of cutaneous squamous cell carcinoma have been reported.[49a] A water moccasin (*Agkistrodon piscivores*) with a 1-cm spherical mass attached to the lower left mandible was histologically diagnosed as having a squamous cell carcinoma.[50]

Papillomas and Fibropapillomas

Papillomas, fibromas, and fibropapillomas were first described in captured adult green turtles (*Chelonia mydas*) 50 years ago.[51,52] Fibropapillomas are distributed over the dorsal cervical region, axillary regions of the hind legs, eyelids, and conjunctivae (Figure 21). These lesions ranged from papillary projections of hyperplastic keratinized epithelium supported by a fibrous core to smooth round fibrous tumors composed of dense connective tissue covered by thickened epithelium. Today fibropapillomas are well established in populations of green turtles in the Indian River lagoon system of east central Florida, the Florida Keys, and the Hawaiian Islands. Although detailed pathologic studies have been done no specific agent has been incriminated. From a comparative standpoint a viral agent seems most likely.

Occasionally, particles with electron-dense centers and measuring 155 to 190 nm were observed in intracytoplasmic vacuoles in epidermal cells of the stratum basale. Their identity remains unknown.

As discussed in the section Viral Skin Diseases, cutaneous papillomas have been commonly seen in the European emerald lizard (*Lacerta viridis*) and several types of viral particles have been found in these lesions. Cutaneous papillomas have also been described for the sand lizard (*Lacerta agilis*) and the European wall lizard (*Lacerta muralis*). Relatively few cases of cutaneous papillomas have been described in snakes.

Pigment Cell Tumors

At least four varieties of pigment cells are found in the integument of reptiles: two kinds of melanophores containing melanin; xanthophores or erythrophores containing pteridines and carotenoids; and iridophores (guanophores) containing reflecting platelets of guanine, adenine, hypoxanthine, and uric acid. Three of these pigment cell types are uniquely located in the dermis, and it is only the epidermal melanophore (melanocyte) that is found in the epidermis.

A variety of pigment cell tumors have been described for snakes. Multiple skin melanomas were reported for each of two reticulated pythons (*Python reticulatus*),[54] and a malignant melanoma was described in each of a caged pair of pine snakes (*Pituophis melanoleucus*).[55] A new neoplasm, a chromatophoroma, was described in a western terrestrial garter snake (*Thamnophis elegans terrestris*),[56] and a malignant chromatophoroma consisting of mosaic chromatophores with pigment particles typical of more than one type of chromatophore was reported for a gopher snake (*Pituophis catenifer sayi*). Combined iridophoroma and melanophoroma was recently described in a northern pine snake (*P. melanoleucus melanoleucus*) with metastases of malignant iridophores to multiple visceral sites.[58]

Fibrosarcoma

I have seen several cases of fibrosarcoma involving the integumentary system of snakes. These neoplasms generally appear as subcutaneous swellings with or without necrosis of the overlying skin, and often spread into surrounding tissues making it difficult to determine the tumor margins. Histologically, fibrosarcomas range from

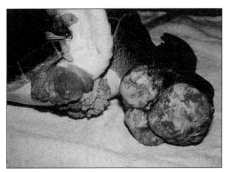

Figure 21—Large fibropapillomas covering the right eye of a juvenile green turtle.

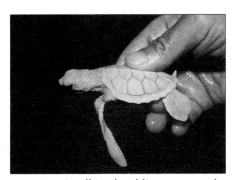

Figure 22—An albino hatchling green turtle.

populations of undifferentiated anaplastic to well-differentiated cells producing abundant collagen.

Treatment/Management of Neoplastic Conditions

Treatment depends on many factors, including the age, species, and physical condition of the individual; type of neoplasm; system affected; and usually the cost of the procedure. Early diagnosis is necessary for the best success. Any unusual skin lesions and internal masses should be biopsied as soon as identified. Once a neoplasm has metastasized the prognosis is grave. Often these metastatic lesions are only diagnosed at necropsy. Although a variety of treatment regimens have been developed for the various cutaneous neoplasms found in mammals, there are few reports of their use in reptiles. The most successful treatment is that of surgical removal. In green turtles with cutaneous fibropapillomas, early lesions that were surgically removed did not recur at the surgical site. Such neoplasms as melanomas and chromatophoromas should have wide surgical margins because they often diffusely infiltrate surrounding tissue. After removal neoplasms should be submitted for histopathology to determine if neoplastic cells extend to the margins of the incised mass.

Congenital Abnormalities

A variety of congenital skin anomalies are described for reptiles. Various abnormalities with regard to coloration have been reported for all groups of reptiles. As mentioned earlier, most reptiles have an array of different pigment cells in the dermis, the various combinations of which give each species its distinctive coloration. Albinism, melanism, and other coloration anomalies have been seen (Figure 22). Many private breeders of snakes are selecting for various colors and patterns that are in demand by the pet trade. The more unusual the color and pattern, the greater the price for the animals. Turtles with above-normal numbers of scutes on their carapace and plastron and scaleless snakes have been reported. Snakes with scales pointing rostrally instead of the normal caudal orientation have also been seen.

Many of the congenital defects in reptiles have been attributed to improper incubation conditions of eggs. Incubation temperatures above or below optimum may result in malformations in the developing embryo. Many of the color and pattern anomalies, however, have a genetic basis, and reptiles can be selectively bred for these traits.

DERMATOLOGIC DIAGNOSTIC TECHNIQUES

The key to evaluating skin lesions of reptiles is collecting and properly evaluating a good biopsy specimen for histologic evaluation, cytology, and microbial culture. Microbial culture by itself is often misleading, however, because many microbes often secondarily colonize skin lesions.

Chelonians

Of all the reptiles, chelonians present the greatest challenge for biopsy especially when lesions involve the shell. As mentioned earlier, the reptile shell is a very hard biologic structure that makes biopsy somewhat difficult. A rotary power saw (Dremel Mototool®—Dremel Mfg. Co.) can be used to cut a wedge out of the shell. For anesthesia ketamine hydrochloride can be administered at 20 to 40 mg/kg body weight given intramuscularly in a forelimb. Ideally, the biopsy should include normal tissue along with the diseased component. A piece should be fixed in neutral buffered 10% formalin for histopathologic evaluation and a piece (with the most superficial contaminated portion removed) submitted for microbial culture. The defect created in the shell should be filled with calcium hydroxide dental paste (RootCal®—Ellman International Mfg.) and covered over with a methacrylate resin (Cyanoveneer®—Ellman International Mfg.). This technique is routinely used in repair of the chelonian shell.

For biopsy of soft tissue a 2% xylocaine block is satisfactory and can be infiltrated around the biopsy site. A biopsy punch can be used for collecting the sample. After biopsy the skin may require a single suture for closure. Monofilament nylon is routinely used.

Crocodilians and Lizards

A full-thickness biopsy may be difficult in those areas of the crocodilian integument having osteoderms. Small crocodilians and most lizards can be manually restrained, whereas large crocodilians and large monitors must be chemically immobilized. The area around the biopsy site should be infiltrated with 2% xylocaine and a full-thickness skin incision taken with a biopsy punch. As with chelonians at least two biopsies should be taken, one for histopathology and one for microbiology. For microbial culture the lesions should be ground in a sterile mortar and pestle and samples applied to the appropriate media. This appears to be particularly important for isolation of fungi from reptile skin lesions.

Snakes

Snakes are ideally suited for skin biopsy. Harmless species can be manually restrained, and poisonous species can be guided into a Plexiglas tube for restraint.

Affected scales can be removed with a scalpel blade, or a sterilized one-hole paper punch can be used for biopsies of individual scales. In certain skin diseases, such as vesiculating skin lesion, larger samples may be needed. In such cases the area around the lesion should be infiltrated with 2% xylocaine hydrochloride and the skin sutured after removal of the specimen. Similarly, for sampling subcutaneous masses 2% xylocaine can be infiltrated subcutaneously around the mass. Once removed the mass should be split in half for both histologic evaluation and microbial culture.

ACKNOWLEDGMENTS

Sections of this chapter were taken from Jacobson ER: Parasitic diseases of reptiles. In: Fowler ME (ed): *Zoo and Wild Animal Medicine.* Philadelphia, WB Saunders Co, 1986, pp 162-181; and Jacobson ER: Reptiles. *Vet Clin North Am [Small Anim Pract]* 17:1203–1225, 1987, with permission.

REFERENCES

1. Zangerl R: The turtle shell, in Gans C (ed): *Biology of the Reptilia*, vol 1. New York, Academic Press, 1969, pp 311–346.
2. Magliola L: The effects of estrogen on skeletal calcium metabolism and on plasma parameters of vitellogenesis in the male, three-toed box turtle (*Terrapene carolina triunguis*). *Gen Comp Endocrinol* 54:162–170, 1983.
3. Rainey WE: *Guide to Sea Turtle Visceral Anatomy.* NOAA Technical Memorandum, NMFS-SEFC-82, 1981.
4. Matoltsy AG, Huszar T: Keratinization of the reptilian epidermis: An ultrastructural study of the turtle skin. *J Ultrastruct Res* 38:87–101, 1972.
4a. Rossi JV: Dermatology, in Mader DR (ed): *Reptile Medicine and Surgery.* Philadelphia, WB Saunders, 1995, pp 104–117.
5. Maderson PFA: Histological changes in the epidermis of snakes during the sloughing cycle. *J Zool* 146:98–113, 1965.
6. Maderson PFA: Some developmental problems of the reptilian integument, in Gans C, Billet F, Maderson PFA (eds): *Biology of the Reptilia.* New York, John Wiley and Sons, 1985, pp 523–598.
7. Schumacher J: Viral diseases, in Mader DR (ed): *Reptile Medicine and Surgery.* Philadelphia, WB Saunders, 1995, pp 224–234.
8. Haines H, Kleese WC: Effect of water temperature on a herpes-virus infection in sea turtles. *Infect Immun* 15:756–759, 1977.
9. Jacobson ER, Popp J, Shields RP, et al: Pox-like virus associated with skin lesions in captive caimans. *JAVMA* 175:937–940, 1979.
10. Foggin CM: Diseases and disease control on crocodile farms in Zimbabwe, in Webb GJW, Manolis SC, Whitehead PJ (eds): *Wildlife Management, Crocodiles and Alligators.* New South Wales, Australia, Surrey Beatty and Sons Pty Limited, 1987, pp 351–362.
11. Horner RE: Poxvirus in farmed Nile crocodiles. *Vet Rec* 7:459–461, 1988.
12. Frye FL: *Biomedical and Surgical Aspects of Captive Reptile Husbandry.* Edwardsville, KS, Veterinary Medicine Publishing Co, 1981, p 167.
13. Jacobson ER, Gaskin JM, Clubb SL: Papilloma-like virus infection in Bolivian side-neck turtles. *JAVMA* 181:1325–1328, 1982.

14. Raynaud MMA, Adrian M: Lesions cutanees a structure papillomateuse associees a des virus chez le lizard (*Lacerta viridis* Laur). *CR Acad Sci Paris* 283:845–847, 1976.

14a. Schumacher J: Viral diseases, in Mader DR (ed): *Reptile Medicine and Surgery.* Philadelphia, WB Saunders, 1995, pp 224–234.

15. Jackson CG, Fulton M: A turtle colony epizootic apparently of microbial origin. *J Wildl Dis* 6:446–468, 1970.

16. Wallach JD: The pathogenesis and etiology of ulcerative shell disease in turtles. *J Zoo Anim Med* 6:11–13, 1972.

17. Jackson CG Jr, Fulton M, Jackson MM: Cranial asymmetry with massive infection in a box turtle. *J Wildl Dis* 8:275–277, 1972.

18. Duran-Reynals F, Clausen HJ: A contagious tumor-like condition in the lizard (*Anolis equestris*) as induced by a new bacterial species, *Serratia anolium* (Sp.N.). *J Bacteriol* 33:369–379, 1937.

19. Boam GW, Sanger VL, Cowan DF, Vaughan DP: Subcutaneous abscesses in iguanid lizards. *JAVMA* 157:617–619, 1975.

20. Plowman CA, Montali RJ, Phillips LJ, et al: Septicemia and chronic abscesses in iguanas (*Cyclura cornuta and Iguana iguana*) associated with *Neisseria* species. *J Zoo Anim Med* 18:86–93, 1987.

21. Rosenthal KR, Mader DR: Microbiology, in Mader DR (ed): *Reptile Medicine and Surgery.* Philadelphia, WB Saunders, 1995, pp 117–125.

22. Dogget RG: Microbiology of *Pseudomonas aeruginosa* in Dogget RG (ed): *Pseudomona aeruginosa: Clinical Manifestations of Infection and Curr Ther.* New York, Academic Press, 1979, pp 1–7.

23. Murphy JB, Armstrong BL: *Maintenance of Rattlesnakes in Captivity.* Lawrence, KS, University of Kansas Publications, Museum of Natural History, 1978.

24. Jacobson ER: *Pseudomonas,* in Hoff GL, Frye FL, Jacobson ER (eds): *Diseases of Amphibians and Reptiles.* New York, Plenum Press, 1984, pp 37–47.

25. Jacobson ER, Ingling AL: Pyloroduodenal resection in a Burmese python. *JAVMA* 169:985–987, 1976.

26. Shotts EB, Gaines JL, Martin C, Prestwood AK: *Aeromonas* induced death among fish and reptiles in a eutrophic inland lake. *JAVMA* 161:603–607, 1972.

27. Brownstein DG: Mycobacteriosis, in Hoff GL, Frye FL, Jacobson ER (eds): *Diseases of Amphibians and Reptiles.* New York, Plenum Press, 1984, pp 1–23.

28. Quesenberry KE, Jacobson ER, Allen JL, Cooley AJ: Ulcerative stomatitis and subcutaneous granulomas caused by *Mycobacterium chelonei* in a boa constrictor. *JAVMA* 189:1131–1132, 1986.

29. Montali FJ, Smith EE, Davenport M, Bush M: Dermatophilosis in Australian bearded lizards. *JAVMA* 167:553–555, 1975.

30. Anver MR, Park JS, Rush HG: Dermatophilosis in the marble lizard (*Calotes mystaceus*). *Lab Anim Sci* 26:817–823, 1976.

31. Simmons GC, Sullivan ND, Green PE: Dermatophilosis in a lizard (*Amphibolurus barbatus*). *Aust Vet J* 48:465–467, 1972.

32. Klingenberg RJ: Therapeutics, in Mader DR (ed): *Reptile Medicine and Surgery.* Philadelphia, WB Saunders, 1995, pp 299–321.

32a. Stein G: Reptile and amphibian formulary, in Mader DR (ed): *Reptile Medicine and Surgery.* Philadelphia, WB Saunders, 1995, pp 465–472.

32b. Rossi JV: Dermatology, in Mader DR (ed): *Reptile Medicine and Surgery.* Philadelphia, WB Saunders, 1995, pp 104–117.

33. Frank W: Mycotic infections in amphibians and reptiles, in Page LA (ed): *Wildlife Diseases.* New York, Plenum Press, 1976, pp 73–88.

34. Hunt TJ: Notes on diseases and mortality in testudines. *Herpetologica* 13:19–23, 1957.

35. Jacobson ER, Calderwood MB, Clubb SL: Mucormycosis in hatchling Florida softshell turtles. *JAVMA* 177:835–837, 1980.

36. Migaki G, Jacobson ER, Casey HW: Fungal diseases in reptiles, in Hoff GL, Frye RL, Jacobson ER (eds): *Diseases of Amphibians and Reptiles.* New York, Plenum Press, 1984, pp 183–204.

37. Jacobson ER: Necrotizing mycotic dermatitis in snakes: Clinical and pathologic features. *JAVMA* 177:838–841, 1980.

38. Jacobson ER: Chromomycosis and fibrosarcoma in a mangrove snake. *JAVMA* 185:1428–1430, 1984.

39. McKenzie RA, Green PE: Mycotic dermatitis in carpet snakes. *J Wildl Dis* 12:405–408, 1976.

40. Page CD, Mautino M, Meyter JR, Mechlinski W: Preliminary pharmacokinetics of ketoconazole in gopher tortoises (*Gopherus polyphemus*), in *Proceed Joint Conference, American Assoc Zoo Veterinarians Amer Assoc Wildlife Veterinarians,* Toronto, Ontario, Canada, 1988, p 63.

41. Wright K, Tousignant A, Overstreet R, et al: *Mesocercariae* infections in a Texas indigo snake and red-sided garter snakes, in *Third International Colloquium on the Pathology of Reptiles and Amphibians.* Orlando, Florida, 1989, p 54.

42. Frank W. Die pathogenen Wirkungen von *Macdonaldius oschei* Chaubaud et Frank 1961 (Filaroidea, Onchocercidae) bei ver schiedenen arten von schlangen (Reptilia, Ophidia). *Z Parasitenkd* 24:249, 1964.

43. Hull RW, Camin JH: *Macdonaldius seetae* Khanna, 1933 in captive snakes. *Trans Am Micros Soc* 78:323, 1959.

44. Telford SR Jr: Some observations on the effects of varying ambient temperatures in vivo on filarial worms of snakes. *Jpn J Exp Med* 35:291, 1965.

45. Jacobson ER, Greiner EC, Clubb SL, Harvey-Clarke C: Pustular dermatitis caused by subcutaneous dracunculiasis in snakes. *JAVMA* 189:1133–1134, 1986.

46. Lichtenfels JR, Lavies B: Mortality in red-sided garter snakes, *Thamnophis sirtalis parietalis,* due to larval nematode, *Eustrongylus* sp. *Lab Anim Sci* 26:465, 1976.

47. Vosburgh KM, Brady PS, Ullrey DE: Ascorbic acid requirements of garter snakes: Plains (*Thamnophis radix*) and eastern (*T. sirtalis sirtalis*). *J Zoo Anim Med* 13:38–42, 1982.

48. Cowen DF: Disease of captive reptiles. *JAVMA* 153:848–859, 1968.

49. Schwartz E: Ueber swei geschwuelste bei kaltbluetern. *Z Krebsforsch* 20:353–357, 1923.

49a. Done LB: Neoplasia, in Mader DR (ed): *Reptile Medicine and Surgery.* Philadelphia, WB Saunders, 1995, pp 125–141.

50. Wadworth JR: Tumors and tumor-like lesions in snakes. *JAVMA* 137:419–420, 1960.

51. Lucke B: Studies on tumors in cold-blooded vertebrates. *Ann Tortugas Lab* (Carnegie Institute, Washington, DC), 1938.

52. Smith GM, Coates C: Fibro-epithelial growths of the skin in large marine turtles, *Chelonia mydas* (Linnaeus). *Zoologica (New York)* 24:379–382, 1938.

53. Jacobson ER, Mansell JL, Sundberg JP, et al: Cutaneous fibropapillomas of green turtles (*Chelonia mydas*). *J Comp Pathol* 101:39–52, 1989.

54. Schlumberger HG, Lucke B: Tumors of fishes, amphibians and reptiles. *Cancer Res* 8:657–753, 1948.

55. Ball HA: Melanosarcoma and rhabdomyoma in two pine snakes (*Pituophis melanolecus*). *Cancer Res* 6:134–138, 1946.

56. Frye FL, Carney J, Harshbarger J, Zeigel R: Malignant chromatophoroma in a western garter snake. *JAVMA* 167:557–558, 1975.

57. Ryan MJ, Hill DL, Whitney CD: Malignant chomatophoroma in a gopher snake. *Vet Pathol* 18:827–829, 1981.

58. Jacobson ER, Ferris W, Bagnara JT, Iverson WO: Chromatophoromas in a pine snake. *Pigment Cell Res* 2:26–33, 1989.

A Color Atlas of Blood Cells of the Yellow Rat Snake*

University of Tennessee
Thomas K. Dotson, DVM
Edward C. Ramsay, DVM

University of Georgia
Denise I. Bounous, DVM, PhD

Definitive identification of peripheral blood cells is a fundamental problem in reptile hematology. Accurate differential cell counts are best done by individuals familiar with the white blood cell morphology for a particular species,[1] but the plethora of species presented in any clinical practice and the lack of comprehensive reference material for reptile hematology preclude many individuals from gaining this expertise.

The problems of differences in blood cell morphology among taxa are further compounded by the lack of standardized nomenclature for circulating leukocytes. Although some investigators have attempted to simplify leukocyte nomenclature,[2,3] considerable controversy regarding names and grouping remains.[4,5] Even the presence of certain cells in peripheral blood, such as eosinophils in the Squamata, remain under question.[6] Cytochemical studies of individual species are beginning to answer some of these questions, but few species have been studied.[7-9]

Several texts offer color photomicrographs of peripheral blood cells of reptiles[4,10]; however, few reports depict all the peripheral blood cells for one species.[7,8] This article provides a pictorial guide, with descriptions, of the peripheral blood cells of a single snake species—the yellow rat snake. The illustrations serve as a guide for clinicians and technicians evaluating snake hematology.

ANIMALS AND TECHNIQUES

Blood was collected by cardiocentesis from wild-caught, unanesthetized, captive yellow rat snakes *(Elaphe obsoleta quadrivittata)* that were generally in good health. The blood was placed in tubes with ethylenediaminetetraacetic acid (EDTA). Smears were stained with an aqueous-based Romanowsky's stain. Identification of cells was based on the nomenclature scheme used by Hawkey.[10]

*This work was supported by grants from the Center of Excellence, College of Veterinary Medicine, The University of Tennessee and The University of Georgia Veterinary Medical Experiment Station fund.

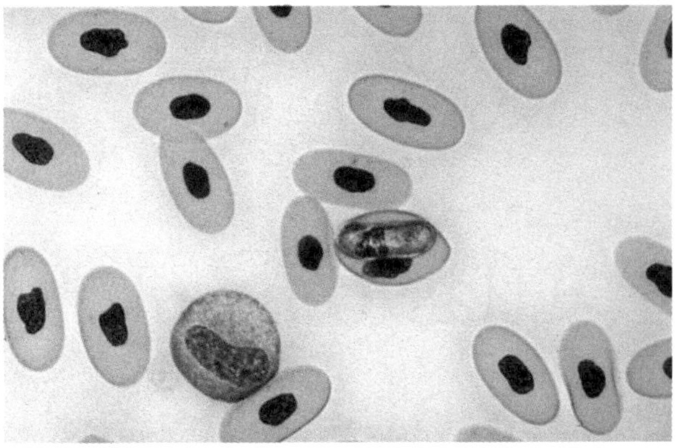

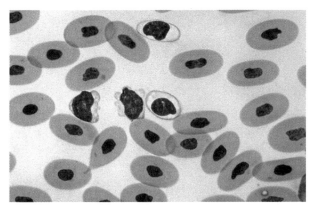

Figure 1—Erythrocytes and an azurophil from a yellow rat snake. One erythrocyte has an intracellular haemogregarine parasite. (EDTA; original magnification, ×330)

Figure 2—Two thrombocytes *(right)* and two small lymphocytes *(left)* from a yellow rat snake. (EDTA; original magnification, ×330)

CELL DESCRIPTIONS
Erythrocytes

Erythrocytes are the most abundant cell type seen in peripheral blood smears. They are elliptic and have a centrally located, basophilic nucleus (Figure 1). The long axis of the nucleus is parallel to that of the cell. The nucleus may be irregularly shaped but tends to be oval with a finely stippled-to-clumped chromatin pattern. In mature erythrocytes, there is a high nucleus-to-cytoplasm ratio. The homogeneous cytoplasm is translucent and consistently light pink-orange. Occasionally, a single small vacuole may be observed adjacent to the nucleus.

Erythroblasts have a greater width-to-length ratio than do mature erythrocytes. Erythrocytes also possess a larger, rounder nucleus. The nucleus of erythroblasts is dark purple with more prominent chromatin clumping. Erythrocytes have a larger nucleus-to-cytoplasm ratio and more basophilic cytoplasm than erythrocytes. Basophilic erythroblasts are spheric with a thin rim of deeply basophilic cytoplasm.

Degenerate erythrocytes (i.e., those approaching senescence) appear swollen but still retain an elliptic shape. The appearance of such erythrocytes can vary from having faded cytoplasm and an enlarged, amorphous, pinkish purple nucleus to a colorless cytoplasm with a pyknotic, deeply basophilic nucleus.

Anomalies of erythrocytes commonly observed in smears include cells twisted and folded onto themselves, spindle-shaped cells, and ruptured cells. Intraerythrocytic parasites were common in the snakes studied (Figure 1).

Thrombocytes

Snake thrombocytes are nucleated and generally assume two shapes (Figure 2). One form is smooth edged and elliptic (much like an erythrocyte), with the long axis of the nucleus parallel to that of the cell;

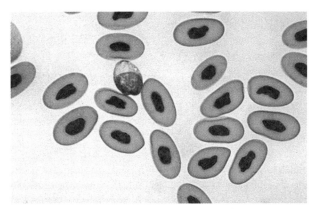

Figure 3—A large lymphocyte from a yellow rat snake. (EDTA; original magnification, ×330)

the other form is generally round, although sometimes misshapen, with irregular edges. In both forms, the nuclei are centrally located and tend to conform to the cell membrane. The nuclei are deeply basophilic with a clumped or smudged chromatin pattern. The cytoplasm is frequently colorless to the extent that the cell membrane is difficult to discern, particularly in the round thrombocytes. Occasionally, the cytoplasm is a very faint blue. A larger nucleus-to-cytoplasm ratio exists for the round thrombocytes than for the elliptic forms. Thrombocytes are often found aggregated or clumped, particularly in the outer edges of the smear. Occasionally, spindle-shaped thrombocytes or thrombocytes with vacuolated or foamy cytoplasm are observed.

Lymphocytes

Reptile lymphocytes are typically described as large or small; small lymphocytes are the most common in the yellow rat snake (Figures 2 and 3). Small lymphocytes are typically round but often have irregular cell outlines. Centrally or eccentrically located nuclei

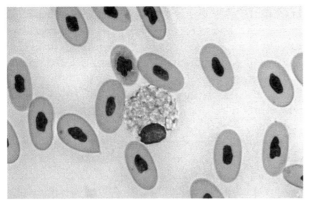

Figure 4A

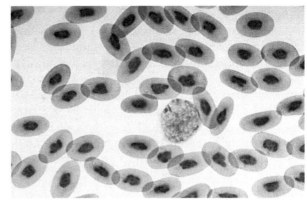

Figure 4B

Figure 4—(**A**) A heterophil and an immature erythrocyte *(above)* from a yellow rat snake. (aqueous-based Romanowsky's stain; original magnification, ×330) (**B**) A heterophil. (alcohol-based Romanowsky's stain; original magnification, ×330)

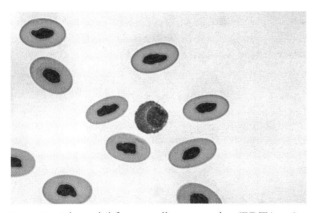

Figure 5—A basophil from a yellow rat snake. (EDTA; original magnification, ×330)

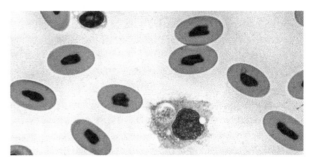

Figure 6—A monocyte-like cell from a yellow rat snake. A thrombocyte is also present. (EDTA; original magnification, ×330)

nearly fill the cell. When the nuclei contact the cell membrane, they follow the contour of the cell shape. Nuclear shape varies from round to polygonal; some nuclei have a small indentation.

Cytoplasm is finely granular, lightly basophilic, and scant, often appearing as a thin rim that surrounds the nucleus. Nuclei are light purple with a smudged chromatin pattern. Cells are occasionally seen with vacuolated or foamy cytoplasm. Aside from size, large lymphocytes differ from small ones by having a more pleomorphic nucleus, more basophilic cytoplasm, and a lower cytoplasm-to-nucleus ratio. Large lymphocytes are often nearly the same size as azurophils and heterophils.

Heterophils

Heterophils are typically the largest cell found in the peripheral blood of the yellow rat snake (Figure 4). Heterophils are round cells with an oval-to-lenticular nucleus eccentrically located in the cell. The nuclei vary in color from light blue to dark pink or purple and, if nuclear detail is discernible, they possess a

clumped chromatin pattern. The nucleus-to-cytoplasm ratio is very small. The pale pink cytoplasm is filled with eosinophilic, pleomorphic granules that give it a homogeneous appearance. Granule shape is best observed near cells that have ruptured. Heterophil anomalies include cells with folded edges, ruptured cells, and degranulated cells.

Azurophils

Mature azurophils are similar in size to heterophils. Azurophils vary in shape from round to monocytoid in appearance (Figure 1). The smaller cells have a greater tendency to be round. The nuclei are generally eccentrically placed and basophilic, with a clumped-to-smudged chromatin pattern. Nuclei vary in shape from round to lenticular, and some are indented, scalloped, or segmented. The nucleus-to-cytoplasm ratio is small in mature cells. The cytoplasm is bluish gray, with a coarsely to finely granular appearance. Characteristic azurophilic, intracytoplasmic granules are present. The granules may be discernible as discrete round structures or may merely impart a purplish hue to the cytoplasm. Occasionally, azurophils are observed with vacuolated cytoplasm.

Basophils

Basophils are infrequently observed in the yellow rat snake. These cells are small and round cells with an oval-to-lenticular–shaped nucleus (Figure 5). The nuclei are eccentrically located in the cell, very dark blue to purple in color, and have a clumped-to-smudged chromatin pattern. Basophils have a large nucleus-to-cytoplasm ratio. The cytoplasm is filled with intensely basophilic, round granules that often obscure the nucleus. The granules give the contour of the cell a cobblestone appearance.

Monocytes

Monocytes are not routinely observed in peripheral blood smears of healthy yellow rat snakes (Figure 6). The lightly basophilic nuclei are eccentrically located and pleomorphic and are often indented with a finely stippled chromatin pattern. The pale bluish gray cytoplasm is finely to moderately granular and may be vacuolated.

DISCUSSION

From comparisons made in our laboratory, EDTA seems to be a suitable anticoagulant for preserving blood of the yellow rat snake. Smears made from blood mixed with EDTA stained well with an aqueous-based Romanowsky's stain and did not exhibit artifacts, such as the rouleauxlike stacking of erythrocytes seen with snake blood mixed with sodium heparin. When an aqueous-based Romanowsky's stain is used, a slightly longer staining time (such as that which is commonly used for cytology preparations) makes azurophilic granules appear more prominent in cells. Differences that may be observed with an alcohol-based stain include heterophil granules, which are more eosinophilic, and lymphocyte cytoplasm, which is more basophilic.

We found reptile leukocytes to be fragile; as a result, proper technique in the preparation of blood smears is critical in obtaining valid differential cell count results. Heterophils seem to be particularly prone to rupture. Derived total white blood cell count methods, such as the eosinophil count method,[11] depend on the percentage of heterophils in the white blood cell differential count to calculate the total white blood cell count. When these methods are used, rupture of significant numbers of heterophils or sequestration of these cells in one area of the peripheral smear can greatly affect the accuracy of both the differential and total white cell counts.

While the presence of the eosinophil in members of the Squamata has been speculated,[5] no eosinophils were found in the snakes of the present report. Similarly, monocytes were not observed in peripheral blood of healthy snakes; however, cells resembling mammalian monocytes do appear in yellow rat snakes with severe bacterial infections.[a] We speculate that these monocyte-like cells are azurophils undergoing infection-related changes or possibly inflammatory activation.

The greatest difficulty in performing differential white blood cell counts is distinguishing between thrombocytes and small lymphocytes. Often, the only visible difference is the light blue tinge imparted to the cytoplasm of the lymphocytes, and slight alterations in staining techniques may affect the color of the cytoplasm. The inability to accurately differentiate between these two types of cells raises important questions about the differential leukocyte counts in snakes. Continued work is needed regarding blood cell morphology of individual species of reptiles.

ACKNOWLEDGMENT

We thank Ms. Doris Millsaps and Dr. C. S. Patton for technical assistance.

About the Authors
Drs. Dotson and Ramsay are affiliated with the Department of Comparative Medicine, College of Veterinary Medicine, University of Tennessee, Knoxville, Tennessee. Dr. Bounous is affiliated with the Department of Pathology, College of Veterinary Medicine, University of Georgia, Athens, Georgia. Dr. Ramsay is a Diplomate of the American College of Zoological Medicine, and Dr. Bounous is a Diplomate of the American College of Veterinary Pathology.

REFERENCES

1. Marcus LC: *Veterinary Biology and Medicine of Captive Amphibians and Reptiles.* Philadelphia, Lea & Febiger, pp 18–22, 1980.
2. Pienaar U de V: Problems of terminology including the naming of cells, in *Haematology of Some South African Reptiles.* Johannesburg, South Africa: Witwatersrand University Press, 1962, pp 27–33.
3. Saint Girons MC: Morphology of the circulating blood cells, in Gans C, Parsons TS (eds): *Biology of the Reptilia,* vol 3. New York, Academic Press, 1970, pp 73–91.
4. Frye FL: *Biomedical and Surgical Aspects of Captive Reptile Husbandry,* vol 1, ed 2. Malabar, FL, Krieger Publishing Company, 1991, pp 209–279.
5. Sypek J, Borysenko M: Reptiles, in Rowley AF, Ratcliffe NA (eds): *Vertebrate Blood Cells.* Cambridge, Cambridge University Press, 1988, pp 211–256.
6. Montali RJ: Comparative pathology of inflammation in the higher vertebrates (reptiles, birds, and mammals). *J Comp Pathol* 99:1–26, 1988.
7. Mateo MR, Roberts ED, Enright FM: Morphological, cytochemical, and functional studies of peripheral blood cells of young healthy American alligators *(Alligator mississipiensis). Am J Vet Res* 45:1046–1053, 1984.
8. Alleman AR, Jacobson ER, Raskin RE: Morphologic and cytochemical characteristics of blood cells from the desert tortoise *(Gopherus agassizii). Am J Vet Res* 53(9):1645–1651, 1992.

[a]Dotson TK, Ramsay EC: Personal observation, 1995.

9. Canfield PJ: Characterization of the blood cells of Australian crocodiles (*Crocodylus porosus* [Schneider] and *C. johnstoni* [Krefft]). *Zbl Vet Med C Anat Histol Embryol* 14:269–288, 1985.

10. Hawkey CM, Dennett TB: *Color Atlas of Comparative Veterinary Hematology*. Ames, IA, Iowa State University Press, 1989.

11. Campbell TW: Hematology of exotic animals. *Compend Contin Educ Pract Vet* 13(6):950–956, 1991.

12. Mader DR: *Reptile Medicine and Surgery*. Philadelphia, WB Saunders Co, 1996, pp 248–257.

Rodents and Hedgehogs (*continued from page 144*)

BIBLIOGRAPHY

Bauck L: Common diseases of the guinea pig. *Small Mammal-Reptile Medicine and Surgery for the Practitioner*. Fifth Annual Conference, 1993.

Bennett RA: Rabbit and rodent orthopedics. *Proc North Am Vet Conf*, 7: 798–790, 1993.

Boll RA, Suckow MA, Hawkins EC: Bilateral ureteral calculi in a guinea pig. *Jrnl Small Exot Anim Med* 2:60–63, 1991.

Brown SA: African Hedgehogs: Husbandry and restraint. *Small Mammal-Reptile Medicine and Surgery for the Practitioner*. Sixth Annual Conference, 1994, pp 57–59,

Burgmann PM: Restraint techniques and anesthetic recommendations for rabbits, rodents, and ferrets. *Jrnl Small Exot Anim Med* 3:113–114, 1992.

Donnelly TM: Emerging viral diseases of rabbits and rodents: Viral hemorrhagic disease and hantavirus infection. *Sem in Avian and Exotic Pet Med* 2:83–91, 1995.

Donnelly TM: Functional anatomy of rodents. *Proc North Am Vet Conf*, 10:855–857, 1996.

Duncan JR, Prasse KW: *Veterinary Laboratory Medicine: Clinical Pathology*. Ames, Iowa, Iowa State University Press, 1986.

Frye, FL: Apparent spontaneous ergot-induced necrotizing dermatitis in a guinea pig. *Jrnl Small Exot Anim Med* 4:165–166, 1994.

Gibson SV, Wagner JE: Cryptosporidiosis in guinea pigs: A retrospective study. *JAVMA* 9:1033–1034, 1986.

Ginsberg, S: Hedgehogs: Prickly Pets Pique Interest. *Exotics Marketplace*.

Harrenstein L: Critical care of ferrets, rabbits, and rodents. *Sem in Avian and Exotic Pet Med* 4:217–228, 1994.

Harvey C: Rabbit and rodent skin diseases. *Sem in Avian and Exotic Pet Med* 4:195–204, 1995.

Hoefer HL: Guinea pig urolithiasis. *Proc North Am Vet Conf*, 10:675, 1996.

Hoyt R: *Atelerix albiventris*. AAZPA 1986 Annual Proceedings, pp 85–89, 1996.

Hsu WH, Bellin SI, Dellmann-Dieter H, Hanson CE: Xylazine-ketamine-induced anesthesia in rats and its antagonism by yohimbine. *JAVMA* 9:1040–1043, 1986.

Hutchkiss CE: Effect of surgical removal of subcutaneous tumors on survival of rats. *JAVMA* 10:1575–1579, 1995.

Kleisius PH, Haynes TB, Malo LK: Infectivity of *Cryptosporidium* sp isolated from wild mice for calves and mice. *JAVMA* 2:192–193, 1986.

Lobprise HB: Oral radiology, rodents and lagomorphs. *Proc North Am Vet Conf*, 10:675, 1996.

Mader DR: Ectoparasites of rodents and lagomorphs. *Proc North Am Vet Conf*, 10:865–866, 1996.

Moody KD, Griffith JW, Lang CM: Fungal meningoencephalitis in a laboratory rat. *JAVMA* 9:1152–1153, 1986.

Morrisey JK: Parasites of ferrets, rabbits, and rodents. *Sem in Avian and Exotic Pet Med* 2:106–113, 1996.

Motzel SL, Gibson SV: Tyzzer disease in hamsters and gerbils from a pet store supplier. *JAVMA* 9:1033–1034, 1986.

Ness R: Hypovitaminosis C in the guinea pig. *Jrnl Small Exotic Anim Med* 1:4–5, 1991.

Perez G, Evans R: Early birth in East African hedgehog (*Atelerix albiventris*). *Animal Keepers' Forum* 3:94, 1993.

Radin M, Fettmann J, Martin J, Wilke WL: Single-injection method for evaluation of renal function with ^{3}H-insulin and ^{14}C-tetraethylammonium bromide in conscious unrestrained Sprague-Dawley rats. *JAVMA* 9:1044–1046, 1986.

Rich GA: Cutaneous lymphosarcoma in a Syrian hamster. *Jrnl Small Exotic Anim Med* 3:113–114, 1992.

Rosenthal, Karen: Hemangiosarcoma in a hamster. *Jrnl Small Exotic Anim Med* 1:15, 1991.

Schmidt RE: Protozoal diseases of rabbits and rodents. *Sem Avian and Exotic Pet Med* 3:126–130, 1995.

Storer P: *Everything You Wanted to Know About Hedgehogs, but You Didn't Know Who to Ask*. Milwaukee, WI, Country Store Enterprise Publisher, 1994.

Swindle MM: Introduction to surgery of rabbits and rodents. *Proc North Am Vet Conf*, 7: 789–790, 1993.

Toft JD: Commonly observed spontaneous neoplasms in rabbits, rats, guinea pigs, hamsters, and gerbils. *Sem Avian and Exotic Pet Med* 2:80–92, 1992.

Williams BH: Diseases of rabbits and guinea pigs. *Proc North Am Vet Conf*, 10: 688–689, 1996.

Williams BH: Diseases of rodents. *Proc North Am Vet Conf*, 10: 690–692, 1996.

Hematology of Exotic Animals

KEY FACTS

- Erythrocytes of lower vertebrates are nucleated and elliptic; with a few exceptions, erythrocytes of mammals are disks that are anucleated and biconcave.
- Granulocytes of mammals, amphibians, and bony fish are known as neutrophils, eosinophils, and basophils; granulocytes of birds and reptiles are known as heterophils, eosinophils, and basophils.
- Although the term *eosinophil* describes granulocytes of both mammals and lower vertebrates, functional or morphologic homology is not necessarily implied.
- Mononuclear leukocytes evidently vary little in form and function among the classes of vertebrates.
- Thrombocytes of all vertebrates (except mammals) are nucleated cells that are derived from mononuclear precursors in hematopoietic tissue.

Colorado State University
Fort Collins, Colorado
Terry W. Campbell, DVM, PhD

EVALUATING the hemogram and peripheral blood smear is often part of a routine diagnostic evaluation of exotic animals. Hematologic data provide clues to the presence of conditions that affect cellular components of peripheral blood, thereby allowing detection and assessment of such conditions as anemia, inflammation, parasitemia, hematopoietic neoplasia, and disorders of hemostasis. This presentation discusses the evaluation of peripheral blood smears from exotic animals.

ERYTHROCYTES

Evaluating erythrocytes includes determining the packed cell volume (PCV), total erythrocyte count, and hemoglobin content of the blood. To obtain a packed cell volume in exotic animals, either the microhematocrit method or calculated erythrocyte mass (which is determined by electronic counters that are accurately adjusted for species differences in sizes of red blood cells) can be used. Hemoglobin concentrations usually are determined by spectrophotometric methods. The cyanmethemoglobin method is preferred in testing blood with nucleated erythrocytes as soon as the free nuclei from lysed red blood cells are removed by centrifugation of the cyanmethemoglobin reagent-blood mixture before obtaining the optical density value. A total erythrocyte count can be determined using

automated or manual procedures. Mean corpuscular values (mean corpuscular volume [MCV], hemoglobin [MCH], and hemoglobin concentration [MCHC]) can be calculated to assess morphologic characteristics of the erythron.

All mammals have round, anucleated erythrocytes with the exception of the members of the family Camelidae, which have oval or elliptic, anucleated erythrocytes. Birds, reptiles, amphibians, and fish have oval or elliptic, nucleated erythrocytes (although a few species of amphibians are reported to have anucleated erythrocytes). Avian erythrocytes are shown in Figure 1. The relatively small size of anucleated mammalian erythrocytes compared with the larger nucleated cells of other vertebrates most likely aids in the transport of cells through blood vessels and allows for greater gaseous exchange.[1] Nuclei of normal, mature red blood cells of lower vertebrates have shapes that generally follow the shape of the cell, are centrally positioned, and contain clumped chromatin that becomes increasingly condensed as the cell matures. In smears stained with Wright's stain, cytoplasm of red blood cells stains orangish pink because of the hemoglobin content. Nuclei of nucleated erythrocytes stain basophilic.

After expulsion of the nucleus during the final stages of maturation of mammalian erythrocytes, the remaining reticulocytes appear polychromatophilic in preparations stained with Wright's stain. The number of circulating polychromatic red blood cells varies by species and may be relatively high (2% to 4%) in small mammals, such as rodents and rabbits; however, polychromatic red blood cells are rare in most large mammals (in equids, reticulocytes do not enter peripheral circulation). Polychromatophilic erythrocytes also are found in blood of lower vertebrates. These apparent reticulocytes, similar to their mammalian counterparts, can be vitally stained using new methylene blue stain. Most circulating erythrocytes from lower vertebrates have varying amounts of reticular material in cytoplasm (which stains blue); however, it generally is accepted that only cells with a distinct band of reticular material encircling the nucleus are true reticulocytes.[2,3] In animals with nucleated red blood cells, reticulocytes and polychromatophilic erythrocytes have larger nuclei with chromatin that is less condensed than that of mature cells. In most species, the response of reticulocytes can be used to evaluate the degree of red blood cell regeneration. Species of the order Perissodactyla (i.e., equids) do not demonstrate peripheral reticulocytosis even in response to severe anemia; however, macrocytic erythrocytes are demonstrated during a regenerative response.[3] In mammals, nucleated red blood cells may be associated with the normal regenerative response and may accompany polychromasia; in lower vertebrates, immature erythrocytes may be associated with the regenerative response. Immature erythrocytes appear round with round, immature nuclei; mature erythrocytes are elliptic.[2]

ABNORMAL-APPEARING erythrocytes may be found in peripheral blood of exotic animals. Erythrocytes in blood smears from lower vertebrates may rupture, thereby resulting in the formation of smudge cells and release of free nuclei. A marked degree of poikilocytosis with red blood cell sickling, which is caused by structural changes in oxygenated hemoglobin, is a common artifact of deer and some species of goats.[3] Rouleaux formation is considered to be normal in blood smears of some mammals (i.e., Perissodactyla) but indicative of inflammation in others (i.e., primates and carnivores). Erythrocytic agglutination is considered to be a pathologic finding in all species.

Punctate basophilia (basophilic stippling) may be seen in erythrocytes as part of a regenerative response to anemia in some species of mammals (i.e., ruminants) and lower vertebrates; on rare occasions punctate basophilia is seen in cases of heavy metal poisoning. Howell-Jolly bodies within erythrocytes are normally found in low numbers in some species of mammals. The numbers may increase during an erythrocytic regenerative response. Heinz bodies can occur in most species of exotic animals exposed to chemical toxins that denature hemoglobin. Heinz bodies

appear as pale blue, blunt projections of the red blood cell membrane when stained with reticulocyte stains, such as new methylene blue. The cytoplasm of erythrocytes from normal reptiles and fish may show vacuolation resulting from autophagic vacuoles, which are created by degenerative changes in the cytoplasm.[4]

LEUKOCYTES

Laboratory evaluation of exotic animals usually involves determining both a total and differential leukocyte count. In mammalian blood, the counts are accomplished either by manual or electronic counting procedures; however, the presence of nucleated erythrocytes and thrombocytes in the blood of lower vertebrates precludes routine methods used to count leukocytes in the blood of mammals. In the blood of lower vertebrates, the sizes of nucleated red blood cells, nuclei of free red blood cells, and thrombocytes are similar to the size of many of the leukocytes and incomplete lysis of erythrocytes often occurs; therefore, alternative manual methods have been developed for determining total leukocyte counts in these animals. A direct method using Natt and Herrick's solution as a stain and diluent can be used to obtain total leukocyte, erythrocyte, and thrombocyte counts in the same charged hemacytometer[2,5] (Figure 2). A disadvantage to the Natt and Herrick's method is that differentiation between small lymphocytes and thrombocytes is often difficult and results in erroneous leukocyte counts. In birds and other animals with heterophils, a semidirect manual method using a phloxine B solution as a stain and diluent is the preferred method to obtain total leukocyte counts[2] (Figure 3). This method is simplified by the Eosinophil Unopette 5877® system (Becton-Dickinson), which is designed to determine the total number of eosinophils in mammalian blood. In this procedure, a total heterophil and eosinophil count is obtained by counting cells that stain distinctly red in a hemacytometer using the standard formula for obtaining total eosinophil counts in mammals. The total leukocyte count is calculated after completing a leukocyte differential using the following formula:

$$\text{Total white blood cells}/\mu l = \frac{(\text{heterophils} + \text{eosinophils}/\mu l) \times 100}{\%\ \text{heterophils and eosinophils}}$$

Granulocytic Leukocytes

The identification, differentiation, and nomenclature of granulocytic leukocytes causes most of the complications when performing leukocytic differentials from various exotic animals. Mammalian granulocytes are classified as neutrophils, eosinophils, and basophils based on staining characteristics in blood smears stained with Romanovsky's stains. Mature neutrophils have polymorphic (lobed) nuclei, colorless cytoplasm, and cytoplasmic granules that show species variation in size, shape, and staining quality. Neutrophilic granules of many exotic species of mammals

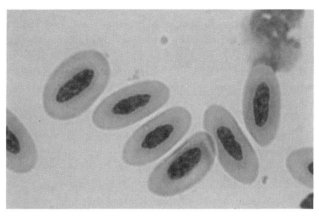

Figure 1—Peripheral blood smear of avian erythrocytes exhibiting polychromasia. (Wright's stain)

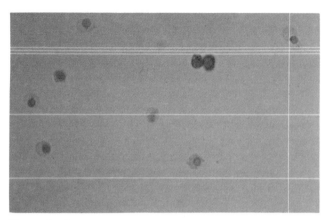

Figure 2—Appearance in a hemacytometer of erythrocytes and leukocytes (dark blue cells) of a shark. (Natt and Herrick's solution)

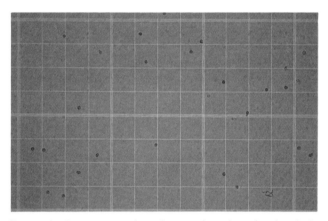

Figure 3—Appearance in a hemacytometer of avian heterophils and eosinophils. (phloxine B)

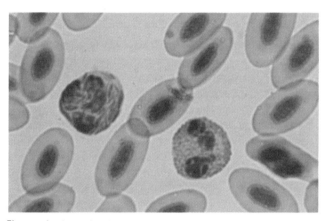

Figure 4—An avian blood smear shows a heterophil (*left*), an eosinophil (*right*), and erythrocytes. (Wright's stain)

are small and stain poorly; neutrophilic granules of some species (i.e., rabbits, guinea pigs, manatees, and hystricomorphic rodents) are large and stain distinctly eosinophilic, thereby resembling avian heterophils. These granules, however, are functionally and biochemically equivalent to the neutrophils of other mammals.[6] Mammalian eosinophils have lobed nuclei; cytoplasm that stains blue; and eosinophilic granules that vary in size, shape, number, distribution, and staining quality among the various species. The appearance of mammalian basophils also varies with the species.

MAMMALIAN neutrophils participate in inflammation and are especially adapted for destruction and removal of microorganisms. Eosinophils and neutrophils behave in a similar manner; however, eosinophils play a more important role in metazoan infections and immune responses, especially those responses associated with mast cell and basophil degranulation.[7-11]

Avian granulocytes are classified as heterophils, eosinophils, and basophils. Typical avian heterophils have lobed nuclei (usually fewer lobes than are present in mammalian neutrophils), colorless cytoplasm, and rod-shaped eosinophilic granules when stained with Wright's stain (Figure 4). Heterophilic granules often have a distinct refractile central body. Typical avian eosinophils have lobed nuclei (which usually stain darker than heterophil nuclei); blue cytoplasm; and round, strongly eosinophilic granules that lack refractile bodies. Some species may have rod-shaped granules. Granules in eosinophils usually stain differently from the granules of heterophils in the same blood smear. Avian basophils have round to oval nuclei and cytoplasmic granules that are deeply basophilic; they often are affected by alcohol fixatives and may appear partially dissolved.

Avian heterophils and mammalian neutrophils are considered to serve the same function. Because avian heterophils lack myeloperoxidase and alkaline phosphatase activity, the microbicidal activity of these heterophils differs from that of mammalian neutrophils.[11-15] The function of avian eosinophils is unknown; however, avian eosinophilic granules are lysosomal and, similar to mammalian eosinophils, contain peroxidase. Unlike eosinophils of mammals, avian eosinophils do not seem to respond to acute hypersensitivity reactions and parasitic antigens.[11] One study suggests that avian eosinophils may even participate in delayed hypersensitivity reactions.[18] Avian and mammalian basophils seem to behave in a similar manner—both release vasoactive amines to initiate vascular changes in areas of inflammation.[19]

The appearance of several types of reptilian blood cells is shown in Figures 5. Granulocytes of reptiles also are classified as heterophils, eosinophils, and basophils.[3,11,20] Reptilian heterophils are large, round cells with nonlobed nuclei (except for certain species of lizards) and prominent granules that are eosinophilic and spicule- or rod-shaped. Reptilian eosinophils and basophils resemble those described for birds, except that reptilian eosinophils exhibit nonlobed nuclei.

Although biochemical differences exist between the cells, reptilian heterophils evidently function in a manner similar to mammalian neutrophils and avian heterophils.[11,20] The function of reptilian eosinophils is unknown; as with many species of birds, peripheral eosinophilia is rare.

AMPHIBIAN GRANULOCYTES are classified as neutrophils, eosinophils, and basophils.[11,21,22] Neutrophils generally are the most numerous granulocytes found in peripheral blood of amphibians. Cytoplasmic granules of neutrophils are small if compared with those of other granulocytes. Variations in size, shape, and staining characteristics occur among the species. Amphibian neutrophils have lobed nuclei; they therefore resemble mammalian neutrophils. In general, eosinophils of amphibians have nuclei with fewer lobes than do neutrophils; amphibian eosinophils also have prominent, round to oval granules. Basophils are rare in some amphibian species but are frequently found in others. Amphibian basophils have nonsegmented nuclei and large metachromatic granules in the cytoplasm.

Neutrophils of amphibians probably serve the same function as the neutrophils of mammals and the heterophils of birds and reptiles.[21] Neutrophils of amphibians seem to have myeloperoxidase activity and show species variation with phosphatase reactions.[22] The precise function of amphibian eosinophils is unknown. There is some evidence that they respond to metazoan parasites.[23] The function of amphibian basophils also is unknown. Type I hypersensitivity reactions have not been demonstrated in amphibians.

Nomenclature and classification of piscine granulocytes differ among classes of fish; therefore, the classes Osteichthyes (bony fish) and Chondrichthyes (cartilaginous fish) are considered separately with regard to their granulocytic leukocytes. Among species of bony fish, there is marked variation in the numbers and staining reactions of granulocytes in the peripheral blood.[4] Granulocytes of bony fish generally are classified as neutrophils, eosinophils, and basophils; reports of the presence of basophils in the peripheral blood of fish do occur but are rare.[4] Neutrophils of goldfish and carp have eccentric, lobed nuclei; pale gray cytoplasm; and small cytoplasmic granules that vary from gray to pale pink when stained with Wright's stain. Neutrophils of channel catfish and certain species of eels contain prominent, rod-shaped eosinophilic granules that resemble the granules of avian heterophils[24] (Figure 6). Piscine eosinophils exhibit round to lobed nuclei; pale blue cytoplasm; and prominent, round- to rod-shaped eosinophilic granules during staining with Wright's stain.

GRANULOCYTES of the peripheral blood of cartilaginous fish also markedly vary in numbers and types among the species. The structure and cytochemistry of granulocytes of the dogfish (*Scyliorhinus canicula*) have been used as models for this group of fish.[4,25] Type I granulocytes (G1) have eccentric, irregular, nonlobed nuclei and round to oval eosinophilic granules in the cytoplasm. Type II granulocytes (G2) have lobed nuclei as well as colorless cytoplasm (when stained with Wright's stain) that lacks distinct granules, thereby resembling mammalian neutrophils. Type III granulocytes (G3) resemble type I granulocytes but generally have lobed nuclei and strongly eosinophilic, rod-shaped granules that stain differently from the granules of type I granulocytes in the same smear stained with Wright's stain. Type IV granulocytes (G4) differ markedly in appearance from the other types of granulocytes of cartilaginous fish. Type IV granulocytes often are elongated with nonlobed nuclei, scant cytoplasm, and many small eosinophilic granules. These granulocytes, which may actually be reactive thrombocytes because they often are found in clusters on the smear, resemble the reactive thrombocytes found in blood smears stained with Wright's stain of birds, reptiles, and other types of fish. Figures 7 and 8 show the appearance of granulocytes of the blood of a shark.

The precise function of piscine granulocytes is unknown; however, they most likely participate in inflammation and microbicidal activity. Whether the granulocytes of fish behave in a manner similar to that of granulocytes of higher vertebrates is unknown; further research therefore is needed to determine whether the function of granulocytes of fish has been preserved in higher vertebrates during the evolutionary process.

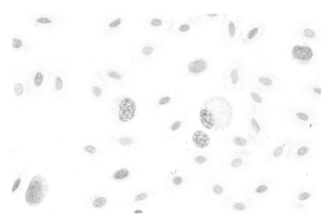

Figure 5—A blood smear of the peripheral blood of a snake shows a heterophil, lymphocyte, monocyte, and thrombocyte as well as several erythrocytes. (Wright's stain)

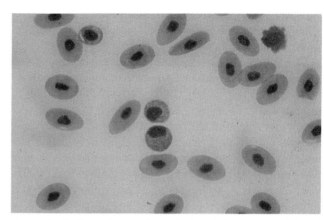

Figure 6—Erythrocytes and two heterophils in the peripheral blood of an eel. (Wright's stain)

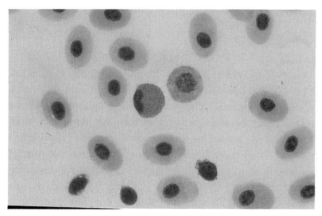

Figure 7—A type I granulocyte (*right*), a type III granulocyte (*left*), thrombocytes, and numerous erythrocytes in the peripheral blood of a shark. (Wright's stain)

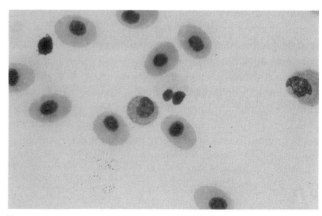

Figure 8—A type I granulocyte (*left*) and a type II granulocyte (*right*) with erythrocytes in the peripheral blood of a shark. (Wright's stain)

Abnormal-appearing granulocytes occasionally are found in the blood of exotic animals. Neutrophils and heterophils may exhibit toxic changes, which are represented by increased cytoplasmic basophilia, vacuolation, abnormal granulation, and degeneration of nuclei.[2] Under severe conditions, immature heterophils and neutrophils are found in the peripheral blood. These cells tend to be larger than the mature cells and have immature-appearing nuclei, cytoplasmic basophilia, and a less-than-normal amount of specific granules. Myeloproliferative disorders do occur but are rare in exotic animals. These disorders are represented by marked numbers of immature granulocytes that sometimes appear abnormal.

Mononuclear Leukocytes

Mononuclear leukocytes of most exotic animals seem to vary little among the species. The appearance and function of lymphocytes and monocytes have evidently changed little during the evolutionary process; therefore, the lympho-cytes and monocytes in blood smears of lower vertebrates resemble the lymphocytes and monocytes of mammals. Lymphocytes of exotic animals typically appear small and mature, although a few larger lymphocytes may be seen in some species. These larger lymphocytes can be round to irregularly shaped (lymphocytes often mold around adjacent cells) with round nuclei. The chromatin clumps heavily; the cytoplasm stains pale blue with Wright's stain. Small, mature lymphocytes have large nuclei and scant cytoplasm. Azurophilic granules are occasionally seen in the cytoplasm of lymphocytes in some species. In lymphocytes of guinea pigs and related species (i.e., capybaras), large basophilic inclusions known as Kurloff's bodies are seen in the cytoplasm[26] (Figure 9). Lymphocytes appear to be involved with cell-mediated (T cell) and humoral (B cell) immunity in all species.

Monocytes typically are the largest leukocytes found in the blood of most animals. These cells have variably shaped nuclei, less nuclear chromatin clumping than oc-

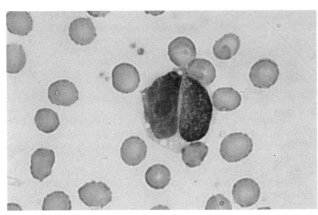

Figure 9—A lymphocyte that contains a Kurloff's body in the peripheral blood of a guinea pig. (Wright's stain)

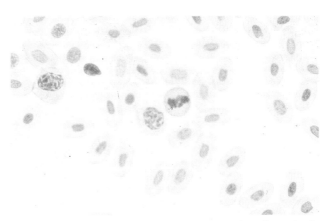

Figure 10—Two azurophils, a mitotic figure, and erythrocytes in the peripheral blood of a snake. (Wright's stain)

curs in lymphocytic nuclei, and abundant bluish-gray cytoplasm that may appear vacuolated or may contain tiny, red granules. Monocytes are the most abundant leukocytes found in the blood of some species. In elephants, monocytes tend to have bilobed nuclei with a fine filament connecting the lobes.[3] Monocytes of exotic animals are phagocytic cells that engulf and destroy microorganisms, foreign or abnormal cells, and foreign material; monocytes also play a major role in the immune process.

Azurophils evidently are a type of mononuclear leukocyte that is unique to reptiles. Azurophils resemble monocytes with fine eosinophilic granulation. They are particularly frequent in the blood of snakes and lizards[3] (Figure 10). The function of these cells is unknown.

PLATELETS AND THROMBOCYTES

Mammalian platelets, which function primarily in hemostasis, are cellular fragments derived from megakaryocytes. Lower vertebrates have thrombocytes, which are true nucleated cells derived from distinct cell lines in hemopoietic tissue. Thrombocytes of birds, reptiles, and amphibians tend to be oval. The round to oval nucleus is centrally located with dense chromatin and a colorless to pale gray cytoplasm during staining with Wright's stain.[2,15,20,22] The cytoplasm may have a reticulated appearance and contains red granules. Thrombocytes of fish occur as round, elongated, or fusiform, depending on the stage of maturity or degree of reactivity.[27] Thrombocytes of lower vertebrates, similar to mammalian platelets, participate in the hemostatic process and tend to clump in blood smears. Thrombocytes also may have limited phagocytic ability.[15]

CONCLUSION

Evaluation of the hemogram of exotic animals can demonstrate the presence of disorders that affect hemic cells. For example, it is necessary to examine the erythron to detect and classify anemia because many species show lit-

tle physical evidence of this condition until it becomes severe. Conditions that affect the absolute numbers of circulating leukocytes reflect the function of these cells. For example, neutrophilic or heterophilic disorders usually are associated with inflammatory conditions, microbial infection, or excess corticosteroids. Physiologic leukocytosis often is present in the hemogram of exotic animals as a result of accelerated blood flow from the struggle of capture and restraint needed for blood collection. Neutropenia and heteropenia usually indicate either an overwhelming peripheral demand for these cells or decreased granulocytopoiesis. Eosinophilia in mammals suggests immune-mediated conditions, helminth infestation, or irritation of tissue with a high concentration of mast cells. It is important to note that eosinophils of lower vertebrates and mammals do not necessarily function in a similar manner and are not necessarily the same types of cells although they are given the same name. Eosinophilia in lower vertebrates therefore may result from different conditions than the conditions that cause eosinophilia in mammals.

Lymphocytosis can be associated with physiologic leukocytosis, recovery from microbial infections, chronic infection, or lymphocytic leukemia. Reactive lymphocytes (large lymphocytes with increased cytoplasmic basophilia) and plasma cells may be seen as a result of chronic stimulation by antigens. Lymphopenia often is associated with glucocorticosteroid excess or infection with specific viruses. Monocytosis frequently is associated with mycotic, mycobacterial, or chlamydial diseases. Although it has not achieved the same level of critical evaluation as has human and domestic mammalian hematology, exotic animal hematology is a useful diagnostic tool.

About the Author
Dr. Campbell is an Associate Professor in Zoological Medicine in the Department of Clinical Sciences at Colorado State University in Fort Collins, Colorado.

REFERENCES

1. Parmley RT: Mammals, in Rowley AF, Ratcliffe HA (eds): *Vertebrate Blood Cells*. Cambridge, Cambridge University Press, 1988, pp 337–424.
2. Campbell TW: *Avian Hematology and Cytology*. Ames, IA, Iowa State University Press, 1988, pp 3–32.
3. Hawkey CM, Dennett TB: *Color Atlas of Comparative Veterinary Hematology*. London, Wolfe Medical Publications Ltd, 1989, pp 9–147.
4. Rowley AF, Hunt TC, Page M, Mainwaring G: Fish, in Rowley AF, Ratcliffe HA (eds): *Vertebrate Blood Cells*. Cambridge, Cambridge University Press, 1988, pp 20–127.
5. Natt MP, Herrick CA: A new blood diluent for counting the erythrocytes and leukocytes of the chicken. *Poult Sci* 31:735–738, 1952.
6. Cohn ZA, Hirsche JG: The isolation and properties of the specific cytoplasmic granules of the rabbit polymorphonuclear leukocytes. *J Exp Med* 112:983–1004, 1960.
7. Weller PF, Goetzle EJ: The human eosinophil, roles in host defense and tissue injury. *Am J Pathol* 100:793–820, 1980.
8. McLaren DJ: The role of eosinophils in tropical disease. *Semin Hematol* 19:100–106, 1982.
9. Litt M: Eosinophils and antigen-antibody fractions. *Ann NY Acad Sci* 116:964–985, 1964.
10. Goetzl EJ: Modulation in human eosinophil polymorphonuclear leukocyte migration and function. *Am J Pathol* 85:419–435, 1976.
11. Montali RJ: Comparative pathology of inflammation in the higher vertebrates (reptiles, birds, and mammals). *J Comp Pathol* 99:1–26, 1988.
12. Brune K, Leffell MS, Spitznagel JK: Microbicidal activity of peroxidaseless chicken heterophil leukocytes. *Infect Immun* 5:283–287, 1972.
13. Brune K, Spitznagel JK: Peroxidaseless chicken leukocytes: Isolation and characterization of anti-bacterial granules. *J Infect Dis* 127:84–94, 1973.
14. Maxwell MH: Histochemical identification of tissue eosinophils in the inflammatory response of the fowl (*Gallus domesticus*). *Res Vet Sci* 37:7–11, 1984.
15. Dieterlen-Lievre F: Birds, in Rowley AF, Ratcliffe MA (eds): *Vertebrate Blood Cells*. Cambridge, Cambridge University Press, 1988, pp 257–336.
16. Maxwell MH: Fine structural and cytochemical studies of eosinophils from fowls and ducks with eosinophilia. *Res Vet Sci* 41:135–148, 1986.
17. Maxwell MH: Ultrastructural and cytochemical studies in normal Japanese quail (*Coturnix japonica*) eosinophils and in those from birds with experimentally-induced eosinophilia. *Res Vet Sci* 41:149–161, 1986.
18. Awadhiya RP, Vegad JL, Kolte GM: Eosinophil leukocytic response in dinitrochlorbenzene skin hypersensitivity reaction in the chicken. *Avian Pathol* 11:187–194, 1982.
19. Carlson HC, Hacking MA: Distribution of mast cells in chicken, turkey, pheasant, and quail and their differentiation from basophils. *Avian Dis* 16:574–577, 1972.
20. Sypek J, Borysenko M: Reptiles, in Rowley AF, Ratcliffe MA (eds): *Vertebrate Blood Cells*. Cambridge, Cambridge University Press, 1988, pp 211–256.
21. David GB, McMullen JM: Quantitative cytochemical observations on the control of respiration in polymorphonuclear neutrophil leukocytes of *Amphiuma tridactylum*. *J Cell Sci* 10:719–747, 1972.
22. Turner RJ: Amphibians, in Rowley AF, Ratcliffe MA (eds): *Vertebrate Blood Cells*. Cambridge, Cambridge University Press, 1988, pp 129–209.
23. Mitchell JB: The effect of host age on *Rana temporaria* and *Gorgoderina vitelliloba* interactions. *Int J Parasitol* 12:601–604, 1982.
24. Cannon MS, et al: An ultrastructural study of the leukocytes of the channel catfish, *Ictalurus punctatus*. *J Morphol* 164:1–23, 1980.
25. Morrow WJW, Pulsford A: Identification of peripheral blood leukocytes of the dogfish (*Scyliorhinus canicula*) by electron microscopy. *J Fish Biol* 17:461–475, 1980.
26. Schalm OW, Jain NC, Carroll EJ: *Veterinary Hematology*. Philadelphia, Lea & Febiger, 1975, pp 233–234.
27. Campbell TW, Murru F: An introduction to fish hematology. *Compend Contin Educ Pract Vet* 12(4):525–533, 1990.

An Introduction to Fish Hematology

KEY FACTS

- The piscine hemogram can be a diagnostic tool.
- The appearances of leukocytes may vary between classes of fish (e.g., cartilaginous and bony fish).
- The piscine hemogram can easily be evaluated in an in-house clinical laboratory.
- Various methods can be used to collect piscine blood for hematologic evaluation.

Colorado State University
Fort Collins, Colorado
Terry W. Campbell, DVM, PhD

Sea World of Florida, Inc.
Orlando, Florida
Frank Murru, BS

HEMATOLOGY has become a valuable routine diagnostic tool in the medical care of humans and domestic mammals and is becoming a useful diagnostic aid in the evaluation of avian patients. Hematology may also provide information that identifies diseases that affect the cells in the peripheral blood of fish.

Veterinary medicine developed from a primary interest in the health of domestic mammals and of birds raised for human consumption. Today, the veterinary profession has a broader scope of interests involving various companion and exotic animals. Veterinarians are involved in commercial fish production (food and ornamental fish), the care of exhibition species in zoos and aquariums, and the care of pet fish.

The 20,000 known piscine species are divided into the following three groups: class Agnatha (jawless fish), class Chondrichthyes (cartilaginous fish), and class Osteichthyes (bony fish).[1] Much of the current knowledge pertaining to fish hematology comes from research involving lampreys and hagfish (class Agnatha), a few species of cartilaginous fish of the subclass Elasmobranchii (i.e., sharks), and a few species of bony fish of the suborder Teleostei (i.e., eels, salmonids, catfish, carp, and goldfish). Fish hematology has lagged behind that of birds and mammals; however, the advancement of hematology as a diagnostic tool in piscine medicine will depend on clinical investigations involving the piscine hemogram.

PISCINE HEMATOPOIETIC TISSUE

All fish lack bone marrow and lymph nodes. The principal hematopoietic tissues of cartilaginous fish include the thymus, the spleen, and the large lymphomyeloid tissues (epigonal organ and organ of Leydig).[1,2] The primary hematopoietic tissues of bony fish are the thymus, spleen, and kidney.[1]

The location and structure of the thymus vary with the species of fish; most of the cells found in the thymus are lymphocytes. In teleosts, the thymus is the major lymphoid organ and during development apparently seeds the kidney and spleen with lymphocytes (probably T lymphocytes).[3,4] The piscine thymus usually is not divided into distinct cortical and medullary zones.[1,4,5] In teleosts, the thymus is closely associated with the pharyngeal epithelium; this association may allow for lymphocytic exposure to antigenic material from the surrounding water as part of immune-related thymic function.

The spleen of cartilaginous fish resembles that of bony fish; in fish of either class, the spleen is usually located on the lateroventral surface of the stomach or adjacent to the stomach or intestines. The spleen of Chondrichthyes species contains white and red pulp areas.[1] The red pulp area contains cells involved in hematopoiesis (erythropoiesis, thrombopoiesis, and lymphopoiesis), plasma cells, macrophages, and mature granulocytes. There are no clear distinctions between red pulp and white pulp in the spleen of

Osteichthyes species, and the areas of erythropoiesis and lymphopoiesis are intermingled.[6] In some teleosts, the spleen contains the only hematopoietic tissue; whereas in other teleosts, it acts as a secondary site of hematopoiesis.[7]

The large lymphomyeloid tissues of cartilaginous fish are the epigonal organ and the organ of Leydig. These organs are associated with granulopoiesis and antibody production. The epigonal organ is associated with the gonad and is the largest lymphomyeloid tissue in some sharks. The organ of Leydig is located in the submucosa of the alimentary tract (i.e., the esophagus) and is similar in structure to the epigonal organ. Both organs contain developing granulocytes, lymphocytes, and plasma cells.[2]

THE KIDNEY is the major blood-forming organ of bony fish and can be divided into two components—the cranial kidney (pronephric or head kidney) and the main kidney (opisthonephric or trunk kidney).[1,7] The hematopoietic tissue of the kidney is the site of erythropoiesis, granulopoiesis, lymphopoiesis, and monocytopoiesis. The kidney is also involved in antigen trapping and antibody formation.

Minor hematopoietic sites in fish include the liver and the peripheral blood. The final stages of erythroid development may occur in the peripheral blood of cartilaginous and bony fish.

BLOOD COLLECTION

Blood from large fish can be collected by various methods.[8] Caudal venipuncture is easily performed on anesthetized or unanesthetized fish. The caudal vein can be approached by inserting a needle (the appropriate size varies with the size of the fish) attached to a syringe into the midventral septum of the caudal peduncle and directing the needle perpendicularly toward the vertebrae. Once the needle has touched a caudal vertebra, it can be slightly withdrawn so that the needle can be properly placed into the caudal vein.

The blood should be aspirated into a plastic syringe. Because piscine blood coagulates rapidly in glass, plastic syringes are recommended.[9] Heparin or ethylenediaminetetraacetic acid (EDTA) are anticoagulants that can be used to coat the needle and syringe before blood collection.

A lateral approach to the caudal vein can be performed by inserting the needle just below the lateral line of the tail and behind the vent.[8] The needle is advanced toward the midline just below the caudal vertebra to reach the vein.

Blood can be collected from the bulbus cordis of teleosts by inserting a needle slightly caudal to the apex of the V-shaped aspect of the fish.[8] A perpendicular angle to the skin is used, and a slight vacuum is applied to the syringe as the needle is advanced toward the bulbus cordis.

Blood from small fish is frequently collected before necropsy when sick fish are sacrificed to determine the nature of a disease involving several fish in a tank or pond. Blood can be collected from the heart by opening the coelomic cavity of an anesthetized fish (various chemical agents can be used to anesthetize fish).[10] Blood can also be collected from the caudal vein after the caudal peduncle is severed; the blood is allowed to drip into a microcollection tube. The disadvantage of this method is the increased chance of contamination of the sample with nonhemic tissue fluids.

The blood of teleosts coagulates easily; and like those of most fish, their blood cells are sensitive to osmotic changes. Hemolysis is therefore common in piscine blood samples. The background of fish blood films often contains a thick, pale, eosinophilic substance that may be related to the degree of hemolysis. The thickness of the background material on stained, air-dried blood films may interfere with the spreading of the cells, thus causing them to appear small and condensed. Cells in blood films with heavy background material may therefore be difficult to identify.

Piscine blood contains nucleated erythrocytes, thrombocytes, lymphocytes, granulocytes, monocytes, and plasma. The plasma contains inorganic ions, sugars, clotting factors, globulins (α, β, and γ), and albumin (except in elasmobranchs). Osmotic balance in teleost blood is maintained by inorganic ions (i.e., Na^+ and K^+); whereas the blood of elasmobranchs is isosmotic with seawater, and urea is retained for osmotic balance.[1] These characteristics may explain the fragility of shark blood cells when they are exposed to anticoagulant. Using blood that contains no anticoagulant may therefore improve the quality of blood films of elasmobranchs.

ERYTHROCYTES

The size and number of erythrocytes in piscine blood vary between species and with physiologic conditions within the same species.[11] Mature piscine erythrocytes in blood films stained with Wright's stain are oval to ellipsoid cells with an abundant pale eosinophilic cytoplasm and centrally positioned nucleus (Figure 1).

The nucleus is usually oval with its long axis parallel to the long axis of the cell. The nucleus may appear round in some species. The densely clumped nuclear chromatin stains dark purple. The cytoplasm of mature erythrocytes of some fish species does not have a homogeneous appearance and often contains a variable amount of rarefied (pale-staining) areas. Prominent cytoplasmic vacuoles may be found in mature erythrocytes viewed through an electron microscope. These vacuoles may be from autophagic vacuoles derived from degenerative mitochondria.[12]

A SLIGHT to moderate amount of polychromasia and anisocytosis is normal in many fish species and suggests that some final maturation of erythrocytes occurs in peripheral blood. Young erythrocytes appear rounded with pale blue cytoplasm and have a vesicular nuclear chromatin in comparison with that of mature erythrocytes.

Early erythrocytes (i.e., erythroblasts and proerythrocytes) are occasionally present in the peripheral blood of fish. These cells are round with a centrally positioned nucleus containing smooth to reticulated chromatin and a scant amount of deeply basophilic cytoplasm. As immature erythrocytes mature, the cytoplasmic basophilia decreases with the progressive increase in hemoglobin content. Immature erythrocytes contain organelles (i.e., Golgi apparatus, mitochondria, ribosomes, centrioles, and smooth and rough endoplasmic reticulum) that are lost in the mature cell.[1,13]

Erythrocytes transport oxygen and carbon dioxide. All fish, except the jawless fish, have erythrocytes that contain hemoglobin with the typical α and β chains that form a tetramer.[14] Just like avian and mammalian hemoglobins, piscine hemoglobin allows the release of oxygen to tissue with a high carbon dioxide concentration.

Abnormal-appearing erythrocytes can be found in the peripheral blood of fish and may indicate erythrocyte pathology. Fish with regenerative anemia often show an increase in polychromasia and the number of immature erythrocytes in the peripheral blood. Environmental stress, such as an increase in population density, can result in microcytic, normochromic anemia.[15] Peroxides produced by microorganisms may damage erythrocytes, thus resulting in microcytic hypochromic anemia with the formation of elongated erythrocytes.[16] Nutritional deficiencies and water pollution may also result in changes in erythrocyte morphology.[17,18]

LYMPHOCYTES

The lymphocyte is the most common leukocyte found in the peripheral blood of many species of fish. The following three types of lymphocytes in the peripheral blood of fish have been described: mature lymphocytes, immature lymphocytes (lymphoblasts), and plasma cells. Mature lymphocytes are small cells that tend to be round but may have an irregular cell outline or mold around adjacent cells (Figure 2). They have a high nucleus-to-cytoplasm ratio, and the nucleus stains dark purple and has coarse chromatin clumping. The round nucleus is surrounded by a thin, homogeneously blue cytoplasm.

The significance of the presence of immature lymphocytes in the peripheral blood of fish is controversial. Some of these cells may represent reactive lymphocytes that are responding to antigenic stimulation. Plasma cells (which are reactive forms of B lymphocytes) are occasionally found in the peripheral blood of fish. Electron micrography of plasma cells reveals swollen, rough endoplasmic reticulum and active Golgi apparatuses involved with immunoglobulin synthesis.[1] Most of the lymphocytes found in the peripheral blood of fish are small and mature.

Whether a lymphatic system exists in fish is also controversial. Cartilaginous fish and some bony fish have a hemolymphatic system because erythrocytes are typically associated with lymphatic fluid.[19] A lymphatic system consisting of four subcutaneous ducts and one or two subvertebral ducts (each of these ducts having smaller connecting vessels and lymph propulsors [heartlike structures]) occurs in some teleosts.[1] Fish do not have lymph nodes or lymphatic vessels that contain valves.[1]

PISCINE LYMPHOCYTES function in cellular and humoral immunity; and contact with antigens leads to lymphocytic proliferation, immunoglobulin production, and T-lymphocyte activation. Most fish produce immunoglobulin that closely resembles the immunoglobulin M of other vertebrates, and evidence suggests that they may produce other classes and subclasses of immunoglobulin.[1,20] The sites of antibody production in cartilaginous fish are primarily in the spleen and lamina propria mucosae of the intestine; minor production occurs in the liver, epigonal organ, and organ of Leydig.[1,21] The kidney and spleen are the major sites for antibody production in teleosts.[22] The mucus coat of fish contains immunoglobulins, agglutinins, and lysozyme, thus making this slime an important protection from parasites and microorganisms.[1]

Exogenous glucocorticosteroids can cause a reduction in the number of circulating lymphocytes in the peripheral blood of fish.[23] Therefore, fish exposed to various stresses (e.g., infectious diseases or adverse environmental conditions) may have low peripheral lymphocyte counts.

GRANULOCYTES

The nomenclature and classification of fish granulocytes are controversial, possibly because of the variation in granulocytes among fish. The confusion may also be complicated by an attempt to classify these cells on the basis of their appearance in blood films stained with a Romanowsky stain and according to the nomenclature used in domestic mammalian hematology. Recent studies involving ultrastructural features, cytochemical evaluation, and leukocytic function tests have begun to remove some of the controversy associated with fish granulocytes. The granulocytes of cartilaginous fish and bony fish must be viewed as two separate types of cells.

There apparently are subpopulations of eosinophilic granulocytes (not to be confused with cells analogous to mammalian eosinophils) in the peripheral blood of elasmobranchs. The granulocyte classification used for dogfish (*Scyliorhinus canicula*) can serve as a model for the classification of granulocytes in cartilaginous fish.

The G_1 (type I) granulocyte is the most common.[1,24,25] This cell has an eccentric, irregular, nonlobed nucleus and prominent round to oval, eosinophilic cytoplasmic granules. The second most common granulocyte, G_4 (type IV), is an elongated cell that contains cytoplasmic granules that are moderately eosinophilic. This cell is often confused with reactive thrombocytes, which tend to be smaller and occur in clumps. A third type of granulocyte found in the dogfish (*Scyliorhinus canicula*) is the G_3 (type III) granulocyte, which has a lobed nucleus and strongly eosinophilic, rod-shaped cytoplasmic granules (Figure 3). The G_2 (type II) granulocyte is often referred to as the neutrophilic granulocyte (Figure 3). It has a slightly indented to lobed nucleus and small heterogeneous cytoplasmic granules. The G_2 granulocyte is the least common of the four in the dog-

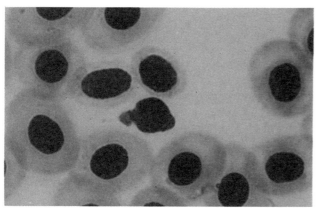

Figure 1—Erythrocytes from a lemon shark (*Negaprion brevirostris*). Note the polychromasia. (Wright's stain)

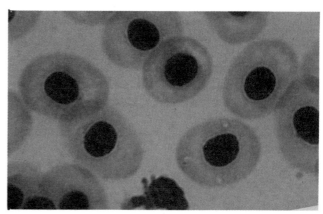

Figure 2—A small mature lymphocyte and two thrombocytes from a lemon shark (*Negaprion brevirostris*). (Wright's stain)

fish (*Scyliorhinus canicula*).

The types of granulocytes present in cartilaginous fish species vary. For example, the nurse shark (*Gingylmostoma cirratum*) has only one population of eosinophilic granulocytes, and rays apparently have two predominant populations (resembling the G_1 and G_3 granulocytes of dogfish) of these cells but completely lack the G_4 type.[13,25]

MOST RESEARCH involving the classification of peripheral blood granulocytes of bony fish comes from studies using cyprinids (goldfish and carp), salmonids (salmon and trout), and ichtalurids (catfish). Goldfish (*Carassius auratus*) have neutrophilic (heterophilic) and eosinophilic granulocytes.[1] The neutrophil has a lobed, eccentric nucleus and a pale gray cytoplasm that contains small granules varying in color from gray to pale pink. Eosinophils tend to be round and smaller than neutrophils (heterophils) and have a round to bilobed nucleus that lies in an eccentric location within the cell. The cytoplasm stains pale blue and contains pale, spherical, or rod-shaped granules.

The granulocytes of carp (*Cyprinus carpio*) are similar to those of goldfish.[26-28] Salmonids have neutrophils (heterophils) as the predominate granulocyte; eosinophilic granulocytes are absent or rare.[1] Channel catfish (*Ictalurus punctatus*) have neutrophils (heterophils) with rod-shaped cytoplasmic granules.[29] The center of mature granules has a crystalline appearance. The nucleus of neutrophils (heterophils) of bony fish shows coarse chromatin clumping and stains dark purple with Wright's stain.

Whether basophils exist in the peripheral blood of fish is controversial. Only a few species have been reported to possess basophils. If basophils are present, they occur in very low numbers.[30,31]

The function of piscine granulocytes resembles that of mammalian neutrophils. They migrate to sites of inflammation, where they participate in phagocytic activity.[32] They also exhibit chemokinetic responses much as mam-

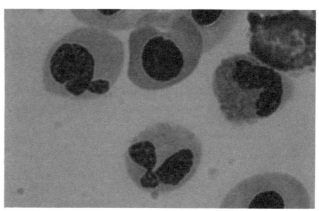

Figure 3—One G_3 granulocyte and two G_2 granulocytes from a lemon shark (*Negaprion brevirostris*). (Wright's stain)

malian neutrophils do. It should, however, be emphasized that although some piscine granulocytes have eosinophilic staining reactions with Romanowsky stains, this finding does not suggest that these cells have the same morphology or function as mammalian eosinophils.

MONOCYTES

Monocytes occur in low numbers in the peripheral blood of most fish (Figure 4). The monocytes are large leukocytes with an abundant blue-gray cytoplasm that lacks granules and is occasionally vacuolated. The nucleus occupies less than 50% of the cell volume, is eccentric in location, and has a variable shape (round to lobed). The nuclear chromatin is coarsely granular to reticulated and lacks the thick clumping that is typical of lymphocyte nuclei. The cell margins may be indistinct or rough because of pseudopodia (protoplasmic projections). The ultrastructure of monocytes indicates similarity among cells of this type from the piscine species studied.[1]

Monocytes participate in inflammatory lesions and are phagocytic.[32] Piscine blood monocytes migrate to areas of inflammation and apparently develop into macrophages. The macrophages isolated from fish are phagocytic and synthesize various secretory products (i.e., interleukin, in-

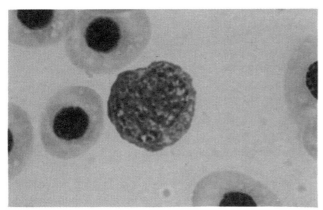

Figure 4—A monocyte from a lemon shark (*Negaprion breviros-tris*). (Wright's stain)

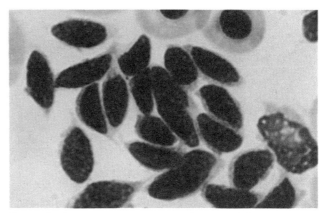

Figure 5—Clumped thrombocytes with eosinophilic cytoplasmic granules indicating reactivity. This sample was from a lemon shark (*Negaprion brevirostris*). (Wright's stain)

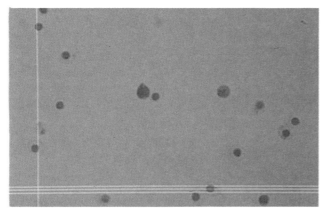

Figure 6—The appearance of erythrocytes and two leukocytes in a hemacytometer. (Natt and Herrick's solution)

terferon, prostaglandin, and leukotriene).[1] Piscine macrophages are also involved in antigen trapping and presentation; therefore, they are an important component of immunologic surveillance in fish.

THROMBOCYTES

Thrombocytes in smears of peripheral blood of fish vary in shape (Figure 2). The three thrombocyte shapes commonly seen in smears stained with a Romanowsky stain are round, elongated, and fusiform. The shape may vary with the stage of maturity or degree of reactivity. The ultrastructure of fish thrombocytes has features that resemble mammalian platelets.[1] Like mammalian platelets, thrombocytes tend to clump in the smear (Figure 5).

The shape of the thrombocyte nucleus follows the shape of the cell. The nucleus stains dark purple and contains dense chromatin. The cytoplasm is colorless to pale blue.

FISH THROMBOCYTES participate in blood coagulation, which is similar to the blood coagulation in birds and mammals.[33] The mechanism of thrombocyte aggregation,

however, may not be the same as in mammalian platelet aggregation.

CLINICAL PISCINE HEMATOLOGY

Hematology involves the evaluation of erythrocytes, leukocytes, and thrombocytes in samples of peripheral blood. The packed cell volume (PCV) is a simple, rapid test used to evaluate the status of erythrocytes in birds and mammals. The packed cell volume of fish varies among species and within a single species. Because of this variation, the value of packed cell volume in the evaluation of the health of fish has been debatable.[1,34-38]

Various methods can be used to determine the hemoglobin concentration of piscine blood. The cyanmethemoglobin method apparently provides more consistent results than do other methods.[39] After the erythrocytes are lysed, the sample should be centrifuged to remove the free erythrocyte nuclei before the spectrophotometer reading for hemoglobin concentration is obtained.

Total erythrocyte counts can be obtained by manual methods using various diluting solutions and a hemacytometer (Figure 6). The blood can be diluted using the erythrocyte Unopette® system (Becton-Dickinson) or by using an erythrocyte diluting pipette (red blood cell pipette) and a dilution fluid, such as Natt and Herrick's solution (see the box on page 228). Both systems make a 1:200 dilution, and the diluted blood is used to fill both sides of an improved Neubauer hemacytometer (American Optical).

The erythrocytes in the four small corner squares and the central square of the hemacytometer chamber are counted on both sides. The average number of erythrocytes obtained from both sides of the hemacytometer is calculated and multiplied by 10,000 to obtain the total erythrocyte count per cubic millimeter of blood. The erythrocyte morphology is determined by the appearance of the cells in a blood smear stained with Wright's stain.

A total leukocyte count can be obtained by using various diluting and staining fluids, such as Shaw's solution, Rees-Ecker fluid, Dacie's fluid, and Natt and Herrick's solution.[40-44] A diluting and staining fluid, such as Natt and

Natt and Herrick's Solution[40]

Constituents

NaCl	3.88 g
Na_2SO_4	2.50 g
$[Na_2HPO_4][H_2O]_{12}$	2.91 g
KH_2PO_4	0.25 g
Formalin (37%)	7.50 ml
Gentian violet 2B	0.10 g

Preparation

The chemicals are dissolved in distilled water to make a total volume of one liter. The solution is allowed to stand overnight and is filtered through Whatman No. 2 filter paper before use.

Herrick's solution, can enable the same charged hemacytometer to provide total erythrocyte, leukocyte, and thrombocyte counts.

WHEN A TOTAL leukocyte count is performed with the same 1:200 dilution used to obtain the erythrocyte count, the leukocytes in all nine large squares in both sides of the hemacytometer chamber are counted. The average number of leukocytes per nine large squares plus 10% of that number is multiplied by 200 to obtain the total leukocyte count per cubic millimeter of blood:

$$\text{white blood cells/mm}^3 = (\text{number of white blood cells in nine large squares} + 10\%) \times 200$$

With Natt and Herrick's solution, the leukocytes appear blue and stain darker than the erythrocytes. The erythrocytes are typically oval and have a small, dark-blue nucleus surrounded by a colorless or faint-pink cytoplasm. Granulocytic leukocytes have a granular cytoplasm. The evaluation of the leukocytes is completed after a leukocyte differential is obtained from a stained peripheral blood smear.

A TOTAL THROMBOCYTE count can be obtained from the same hemacytometer charged with blood diluted with the same solution used for obtaining the total erythrocyte and leukocyte counts. When Natt and Herrick's solution is used, the thrombocytes resemble the erythrocytes but are much smaller and have a greater nucleus-to-cytoplasm ratio. To obtain a total thrombocyte count, the thrombocytes in all of the small squares in the central large square in both sides of the hemacytometer chamber are counted. The average number of thrombocytes in one large

hemacytometer square is calculated and multiplied by 2000 to obtain the total number of thrombocytes in each cubic millimeter of blood.

CONCLUSION

Clinical hematology has proven to be a valuable diagnostic tool in avian, mammalian, and human medicine. Numerous researchers have made a commitment to the study of the morphology and function of piscine blood cells. It is the responsibility of the veterinary profession to develop clinical applications for this valuable information. This goal can be accomplished by applying clinical hematologic techniques to piscine patients (normal and abnormal) and observing the cellular changes that occur in the peripheral blood.

About the Author

Dr. Campbell is an Associate Professor in Zoological Medicine in the Department of Clinical Sciences at Colorado State University in Fort Collins, Colorado. Mr. Murru is General Curator, Sea World of Florida.

REFERENCES

1. Rowley AF, et al: Fish, in Rowley AF, Ratcliffe HA (eds): *Vertebrate Blood Cells.* New York, Cambridge University Press, 1988, pp 19–127.
2. Fange R, Pulsford A: Structural studies on lymphomyeloid tissues of the dogfish, *Scyliorhinus canicula* L. *Cell Tissue Res* 230:337–351, 1983.
3. Grace MF, Manning MJ: Histogenesis of the lymphoid organs in rainbow trout, *Salmo gairdneri. Dev Comp Immunol* 4:255–264, 1980.
4. Bly JE: The ontogeny of the immune system in the viviparous teleost *Zoarces viviparous* L., in Manning MJ, Tatner MF (eds): *Fish Immunology.* New York, Academic Press, 1985, pp 327–341.
5. Manning MJ: A comparative view of the thymus in vertebrates, in Kendall MD (ed): *The Thymus Gland.* New York, Academic Press, 1981, pp 7–20.
6. Takashima F: Spleen, in Hibiya T (ed): *An Atlas of Fish Histology. Normal and Pathological Features.* Tokyo, Kodansha Ltd, 1985, pp 62–64.
7. Catton WT: Blood cell formation in certain teleost fishes. *Blood* 6:39–60, 1951.
8. Campbell TW: Fish cytology and hematology. *Vet Clin North Am [Small Anim Pract]* 18(2):349–364, 1988.
9. Smith GC, Lewis WM, Kaplan HM: A comparative morphologic and physiologic study of fish blood. *Prod Fish Cult* 14:169–172, 1952.
10. Brown LA: Anesthesia in fish. *Vet Clin North Am [Small Anim Pract]* 18(2):317–330, 1988.
11. Yokote M: Blood, in Hibiya T (ed): *An Atlas of Fish Histology. Normal and Pathological Features.* Tokyo, Kodansha Ltd, 1985, pp 64–72.
12. Stokes EE, Firkin BG: Studies of the peripheral blood of the Port Jackson shark (*Heterodontus portusjacksoni*) with particular reference to the thrombocyte. *Br J Haematol* 20:427–435, 1971.
13. Hyder SL, Cayer ML, Pettey CL: Cell types in peripheral blood of the nurse shark: An approach to structure and function. *Tissue Cell* 15:437–455, 1983.
14. Coates ML: Hemoglobin function in the vertebrates: An evolutionary model. *J Mol Evol* 6:285–307, 1975.
15. Murray SA, Burton CB: Effects of density on goldfish blood—II.

Cell morphology. *Comp Biochem Physiol* 62A:559–562, 1979.

16. Sanchez-Muiz FJ, De LaHigurea M, Varela G: Alterations of erythrocytes of the rainbow trout *Salmo gairdneri* by the use of *Hansenula anomola* yeast as sole protein source. *Comp Biochem Physiol* 72A:693–696, 1982.

17. Ellis AE: Bizarre forms of erythrocytes in a specimen of plaice, *Pleuronectes platessa* L. *J Fish Dis* 7:411–414, 1984.

18. Eiras JC: Erythrocyte degeneration in the European eel, *Anguilla anguilla*. *Bull Eur Assoc Fish Pathol* 3:8–10, 1983.

19. Hildebrand M: *Analysis of Vertebrate Structure*, ed 2. New York, J Wiley & Sons, 1982.

20. Litman GW: Physical properties of immunoglobulins of lower species: A comparison with immunoglobulins of mammals, in Marchalonis JJ (ed): *Comparative Immunology*. Oxford, Blackwell Scientific, 1976, pp 239–256.

21. Tomonaga S, et al: Two populations of immunoglobulin-forming cells in the skate, *Raja kenojei*: Their distribution and characterization. *Dev Comp Immunol* 8:803–812, 1984.

22. Rykers GT, et al: The immune system of cyprinid fish. Kinetics and temperature dependence of antibody-producing cells in carp (*Cyprinus carpio*). *Immunology* 41:91–97, 1980.

23. McLeay DJ: Effects of cortisol and dexamethasone on the pituitary-interrenal axis and abundance of white blood cell types in juvenile coho salmon, *Oncorhynchus kisutch*. *Gen Comp Endocrinol* 21:441–450, 1973.

24. Mainwaring G, Rowley AF: Separation of leucocytes from the dogfish (*Scyliorhinus canicula*) using density gradient centrifugation and differential adhesion to glass coverslips. *Cell Tissue Res* 241:283–290, 1985.

25. Mainwaring G, Rowley AF: Studies on granulocyte heterogeneity in elasmobranchs, in Manning MJ, Tatner MF (eds): *Fish Immunology*. Orlando, FL, Academic Press, 1985, pp 57–69.

26. Bielek E: Developmental stages and localization of peroxidatic activity in the leucocytes of three teleost species (*Cyprinus carpio* L.; *Tinca tinca* L.; *Salmo gairdneri* Richardson). *Cell Tissue Res* 220:163–180, 1981.

27. Cenini P: The ultrastructure of leucocytes in carp *(Cyprinus carpio)*. *J Zool* 204:509–520, 1984.

28. Weinreb EL: Studies on the fine structure of teleost blood cells in peripheral blood. *Anat Rec* 147:219–238, 1963.

29. Cannon MS, Mollenhauer HH, Eurell TE, et al: An ultrastructural study of the leucocytes of the channel catfish, *Ictalurus punctatus*. *J Morphol* 164:1–23, 1980.

30. Ellis AE: The leucocytes of fish: A review. *J Fish Biol* 11:453–491, 1977.

31. Saunders DC: Differential blood cell counts of 121 species of marine fishes of Puerto Rico. *Trans Am Microscop Soc* 85:427–449, 1966.

32. Finn JP, Nielsen NO: The inflammatory response of rainbow trout. *J Fish Biol* 3:463–478, 1971.

33. Doolittle RF, Surgenor DM: Blood coagulation in fish. *Am J Physiol* 203:964–970, 1962.

34. Burton CB, Murray SA: Effects of density on goldfish blood—I. Hematology. *Comp Biochem Physiol* 62A:555–558, 1979.

35. Haws GT, Goodnight CJ: Some aspects of the hematology of two species of catfish in relation to their habitats. *Physiol Zool* 35(1):8–17, 1962.

36. Kamra SK: Effect of starvation and refeeding on some liver and blood constituents of Atlantic cod. *J Fish Res Board Can* 23(7):975–982, 1966.

37. Sano T: Hematological studies of the culture fishes in Japan. *J Tokyo Univ Fish* 46:68–87, 1960.

38. Summerfelt RC: Measurement of some hematological characteristics of goldfish. *Prog Fish Cult* 29(10):13–20, 1967.

39. Larsen HN, Snieszko SF: Comparison of various methods of determination of hemoglobin in trout blood. *Prog Fish Cult* 23:8–17, 1961.

40. Natt MP, Herrick CA: A new blood diluent for counting the erythrocytes and leucocytes of the chicken. *Poultry Sci* 31:735–738, 1952.

41. Blaxhall PC, Daisley KW: Routine hematological methods for use with fish blood. *J Fish Biol* 5:771–781, 1973.

42. Shaw AE: A direct method for counting the leucocytes, thrombocytes, and erythrocytes of bird blood. *J Pathol Bacteriol* 32:833–835, 1930.

43. Dacie JV, Lewis K: *Practical Hematology*, ed 4. New York, Churchill Livingstone, 1968.

44. Campbell TW: *Avian Hematology and Cytology*. Ames, IA, Iowa State University Press, 1988.

Common Disorders of Marine Fish

KEY FACTS

- Common disorders of marine fish often manifest during periods of stress.
- Poor environmental conditions predispose marine fish to stress and, therefore, disease.
- Infectious agents of marine aquaria include bacteria, viruses, chlamydia, fungi, protozoa, helminths, and crustaceans.
- Skin scraping and gill biopsy provide the practitioner with quick and powerful diagnostic techniques that are helpful in differentiating among many common diseases of marine fish.

The National Aquarium in Baltimore
Baltimore, Maryland
Brent R. Whitaker, MS, DVM

A UNIQUE challenge faces the practitioner when presented with a marine fish patient. Many of the same principles that are applied to familiar species can be modified to diagnose disease in fish. A basic understanding of husbandry techniques, fish physiology, and common diseases of marine fish facilitates this endeavor.

The Marine Patient

As with any patient, obtaining a complete history from the client is essential. A complete history includes a description of the diseases as well as general information regarding the fish. Water quality parameters, social structure, nutritional plan, quarantine protocol, and any changes made by the client before the outbreak of disease should be evaluated.

Physical examination begins with observation. Condition of the scales and fins, clarity of the eyes, rate of respiration, body weight, and behavior of the patient should be noted. Hemorrhagic scales or fins, exophthalmus, cloudy eyes, elevated scales, skin ulcerations, white spots, increased respiration, loss of equilibrium, and scratching are indicators that further diagnostic techniques should be undertaken.

Skin scraping and biopsy of gills and fins are easily performed procedures that, in many cases, enable the clinician to diagnose the disorder. Blood sampling, fecal analysis, paracentesis, radiography, and microbial cultures also may be incorporated into diagnostic procedures. Anesthesia re-

duces the stress of sample collection for the patient.

Tricaine methanesulfonate (MS-222) is an excellent anesthetic agent for most marine fish. When the agent has dissolved, the acidic solution should be buffered and used as a bath at 50 to 100 parts per million (ppm).[1] To prevent damage to the protective mucus layer, latex gloves are worn when handling a fish.

Disease in a marine aquarium is rarely limited to one individual. When a large population is at risk, necropsy of select animals is beneficial. Squash preparations, made by pressing a small piece of tissue between a coverslip and glass microslide, may provide immediate diagnosis. Tissue also should be collected for histopathologic examination. Culture and sensitivity tests performed on the liver, kidneys, and brain as well as any other affected organs may guide the practitioner in administering specific therapeutic agents for remaining fish.

When a diagnosis has been made, the goals of the practitioner should be to provide appropriate therapy and to educate the client. Few pharmacologic studies have been carried out in marine fish, and most drug doses are empirical (Table I). Drugs may be administered topically, by injection, or in the water or food. Each route has advantages and disadvantages that require careful analysis of the individual case.

Disease Related to Environment

In the wild, marine fish live within a delicately balanced

TABLE I
Selected Medications for Use in Marine Fish

Medication	Dosage	Indication	Comments
Antibiotics			
Oxytetracycline	50–75 mg/kg daily, orally 400 mg/gallon Dip 1 hour daily for 5 days	Systemic bacterial infection; fish eating	Binds to calcium in diet
Gentamicin	3 mg/kg every other day, intraperitoneally or intramuscularly, three treatments	Resistant gram-negative infections; serious infections	Nephrotoxic
Chloramphenicol sodium succinate	40 mg/kg daily, intramuscularly or orally	*Myxobacteria* and *Vibrio* infection	Anorexia
Sulfadiazine-trimethoprim	30–50 mg/kg daily for 5–10 days	Coccidial and bacterial infections	Sulfas may be toxic to some fish
Sulfamethoxazole-trimethoprim	960 mg per 10 gallons for 6-hour bath daily for 7–10 days	Coccidial and bacterial infections	Crushed tablets do not completely dissolve
Nitrofurazone	50 mg/kg daily, orally	Systemic bacterial infection	None
Antifungal Agents			
Formalin (Formaldehyde gas 37%)	25 ppm (1 ml per 10 gallons tank water) indefinitely	External fungal and parasitic infections	Carcinogenic; must be handled with care Aerate well during treatment Avoid if larger, open lesions are present
Povidone-iodine preparation	1:10 dilution, topically	Localized fungal infection	Potential toxicity, may burn skin
Antiparasitic Agents			
Chloroquine	50 mg/kg orally, twice a week for 3 weeks 10–20 ppm for 48 hours weekly for 4 weeks	Protozoal infections	Invertebrates and some fishes may be sensitive; drug is light sensitive
Copper sulfate	0.18–0.22 mg/L for 14 to 21 days	External ciliates, dinoflagellates, some monogenea	Toxicity Decreased immunologic function
Fenbendazole	50 mg/kg orally once a week for three weeks	Nematodes	
Formalin (Formaldehyde gas 37%)	25 ppm (1 ml per 10 gallons tank water) indefinitely or 100 ppm (4 ml per 10 gallons tank water) to 250 ppm (1 ml per gallon tank water) for up to 1 hour, every other day	External ciliates and flagellates; some monogenea and copepods	Same as for antifungal agents
Metronidazole	250 mg/10 gallons for 6 to 8 hours or 625 mg/100 g food for 5 days, orally	Flagellates, possibly *Uronema*	Anaerobic bacterial infections
Praziquantel	10 mg/L for up to 3 hours or 400 mg/100 g food for 3 to 5 days	Cestodes and trematodes	May cause central nervous system dysfunction (terminate dip)
Trichlorfon	0.5 mg/L for up to 1 hour	External trematodes, copepods, and leeches	Organophosphate toxicity
Anesthetic Agents			
Ketamine hydrochloride	30–40 mg/lb, intramuscularly	—	Anesthetic effect lasts for 15 to 20 minutes: Duration and extent of effect is highly species specific
Tricaine methanesulfonate (MS-222)	50–200 mg/L	Approved for use in food fish	Can regulate depth of anesthesia

ecosystem. Re-creation and maintenance of this environment is essential to the health of the fish. Suboptimum conditions cause stress in fish. As in other animals, stress induces a catecholamine and corticosteroid release and subsequent disruption of osmoregulation, reduced immune function, and altered biochemical and hematologic parameters. Disease as well as diminished growth rate and decreased levels of reproduction are recognized (see Response to Stress in Fish).

Most diseases that occur in fish acquired by a new hobbyist are related to improper water quality. Secondary bacterial and parasitic infection are commonly recognized and treated but recur unless the primary cause is eliminated. Temperature, salinity, pH, dissolved oxygen, ammonia, nitrite, and nitrate should be frequently monitored in the marine aquarium. Home test kits are available for this purpose.

TEMPERATURE requirements are species specific. Both cold water fish and warm water tropical fish require consistent temperatures. Abrupt alterations in temperature are detrimental to the health of the fish. Like reptiles, fish depend on environmental temperature to maintain metabolic processes. Temperatures that fall below those for which an animal is adapted retard metabolic processes, including immunologic function, digestion, drug absorption, and drug utilization.

The environment of marine fish contains a higher concentration of osmotically active ions than do the body fluids of the fish. Salinity of the water is a measure of its ionic concentration. Marine fish prevent dehydration in several ways. Their scales, intact epithelium, and mucus layer provide a physical barrier to the environment. They also drink large quantities of seawater; healthy fish maintain homeostatic mechanisms that eliminate excess salts. Although gradual changes in salinity are tolerated, sudden modifications disrupt these mechanisms.

Oxygen is essential to the survival of fish, important aerobic nitrifying bacteria, and heterotrophic organisms. The amount of dissolved oxygen in water is determined by salinity, temperature, and atmospheric pressure. Increased salinity or temperature reduces saturation of the water with oxygen. Low levels of dissolved oxygen result in hypoxia. Increased opercular movements (gilling) indicate respiratory distress. Providing 1.5 to 2.0 liters of air per hour for each liter of water should allow sufficient levels of dissolved oxygen.[2] On the other hand, supersaturation of the water with oxygen may result in gas bubble disease. Diagnosis is made by observation of gas bubbles in the fins, gill lamellae (Figure 1), eyes, and skin. Gas bubble disease often is caused by cavitating pumps that force air into solution. Agitating the water and stirring the substrate of the tank helps to release dissolved gas from the water.

Response to Stress in Fish[a]

Primary response–The endocrine system
  Corticotropin-releasing factor from the hypothalamus
  Corticotropin release from the pituitary
  Cortisol release from the interrenal tissue
  Epinephrine release from chromaffin tissue in head kidney

Secondary response–Blood and tissue alterations
  Increase branchial blood flow and gill permeability
  Diuresis
  Diminished osmoregulatory ability
  Electrolyte imbalance
  Interrenal vitamin C depletion
  Reduced clotting time
  Hyperglycemia
  Hemoconcentration

Tertiary response–Whole-animal and population
  Decreased growth
  Decreased immune function
  Decreased reproduction

[a]From Wedemeyer GA, Barton BA, McLeay DJ: Stress and acclimation, in Schrech CB, Moyle PB (eds): *Methods for Fish Biology.* Bethesda, MD, American Fish Society, 1990, pp 451–490. Modified with permission.

Environmental toxins, such as ammonia, nitrite, heavy metals, chlorine, and chloramines, must always be considered when death or disease occurs within an aquarium. Clinical signs include a darkening in color, excess mucus production, increased respiratory effort, loss of coordination, and loss of equilibrium. Often more than one animal is affected. A squash preparation of a gill biopsy often shows evidence of excess mucus and hypertrophy of epithelial cells. Water quality analysis and submitting liver samples from dead specimens for heavy metal analysis may provide the definitive diagnosis. Treatment consists of removing the offending toxin by changing large volumes of water in the tank and implementing use of filters charged with activated carbon.

Ammonia toxicity is extremely common in newly established systems. This may result from insufficient growth of nitrifying bacteria (i.e., *Nitrosomonas* species and *Nitrobacter* species) or a sudden increase in pH. Un-ionized ammonia (NH_3) is much more toxic than is ionized ammonia (NH_4^+). At a higher pH, the proportion of un-ionized to ionized ammonia is significantly greater.

In the biologic filter, *Nitrosomonas* species use the ammonia that is excreted by fish as well as the ammonia that is produced by heterotrophic bacteria from organic waste to yield less toxic nitrite. Methemoglobinemia occurs in fish, as in other animals, when they are exposed to high levels of nitrite. A healthy population of *Nitrobacter* species prevents methemoglobinemia by consuming nitrite, thereby yielding nitrate, which is relatively harmless and easily removed by routine water changes. The use of medications, especially antimicrobial agents, may significantly alter populations of nitrifying bacteria and result in accumulation of these toxins.

OXIDIZING AGENTS, such as chlorine and chloramines, may be added to local water supplies. These agents destroy blood cells and oxidize the iron that is present in hemoglobin to a stable state, thereby disrupting oxygen transfer.[3]

Copper has been used to treat parasitic infestations in marine aquariums for a long time. Therapeutic levels generally are maintained at 0.18 to 0.22 ppm for 14 to 21 days. At this concentration level, copper is toxic to invertebrates and some sensitive species of fish. A copper test kit should be used to monitor copper levels daily because changes in pH and salinity can result in sudden release of bound copper from substrates. Toxicity also has been reported in small fish fed live accumulators of copper, such as brine shrimp, during copper treatment.[5] Despite its usefulness as a therapeutic agent, copper also may depress immune function[6]; chronic use should be avoided. In houses with copper pipes, leaching of copper into the water can be significant. Water should be flushed through household pipes before collection for water changes.

Exposing fish to nicotine may result in death. This often occurs if an ashtray is placed next to the air pump. Use of pesticides and cleaners should also be closely monitored to prevent contamination of the aquarium environment.

Viral and Chlamydial Disease

The number of identified viral agents that potentially infect fish continues to grow. The development of appropriate cell lines for viral culture and electron microscopy have contributed significantly to the practitioner's understanding of viral diseases in fish. As in higher vertebrates, viruses that infect fish may exist as latent infections that manifest in times of stress.[7] Treatment of infected fish is primarily supportive and directed toward secondary infection.

Lymphocystis, an iridovirus, is the most commonly recognized viral disease of marine and freshwater fish. Grayish, wartlike lesions appear on the dermis and fins of infected fish as a result of hypertrophy of fibroblasts and osteoblasts.[7] Infected cells also may be found in muscle, peritoneum, and membranes that cover internal organs. This chronic disease is principally transmitted by contact[8]; infected individuals therefore should be isolated. Diagnosis is made by visualization of hypertrophic cells from a skin

TABLE II
Bacterial Disease in Marine Fish

Bacteria	General Characteristics
Gram-negative organisms *Vibrio* species *Aeromonas hydrophila* *Pasteurella piscicida* *Edwardsiella tarda* *Pseudomonas punctata*	Hemorrhagic septicemias High mortality
Gram-positive organisms *Streptococcus* species *Renibacterium salmoninarum*	Local and systemic infection
Acid-fast bacteria *Mycobacterium* species *Nocardia kampachi*	Granulomatous lesions Chronic wasting disease Acid-fast positive
Myxobacteria *Flexibacter maritimus*	Necrotic ulcers of skin, fins, and gills
Anaerobic bacteria *Eubacterium tarantellus*	Systemic infection Central nervous system dysfunction

scraping or fin biopsy. Differentiation from epidermal sarcomas may be made by histologic section.

Chlamydial infection (or epitheliocystis) produces hypertrophic epithelial cells within the gills and occasionally the skin, thus differentiating chlamydial infection from lymphocystis (Figure 2). As the infection progresses, respiratory distress and death occur.

Bacterial Disease

Most bacterial agents that affect marine fish are gram-negative opportunistic pathogens, such as *Vibrio* and *Pasteurella*. Myxobacteria, Streptococci, Mycobacteria, Nocardia, and anaerobic organisms have also been isolated[9] (Table II). Definitive diagnosis and treatment of bacterial disease is based on culture and sensitivity tests using specialized medias. Blood as well as cerebrospinal fluid and fluids from the abdomen, liver, and kidneys from moribund fish provide excellent samples for culture.

Vibriosis is the most common and serious bacterial infection of marine fish. The impact of the disease on cultured fish is so great that a vaccine has been developed.[7] Poor environmental conditions, temperature fluctuation, and stress frequently precede an outbreak. Acute septicemia is accompanied by loss of appetite, skin discoloration, epidermal hemorrhage, and erythema of the tail and fins. As the disease progresses, necrotic ulcers extend into the musculature, thereby resulting in loss of body fluids (Figure 3). Congestion and necrosis of the kidneys, liver, and spleen are present at necropsy. Early treatment with such antibiotics as tetracycline may be successful in avoiding extensive loss of fish.

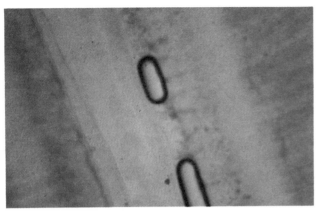

Figure 1—Gas embolism in the gill lamella of a lionfish. (Courtesy of Terry W. Campbell, DVM, PhD, Sea World of Florida, Inc., Orlando, Florida)

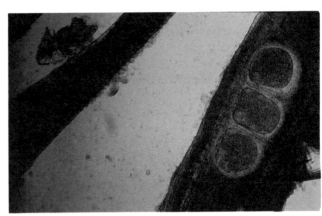

Figure 2—Large chlamydial cysts located in the primary lamellae of a flame angel fish.

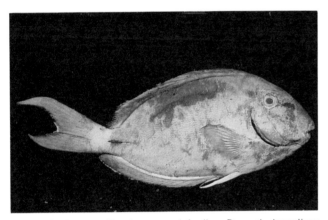

Figure 3—Primary *Cryptocaryon* infection. Dermal ulcerations and erythematous tail and fins resulting from secondary infection with *Vibrio* species are evident.

ACUTE OUTBREAKS of *Pasteurella piscicida* present as a hemorrhagic septicemia similar to vibriosis. Chronic disease, however, manifests as grayish-white granulomatous lesions in the spleen, liver, and kidneys and is called pseudotuberculosis.[9]

Mycobacterial disease is extremely common in aquarium fish. Infection with *Mycobacterium marinum* or *M. fortuitum* results in granulomatous disease that potentially affects all organs of the fish. Clinical signs are not specific but often include emaciation, anorexia, loss of color, exophthalmus, lethargy, and respiratory distress. Secondary infection is common. Diagnosis is supported by a finding of acid-fast bacteria on impression smears or histopathology. Isolation of mycobacteria is possible using Löwenstein-Jensen or brain–heart infusion agar (BHIA).

Treatment with streptomycin or isoniazid with rifampin has been reported.[10] Clients should be educated regarding zoonotic potential of mycobacteria; euthanasia of infected fish should be considered.

Fungal Disease

Poor water quality, stress, and use of antibiotics predispose fish to fungal infection. Reports of fungal disease in marine fish, however, are sporadic with the exception of *Ichthyophonus hoferi* infection.

Fish become infected with *Ichthyophonus* after ingesting food containing viable spores. Systemic dissemination of spores results in formation of white connective tissue nodules throughout affected organs. Necrosis of vital tissue results in death. External lesions may include skin discoloration and multiple whitish papules.[11] Exophthalmus, incoordination, and ascites frequently are associated with infection. Visualization of granulomas containing both round and elliptic cysts confirms the diagnosis.[12] The absence of acid-fast bacteria allows differentiation from piscine tuberculosis. Treatment using systemic antifungal agents is experimental. Prevention includes eliminating fresh fish from the diet and removing moribund fish from the system.

Parasitic Disease

Parasites of marine fish include protozoa, helminths, and crustaceans. External infection may be diagnosed by a simple skin scraping and gill biopsy. Internal parasites can be diagnosed by observation of eggs or larvae in the feces (Figure 4).

Protozoa

Protozoal disease is represented by ciliates, flagellates, microsporidia, myxosporidia, and coccidia. Diagnosis may be difficult because of the presence of different stages of the life cycles (Figure 5). The most frequently recognized ciliated protozoan of captive marine fish is *Cryptocaryon*

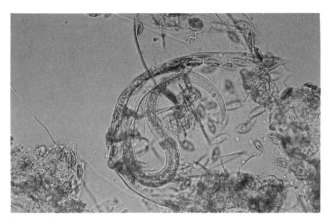

Figure 4A

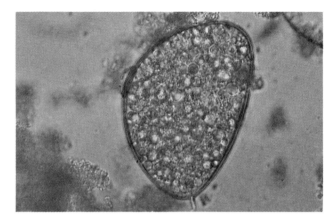

Figure 4B

Figure 4—(**A**) Nematode larvae and (**B**) trematode egg found on routine fecal examination.

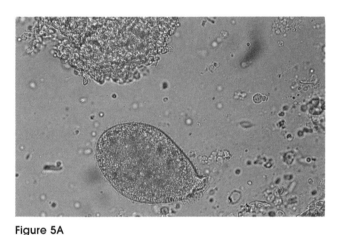

Figure 5A

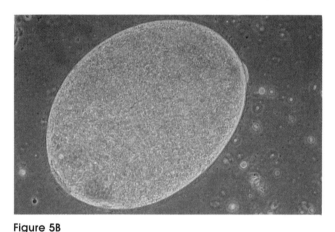

Figure 5B

Figure 5—(**A**) Infective theront and (**B**) burrowing trophont of *Cryptocaryon* species obtained from a skin scraping of an ocean surgeon. (100×)

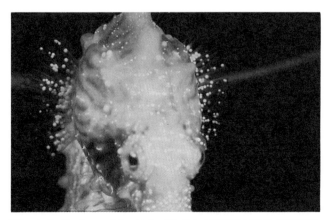

Figure 6—Seahorse infected with the microsporidial organism *Gluglea hiraldi.*

irritans. Mature burrowing trophonts manifest as small, whitish-gray nodules on the skin and gills and subsequently result in scratching, excess mucus production, and in-

creased respiratory effort. After reaching considerable size (500 μm), the ciliated trophonts leave the fish and encyst on the substrate of the tank. Binary fission within the cyst (tomont) produces more than 200 tomites that are released as free-swimming infective theronts.[13] Treatment of *Cryptocaryon* infestation with copper sulfate is directed at preventing infection by eliminating the newly emerged adult and the immature free-swimming stage.

Other ciliated protozoa include *Uronema* species and *Brooklynella hostilis. Uronema* is invasive and, in fish, has been observed in the parenchyma and blood vessels of the liver, stomach, spleen, swim bladder, and gills. Treatment with metronidazole may be effective.[14] *Brooklynella* infection generally is limited to the gills and results in petechiae and hemorrhage.[15] Formalin is the treatment of choice because copper is not as effective.

Amyloodinium ocellatum (which causes velvet disease) is a dinoflagellate with broad tolerance to temperature and salinity. After attaching to skin and gills, free-swimming dinospores send rhizoids into host cells.[7] Death results from destruction of lamellar tissue. Copper sulfate is effective in controlling the disease. Chloroquine administered in food may provide an alternate therapy.[16]

Microsporidial diseases of marine fish include the genera *Glugea, Pleistophora*, and *Nosema*. White spot disease of the seahorse (*Hippocampus erectus*) results from *Gluglea hiraldi* infection (Figure 6). The cysts, or xenomas, are confined to the stratum compactum and contain developing spores. Death usually follows observation.[17] No successful treatment has been reported.

Helminths

Nematodes, cestodes, acanthocephalans, and trematodes are common in fish. Digenetic trematodes, which are commonly found in the digestive tract of fish, require an intermediate host for completion of the life cycle. Monogenea, however, are generally hermaphroditic ectoparasites with a direct life cycle.[18] These ectoparasites are recognized by hooks that allow them to attach to the skin, gills, and fins; they feed on blood, tissue, and mucus. *Gyrodactylus* and *Benedinia* are two highly contagious monogenea that cause corneal ulcers, increased respiration, and scratching. A praziquantel bath at 10 ppm for three hours has been reported to be effective against monogenea[19] and cestodes.

Crustaceans

Parasitic crustaceans can cause gill damage, erosion of scales and skin, and destruction of sensory organs. Secondary infection often is associated with these parasites. The branchiuran *Argulus* (fish louse) creates such problems in captive fish.[7] Organophosphate baths have been used to eliminate copepods, but formalin or freshwater dips may provide a safer alternative for fish and aquarists.

Summary

Diseases of marine fish are numerous but are not always easy to identify. Understanding basic mechanisms and characteristics of specific fish pathogens allow extrapolation from familiar species. Tentative diagnosis can then be made and treatment implemented. Preventive maintenance programs that aim to advance environmental conditions and provide specific nutritional requirements should be developed in order to avoid common diseases of marine fish.

ACKNOWLEDGMENTS

The author thanks George Grall at The National Aquarium in Baltimore, Baltimore, Maryland, for photographing Figures 2 to 6. Thanks are also due to Dr. Terry Campbell of Sea World of Florida, Inc., Orlando, Florida, for providing Figure 1.

About the Author
Dr. Whitaker is a staff veterinarian with The National Aquarium in Baltimore, Baltimore, Maryland.

REFERENCES

1. Brown L: Anesthesia in fish. *Vet Clin North Am [Small Anim Pract]* 18:315–330, 1989.
2. Beleau MH: Evaluating water problems. *Vet Clin North Am [Small Anim Pract]* 18:291–316, 1988.
3. Smith LS: *Introduction to Fish Physiology.* Neptune City, NJ, T.F.H. Publications, 1982.
4. Cardeilhac PT, Whitaker BR: Copper treatments: Uses and precautions. *Vet Clin North Am [Small Anim Pract]* 18:435–448, 1988.
5. Dempster RP, Shipman WH: The use of copper as a medicant for aquarium fishes and as an algicide in marine mammal systems. *Marine Aquarist* 1(2):24, 1970.
6. Elsasser MS, Roberson BS, Hetrick FM: Effects of metals on chemiluminescent response of rainbow trout, *Salmo gairdneri*, phagocytes. *Vet Immunol Immunopathol* 12:243, 1986.
7. Sinderman CJ: *Principal Diseases of Marine Fish and Shellfish*, vol 1, New York, Academic Press, 1990, pp 19, 22, 36.
8. Wolfe K: *Fish Viruses and Fish Viral Diseases.* Ithaca, NY, Cornell University Press, 1988, p 281.
9. Frerichs GN: Bacterial diseases of marine fish. *Vet Rec* 125:315–318, 1989.
10. Oestmann DJ: Environmental and disease problems in ornamental marine aquariums. *Compend Contin Educ Pract Vet [Small Anim Pract]* 7(8):656–668, 1985.
11. Neish GA, Hughs GC: Fungal diseases of fishes, in Snieszko SF, Axelrod HR (eds): *Diseases of Fishes, Book 6.* Neptune City, NJ, T.F.H. Publications, 1980, pp 61–100.
12. Untergasser D: *Handbook of Fish Diseases.* Neptune City, NJ, T.F.H. Publications, 1980.
13. Lom J: Diseases caused by protistans, in Kinne O (ed): *Diseases of Marine Animals. Part 1*, vol. IV, Helgoland, Hamburg, Germany, Biologische Anstalt, 1984, pp 114–168.
14. Whitaker BR, Reimschuessel R, Lipsky MM: A case of systemic parasitism in the John Dory. Vancouver, BC, *IAAAM Proc*: 169–171, 1990.
15. Lom J, Nigrelli RF: *Brooklynella hostilis.* A pathogenic crytophorine ciliate in marine fishes. *J Protozool* 17(2):224–232, 1970.
16. Lewis DH, Wang W, Ayers A, Arnold CR: Preliminary studies on the use of chloroquine as a systemic chemotherapeutic agent for amyloodinosis in the red drum (*Sciaenops ocellatus*). *Cont Marine Sci* 30:183–189, 1988.
17. Vincint CJ: Parasitic infection of the seahorse (*Hippocampus erectus*). A case report. *J Wildl Dis* 25(3):404–406, 1989.
18. Crow GL: A synoptic review of the monogenetic trematodes. *J Aquaculture and Aquatic Sci* V(4):74–78.
19. Schmahl G, Mehlhorn H: Praziquantel effective against monogenea. *Z Parasitenkd* 71:727–737, 1985.

ADDITIONAL READING

Brown L: *Aquaculture for Veterinarians.* New York, NY, Pergamon Press, 1993.
Citino SB: Basic ornamental fish medicine, in Kirk RW, Bonagura JD (eds): *Current Veterinary Therapy X.* Philadelphia, PA, WB Saunders Co, 1989.
Ellis AE: *Fish Vaccination.* New York, NY, Academic Press, 1988.
Ferguson HW: *Systemic Pathology of Fish.* Ames, Iowa, Iowa State University Press, 1989.
Gratzek JB, Matthews JR: *The Science of Fish Health Management—Master Volume.* Morris Plains, NJ, Tetra Press, 1992.
Noga EJ: *Fish Disease Diagnosis and Treatment.* Baltimore, MD, Mosby Year Book 1996.
Stoskopf MK: *Fish Medicine.* Philadelphia, PA, WB Saunders Co, 1993.

Tortoises *(continued from page 64)*

REFERENCES

1. Jacobson ER: Infectious diseases of reptiles, in Kirk RW (ed): *Current Veterinary Therapy. Small Animal Practice*, ed 7. Philadelphia, WB Saunders Co, 1980, pp 625–626.

2. Samour JH, Hawkey CM, Pugsley S, et al: Clinical and pathological findings related to malnutrition and husbandry in captive giant tortoises (*Geochelone* species). *Vet Rec* 118:299–302, 1986.

3. Frye FL: *Biomedical and Surgical Aspects of Captive Reptile Husbandry*. Edwardsville, KS, Veterinary Medicine Publishing Co, 1981.

4. Williams R: Tortoise reproduction at the Jacksonville Zoological Park. *Proc AAZPA*:126–134, 1986.

5. Jarchow JL: Hospital care of the reptile patient, in Jacobson ER, Kollias GV (eds): *Contemporary Issues in Small Animal Practice: Exotic Animals*. New York, Churchill Livingstone, 1988, pp 19–34.

6. Jackson OF: Weight and measurement data on tortoises (*Testudo gracea* and *Testudo hermanni*) and their relationship to health. *J Small Anim Pract* 21:409–416, 1980.

7. Heard DJ, Cantor GH, Jacobson ER, et al: Hyalohyphomycosis caused by *Paecilomyces lilacinus* in an Aldabra tortoise. *JAVMA* 189(9):1143–1145, 1986.

8. Page CD, Jacobson ER, Mechlinski W, et al: Medical management of a debilitated leopard tortoise. *Proc AAZV*:118–119, 1986.

9a. Bennett RA: A review of anesthesia and chemical restraint in reptiles. *Journal of Zoo Wildlife Medicine* 22(3):282, 1991.

10. Jacobson ER: Use of chemotherapeutics in reptile medicine, in Jacobson ER, Kollias GV (eds): *Contemporary Issues in Small Animal Practice: Exotic Animals*. New York, Churchill Livingstone, 1988, pp 38–46.

11. Taylor RW, Jacobson ER: Hematology and serum chemistry of the gopher tortoise, *Gopherus polyphemus*. *Comp Biochem Physiol* 72A(2):425–428, 1982.

12. Jackson OF, Fasal MD: Radiology in tortoises, terrapins and turtles as an aid to diagnosis. *J Small Anim Pract* 22:705–707, 1981.

13. Morgan JP, Silverman S, Zontine WJ: *Techniques of Veterinary Radiography*. Davis, CA, Veterinary Radiology Associates, 1975, pp 269–279.

14. Rosskopf WJ: Shell disease in turtles and tortoises, in Kirk RW (ed): *Current Veterinary Therapy. Small Animal Practice*, ed 9. Philadelphia, WB Saunders Co, 1986, pp 757–758.

15. Jacobson E, Kollias GH, Peters LJ: Dosages for antibiotics and parasiticides used in exotic animals, in *The Compendium Collection: Exotic Animal Medicine in Practice*, Lawrenceville, NJ, Veterinary Learning Systems Co, 1986, p 207.

16. Page CD, Mautino M, Meyer HR, Mechlinski W: Preliminary pharmacokinetics of ketoconazole in the gopher tortoise *(Gopherus polyphenus)*. *J Vet Pharmacol Ther* 11:397–401, 1988.

17. Raphael BL, Papich M, Cook RA: Pharmacokinetics of enrofloxacin after a single intramuscular injection in Indian Star Tortoises *(Geochelone elegans)*. *Journal of Zoo Wildlife Medicine* 25(1):88, 1994.

Environmental and Disease Problems in Ornamental Marine Aquariums*

Daniel J. Oestmann, DVM
Marine Biomedical Institute
University of Texas Medical Branch
Galveston, Texas

With the right education, the tropical fish hobbyist in the United States could become an active part of the veterinarian's clientele. A survey sponsored by the United Nations showed that the United States was the world's largest importer of tropical fish in 1979. Americans spent $272 million buying dogs, followed closely by $234 million for pet fish. Bird owners spend $83 million, and cat owners spent $48 million.[1] Human population trends influence pet ownership. Increasing urbanization favors pets such as caged birds; however, these figures suggest that a client is more likely to have an aquarium than a bird cage in the living room.

Tropical fish come from warm water and equatorial regions, many from East Asia and the Amazon River.[1] Africa and South and Central America also are source areas. Tropical fish can be of freshwater or saltwater origin. Marine fish are from salt water, either warm (tropical) or cold (North Atlantic or North Pacific). Tropical coral reef fish are the most popular in display aquariums because of their bright colors and various forms. Cold water varieties of fish tend to be drab in appearance but hardier; they require expensive chiller units to maintain proper temperature. Veterinary services are sought more often for marine fish, which are more expensive, than for most freshwater tropical fish.

Environment of the Marine Aquarium

Management of the saltwater aquarium, more difficult than that of the freshwater one, requires constant attention and knowledge of the systems involved. The specimens in the tank live in a subtle balance between salinity, ammonia-nitrite-nitrate, pH, temperature, aeration, filtration, and waste (Table I). Most disease problems probably occur secondary to environmental changes within the aquarium.

Population Density

One of the most common environmental problems in display aquariums is population density. Because the natural fish-to-water ratio of the

*Kansas State University Agricultural Experimental Station Journal Series No. 84-295-J. (The research for this article was performed while the author was a student at the College of Veterinary Medicine.)

TABLE I
Parameters of a Marine Aquarium

Size	Easily maintained if over 75 L (20 gal)
Material used	No metal in contact with water; glass sealed with silicone and plastic airflow systems preferred
Filtration capacity	15–23 L (4–6 gal)/hr for each 3.8 L (1 gal) tank capacity
Aeration capacity	5.7–7.6 L (6–8 qt) of air/hr for each 3.8 L (1 gal) water
Population density	Approximately 13 L (3.5 gal)/ medium-sized fish
Temperature	21°–29.4° C (70°–85° F); 24.4° C (76° F) optimal
Water changes	One tenth to one third of capacity each 4–6 weeks
Salinity	34–35 ppt
Specific gravity	1.020–1.025, depending on temperature
pH	8.0–8.3
Ammonia	Less than 0.01 ppm un-ionized ammonia; test kits that measure total ammonium nitrogen should indicate 0.1 ppm or less
Nitrite	Less than 0.1 ppm
Nitrate	Less than 20 ppm

coral reef would be unacceptable for a home aquarium, many people overpopulate a tank without proper compensatory apparatus.

Many public aquariums overcome this problem by having a small display tank, with a high fish-to-water ratio, in circulation with huge filtration tanks that the public never sees. This system is similar to the natural reef environment, in which the surrounding ocean constantly replenishes and cleans the local fish habitat.

Few home hobbyists can afford large filtration tanks. As little as 28 L (7.5 gal) of water can be used, but at least 75 L (20 gal), and preferably more, is recommended for marine fish.[2] A safe number of fish for larger tanks can be estimated as follows: 30 fish 5 to 7.6 cm (2 to 3 inches) in length per 380 L (100 gal) of water, or approximately 13 L (3.5 gal) for one medium-sized fish. If the fish are longer than 7.6 cm, population density must be reduced. No more than 10 fish of 10 to 13 cm (4 to 5 inches) can be maintained safely in 380 L.[3] The capacity of the tank also can be estimated as a function of the surface area of the bacterial filter-bed. Approximately 7.6 cm of fish per 926 cm² (1 ft²) of bed is proper, provided that the gravel is 3/16-inch grain and 7.6 cm deep and that the flow of water is at least 3.8 L (1 gal)/min/926 cm².[4]

Species selection also must be considered because territorial aggression often is more of a limiting factor than tank volume.[a]

Aeration and Filtration

Vigorous aeration and filtration must be maintained to compensate for high fish-to-water ratios in display aquariums. As little as 3.8 to 7.6 L (1 to 2 gal) of water per medium-sized fish is sufficient if there is proper undergravel filtration and heavy aeration and if proper attention is given to species combination. A breakdown in the system can result in rapid loss of fish.[3]

Gas exchange is critical in marine aquariums because salt water, with its dissolved solids, contains approximately 20% less oxygen than fresh water.[5] Most gas exchange occurs at the water-to-atmosphere interface. A long, low tank, which provides a larger interface, is recommended.[4] Aeration is the principal means of moving water in the marine aquarium. Rising columns of air bubbles create water circulation from the bottom of the tank to the top, where gas exchange can occur. To maintain proper aeration, 5.7 to 7.6 L (6 to 8 qt) of air for each 3.8 L of water should be moving through the system.[6] An excess of air probably will do no harm in a home aquarium situation and may be required for high population densities.

With the current equipment, aeration and bacterial filtration can be accomplished with the same undergravel filtration equipment. External power filters provide the necessary mechanical and chemical filtration and rapid flow of water. In such filters, incoming water flows over Dacron™ floss, which removes large particulate matter by trapping it in the mesh.[6] The floss must be changed regularly to prevent plugging of the system and subsequent anaerobic conditions. The resulting bacteria release many by-products that are potentially toxic to the fish. The filter system should circulate approximately 15 to 23 L (4 to 6 gal) of water per 3.8 L of tank capacity per hour.[5]

The water then flows through a bed of activated charcoal. Although the charcoal does not remove ammonia, nitrite, or nitrate, it does absorb the substances that eventually turn the tank yellow.[6] These organic substances, which are in solution, are not removed mechanically by the floss. Other types of chemical filtration—such as airstripping, ozone, and ultraviolet light—are options for very large aquariums.[4]

Ammonia-Nitrite-Nitrate

The third type of filtration is invisible and takes time and expertise to develop and maintain. The biologic filter consists of various populations of bacteria that must be cultured in a new tank. These bacteria exist in and under the gravel bed of the tank as long as enough water is flowing through it to maintain aerobic conditions.

---

[a]Klocek R: Personal communication, John G. Shedd Aquarium, Chicago, Illinois, 1985.

The first group of bacteria, the heterotrophs, perform the process of ammonification. Heterotrophic bacteria use organic matter from excess food, dead organisms, and detritus as an energy source. They decompose this matter to form ammonia and other products.[4]

Ammonia is toxic to aquarium fish and must be removed. This removal is accomplished by nitrifying bacteria, which use ammonia as an energy source. One group of bacteria, the *Nitrosomonas* spp., convert ammonia to nitrite, which, still somewhat toxic, is in turn converted to nitrate by the *Nitrobacter* spp. bacteria.[4]

Aquarium denitrification is accomplished by bacteria that reduce nitrates to nitrous oxide and elemental nitrogen, which are used by diatoms (also called *brown algae*) and green algae.[6] The algae in turn provide oxygen and other products that contribute to the health of the fish when eaten, such as vitamin B_{12}, trace elements that apparently have a tonic effect on fish, and antibiotic substances[6] (Figure 1).

The bacterial culture-bed can be established in a new tank by placing a hardy specimen, such as a hermit crab or a clownfish, in the tank. The crab or fish will start the cycle by excreting ammonia products. Within two weeks the ammonia level should peak at approximately 6 ppm. Slightly later, the nitrite level will peak at the same mark. The nitrite level will gradually decrease as the nitrate level rises (Figure 2). It can take up to two months until the tank is ready to be populated with fish.[4] This should be done slowly to avoid overwhelming the bacterial filter and causing another ammonia spike. The process can be accelerated by as much as a month by adding gravel from a well-established aquarium or by adding a small amount of common garden soil.[6] Care must be taken to avoid adding soil and developing the culture too quickly; excessive heterotrophs will inhibit the growth of denitrifying bacteria.[b]

The tank should be monitored daily during the culturing period. After the tank has been stabilized, the nitrite level should be less than 0.1 ppm and the nitrate level less than 20 ppm.[4] Monitoring test kits are available in pet stores.

Aquarium algae are useful in proper maintenance of the nitrogen cycle, depicted in Figure 1. Fish might stay healthy longer and experience better growth rates in tanks that contain abundant algae growth or that maintain algae filters. The presence of brown or blue-green algae can indicate that the bacterial balance is upset, or that nitrates have accumulated from excess feeding.[a] These algae can survive poor light, low oxygen content, low pH, and low oxidation-reduction potentials.[6] Brown algae are usually the first evident growth, but, if a seed culture is used from an established tank, they should be replaced by green algae within three to four weeks after the tank has been stabilized.

Organic Matter

The bacterial filter can be upset easily and quickly,

[b]Herwig N: Personal communication, Houston Zoological Gardens, Houston, Texas, 1983.

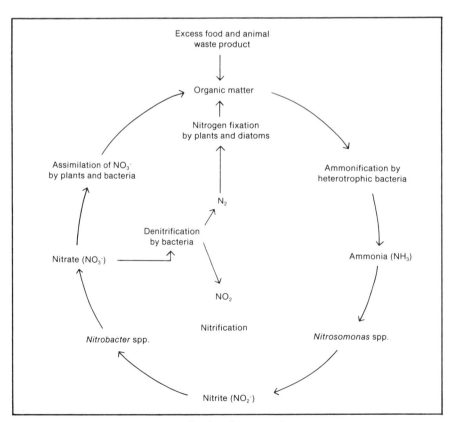

Figure 1—Ammonia-nitrite-nitrate cycle of a saltwater tank.

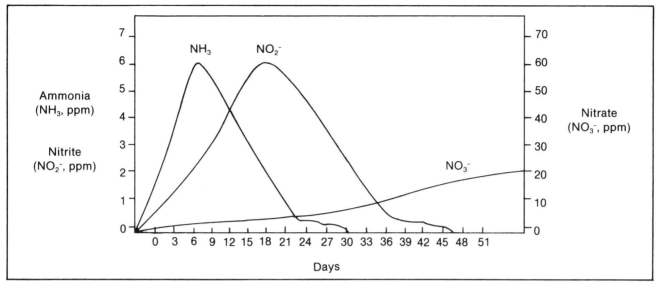

Figure 2—Ammonia, nitrite, and nitrate levels during culture period.

causing disease and death to the fish. If the fish are improperly fed and excess food settles to the bottom and decays or if a specimen dies and is not promptly removed, organic matter floods the tank. *Bacterium coli, Bacterium proteus,* and *Bacterium subtilis* begin to digest these proteins. As metabolic by-products, the bacteria release toxins that even in relatively small concentrations are dangerous to specimens.[6]

These bacteria do not live within the filter system of the aquarium. All excess food and protein should be filtered out by mechanical filtration or hand siphoning. In this way, the *Bacterium* spp. will not be able to act on the proteins because they live on the bottom soil, the stones, the corals, the glass, and the fish.[6]

Amino acids are released when excess protein floods the tank. One group, the sulfurous amino acids, lowers the oxidation-reduction potential, thus decreasing the oxygen capacity of the water. The proliferation of the *Bacterium* spp. also uses large amounts of oxygen and releases much carbon dioxide (CO_2). The release of amino acids and CO_2 into the water lowers the pH, which also contributes to a lower oxygen capacity of the water.[6]

High surface tension (the bubbles from aeration persist for an extended time) and a temporary drop in pH are clues to excess protein in the tank. Other, less dangerous bacteria degrade protein by releasing aromatic amino acids, causing the tank to emit a ripe fruit or onion odor. Still other bacteria degrade amino acids to phenols and cresols, which are dyes that accumulate in the water and turn it yellow or yellowish brown.[6]

pH

The pH of natural sea water normally is 8.0 to 8.3. The aquarium should be kept as close to this as possible; a range of 7.8 to 8.5 is acceptable. The amount of dissolved CO_2, the amounts of magnesium and calcium, and the production of acids and nitrates are major factors affecting aquarium pH.[6]

The effect of CO_2 concentration on pH is illustrated in Figure 3. A pH drop occurs in situations in which CO_2 concentration rises, such as water stagnation, too great an animal load, or bacterial (*Bacterium* spp.) overgrowth resulting from excess protein. Proper aeration can help a tank blow off excess CO_2. This accumulation of CO_2 can be avoided with proper filtration, proper tank population, and proper algae growth levels maintained by harvesting.

Normally, there is scant free CO_2 dissolved in the water. The CO_2 that is present is rapidly used by algae for photosynthesis. When the CO_2 is gone, the algae turn to hydrocarbonates for photosynthetic fuel; this causes the precipitation of carbonates and results in increased pH levels, up to 10.[6]

Phosphates accumulate in the water as an end product of the decomposition of organic matter. When phosphates reach the saturation point, they precipitate as magnesium phosphate and calcium phosphate.[6] The magnesium and the calcium come from the many dissolved seawater salts, primarily calcium sulfate ($CaSO_4$), magnesium sulfate ($MgSO_4$), calcium carbonate ($CaCO_3$), and sodium chloride ($NaCl$). Seawater salts provide dissolved ions, both acid and alkaline, with buffering capacity. This capacity is lost when magnesium and calcium precipitate with phosphates from organic matter decomposition.

Dolomite gravel or oyster shells and coral ornaments can be used as renewable sources of calcium and magnesium.[4] Phosphates will react with the calcium and magnesium of the shells so that the seawater salt ions are not removed from the water. Dolomite and coral sand are dissolved readily by carbonic acid to form calcium hydrocarbons. In this way, CO_2 is removed and the equation in Figure 3 is shifted to the left, keeping the pH high.[6]

The dolomite gravel, composed of magnesium and

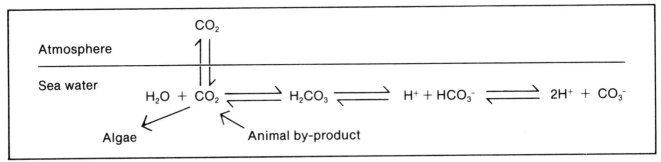

Figure 3—The effect of CO_2 concentration on pH.

calcium carbonate, will form a layer of mineral apatite on its surface resulting from its reaction with phosphates. The apatite layer renders dolomite ineffective as a buffering agent.[a] If the pH level drops for this reason, a mixture of six parts sodium bicarbonate and one part sodium carbonate can be added slowly, while the pH level is monitored until it returns to normal. An additional 5 ml (1 tsp) of the mixture then is added for every 95 L (25 gal) of water.[6] This is a temporary solution; renewal of the saltwater or the buffering gravel is essential.

Ammonia levels must be determined before the pH level is corrected. At pH 6, ammonia is all in the harmless ammonium form. Correcting the pH to 8.3 will cause slightly more than 4% of the ammonium to convert back to toxic ammonia (Table II).[6]

Accumulation of excess organic matter produces organic acids that will lower the pH level. Normally these acids are broken down rapidly and begin to go through the ammonia-nitrite-nitrate cycle; however, excess ammonia accumulation slows down this process, and the organic matter will remain longer in the organic acid form, keeping the pH level low.

Water Changes

Because a steadily falling pH is a sign of water aging, regular pH monitoring is imperative.[6] It is advisable to replace one tenth to one third of the salt water every four to six weeks. If the tank is overpopulated, it might be necessary to replace half of the water.[6] Because of the various interrelating factors, each tank will have distinct needs and care requirements. When cleaning a tank and changing its water, care must be taken to not disturb the bacterial filter-bed because the bacteria can be killed.[6] For this reason, siphoning of superficial detritus that might clog the gravel bed also should be done carefully.[a]

Aquarium cleaning should coincide with water renewal. Harvesting excess algae and scraping it from the sides of the tank should be done at this time. If excess algae are not removed, they can become a major source of excess organic matter when they die.

Water test kits for pH, ammonia, nitrite, nitrate, copper, and other indicators are available from pet stores. Liquid pH indicators are more accurate and more consistent than paper ones.

Temperature

The temperature of the marine aquarium should be as close as possible to that of the fish's natural environment; for most reef fish, this is between 21° and 29.4° C (70° to 85° F). Some sources claim that display fish thrive at 26.7° C (80° F).[3] This temperature provides adequate warmth for metabolism (most fish are cold blooded) and permits proper oxygen content of the water.

A temperature of 26.7° C might be unnecessary, however. A temperature of 23.3°C (74° F) will decrease the replication rate of microbes and will slow the life cycle of parasites. The fish's metabolism also is slowed; although they are not as active, they produce less waste products to contaminate the tank and will live longer.[b] Oxygen content actually is increased at the lower temperature.[6] Water temperature should not fluctuate more than 2.8° C (5° F) during a 24-hour period.[a]

Salinity and Specific Gravity

Because marine animals have a slightly lower salt content in their bodies than that in the water around them, they must maintain hypo-osmoregulation. Freshwater fish are hyperosmoregulatory, that is, their bodies contain *higher* salt concentrations than the surrounding water. The marine fish loses water through its skin to its environment down the osmotic gradient and must constantly drink water, at a rate of 0.2% to 0.5% of its body weight/hr.[4] The excess salts are excreted through the mucus cells in the skin, in the feces, by the kidneys, and particularly by specialized cells in the gills.[4] Because of their constant water loss through the

TABLE II

Conversion of Ammonium to Ammonia at Various pH Values

pH	% Ammonium (NH_4OH)	% Ammonia (NH_3)
6	100	0
7	99	1
8	96	4
9	75	25
10	22	78
11	4	96

skin to the environment, marine fish excrete scant urine —approximately 2 to 4 ml/kg/day. Freshwater fish can excrete 300 ml/kg/day.[6]

Marine fish can endure slight fluctuations in salinity, but abrupt changes can be harmful. The optimum salinity for tropical marine fish is 34 to 35 parts per thousand (ppt). Salinity varies with temperature changes and is directly related to specific gravity, which is measured with a hydrometer. A specific gravity range of 1.021 to 1.025 at 26.7°C is optimum for most ornamental marine fish.[6] The effect of temperature on salinity is crucial. A nomogram can be used to find the proper hydrometer reading to keep the salinity at 34 to 35 ppt at varying temperatures (Figure 4).

A salinity of 20 to 24 ppt and a specific gravity of 1.018 to 1.020 has been recommended[b]; the majority of saltwater pathogens and parasites are obligatory halophils, and reduced salinity endangers them and thus might decrease the likelihood of disease. Reduced salinity is still experimental, and stress on the pathogens also stresses the fish. Lower salinity also slows the fish's metabolism, thus decreasing waste production.

Tank Material

The marine tank itself is a vital consideration. The tank parts and the materials in the tank are subjected to the weight (salt water weighs more than fresh water) and the highly corrosive action of the salt water. Metal salts, which are toxic to the fish, can form if the tank has metal parts or if any metal from the pumps, the heater, the lighting, or the airways is in contact with the water.[5]

All-glass tanks sealed with inert silicone are preferred. Even plastic tubing, air lifts, and siphon tubes can be toxic. To keep the plastic pliable, many contain mollifiers that eventually dissolve into the water and become toxic to the fish. Tygon tubing is recommended for the marine aquarium.[6]

Disease in the Marine Aquarium

Because the ocean is vast, the constant mixing of water in the reef environment causes any change to be diluted quickly. Thus, the changes are, in effect, slight and of short duration. Coral reef fish therefore might never have been exposed to oxygen shortages or various pollutants and probably never have developed adequate adaptive mechanisms to accommodate for environmental stresses.[6] Fish in the marine aquarium change the water and cause it to differ significantly from sea water. These factors are important in considering disease in a marine tank (Table III).

Environmental poisoning can cause signs that resemble those of other diseases. Metal (copper or zinc) poisoning accelerates respiration because of the coagulation of slime on the gills.[6] Rapid respiration is a common sign of protozoal disease, gill flukes, and a lowering pH because of poor water quality. Phenol and ammonia poisoning manifest as sudden, uncoordinated bursts of swimming. A significant water change must be performed to correct the poisoning.[6] This sign, however, also can indicate irritation from crustaceans or protozoa.

There is scant information available about treatment

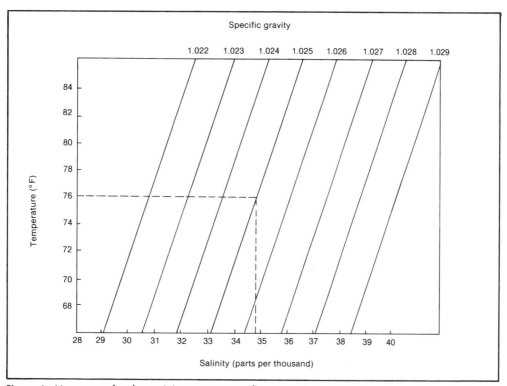

Figure 4—Nomogram for determining proper specific gravity at varying temperatures. (From de Graff F, Spiekman J [trans]: *Marine Aquarium Guide*. Harrison, NJ, Pet Library Ltd, 1973. Modified with permission.)

of specific diseases in marine aquariums. Treatments advocated for tropical freshwater fish often are inadequate and unsuccessful in the marine tank; this is especially true of the use of antibiotics. Penicillin can cause blindness in clownfish, and high doses of broad-spectrum antibiotics, such as chlortetracycline or chloramphenicol, are relatively ineffective in the tank.[3] Sulfa drugs and oxytetracycline also are not recommended because long-term use has created resistance in some bacteria.[7]

Most diseases can be treated and controlled by applying the following principles. A "sick tank" should be established. This tank also can serve to quarantine new arrivals. The tank should be kept in semidarkness and should have some hiding places—clay flowerpots are suitable for this. The temperature must be constant. Biologic and chemical filtration should not be maintained in the sick tank because it will absorb or destroy many of the antibiotics used to treat the fish. The display tank never should be treated with antibiotics, which are nonspecific in their action and can damage the bacterial filter-bed of the tank. Vigorous aeration of the sick tank should be maintained, and ammonia levels should be controlled by water changes, which are required daily for most antibiotics to maintain effective levels.[4]

One theory suggests that the sick tank should be

TABLE III
Disease Problems in a Marine Tank

Disease Condition	Signs	Treatment
Low pH	Sudden darting movements, heavy respiration, milky-white clouding of the skin (sometimes with pinpoint hemorrhages), decreased appetite	Slowly add a mixture of six parts sodium bicarbonate to one part sodium carbonate until pH is normal, then add 5 ml/95 L more; change water or gravel
Metal or ammonia poisoning	Abnormal swimming, darting, heavy or irregular respiration	Control with water changes and proper filtration
Salinity changes	Fish lies on bottom, heavy breathing after transfer to new tank, shock	Prevent with gradual water changes
Viral lymphocystis	Small, cauliflowerlike, white tubercles on fin edges or skin	Heals spontaneously; ozone or ultraviolet light might speed cure
Tuberculosis, *Mycobacterium* spp.	Exophthalmos, fading colors, emaciation, loss of appetite, skin and scale defects with ulceration, fin destruction	Streptomycin, 80 mg/3.8 L (1 gal) for 1 week (usually diagnosed too late to cure)
Red disease, *Vibrio parahaemolyticus*	Inactivity, loss of appetite, skin hemorrhages, discolored skin patches, fin degeneration, cloudy eyes, red cloaca, internal organ distention and congestion	Gentamicin or kanamycin baths, 66 mg/L; or nitrofurazone baths, 25 mg/3.8 L (1 gal)
Fin rot, *Vibrio* or *Pseudomonas ichthyodermis*	Whitening and deterioration of fin tissue	Check water quality; touch area with copper sulfate; nitrofurazone baths, 25 mg/3.8 L (1 gal)
White spot disease, *Cryptocaryon irritans*	Coarse, white to grayish dots on skin, especially fins, cloudy eyes, heavy respiration, some tissue sloughing	Copper sulfate solution in treatment tank, 0.15-0.25 ppm for 2 weeks
Coral fish disease, *Oodinium ocellatum*	Small, white to yellowish dots on skin, especially gills, heavy respiration, cloudy eyes, erratic swimming and rubbing	Copper sulfate solution in treatment tank, 0.15–0.20 ppm for 2 weeks
Brooklynella hostilis and *Uronema marinum*	Lethargy, loss of appetite, excess mucus production and progressive boillike body lesions with skin sloughing	Copper sulfate bath, 0.25 ppm; malachite green bath, 0.15 ppm; 50-min bath of 1 ml of 37% formalin per gal of water
Fungus (external)	Cottonlike growth on skin or wounds; very rare	Touch with copper sulfate, check water quality
Ichthyophonus hoferi	Same as tuberculosis	No known cure
Crustaceans or worms	Immobile or mobile skin parasites, visible to the naked eye, usually oblong	Pull with tweezers; for worms, 15-min bath of 1 ml of 37% formalin per gal of water

maintained at a higher temperature[6] to speed up the life cycle of the pathogen and thus force it into a vulnerable stage in which chemotherapy will be effective against it. This effect might be achieved, but the higher temperature also places additional stress on the already stressed patient; care and close observation therefore are indicated.

Viral Disease

Although there are numerous viral diseases of saltwater fish, only lymphocystis disease has been observed in marine aquarium fish. This wartlike lesion can be removed surgically, but a spontaneous cure usually occurs within approximately two months.[7] Ozone or ultraviolet light can hasten resolution in the sick tank (Figures 5 and 6).[4]

Bacterial Disease

Most bacterial pathogens that affect fish are gram-negative. Fish can be given antibiotics orally in food or parenterally (subcutaneously or intraperitoneally). Intramuscular injections are inappropriate in fish; because fish muscle is poorly vascularized, absorption is slow and sterile abscesses can develop around the injection site.

Piscine tuberculosis caused by *Mycobacterium* spp. is a common bacterial disease of captive marine aquarium fish.[4] Usually, the disease is slowly progressive. External signs include listlessness, rapid respiration, lack of appetite, emaciation, skin and scale defects, exophthalmos if the bacteria infect the eye socket (Figure 7),[6] skin ulceration, and fin destruction.[8] Necropsy findings include grayish, knoblike lesions in and on the internal organs, especially the liver, the spleen, and the intestine.[6] The organism can be isolated from a swab of an infected organ or nodule and is microscopically visible (Figure 8).

If the disease is recognized early, a streptomycin bath at 80 mg/3.8 L (1 gal) for one or more weeks can be beneficial.[6] Isoniazid (Rifamate®—Merrell Dow Pharmaceuticals) and rifampin (Rifadin®—Merrell Dow Pharmaceuticals) also have been recommended.[6] If piscine tuberculosis is diagnosed on necropsy by the presence of acid-fast bacteria in lesions, the patient should be burned or buried with quicklime at a site far from water drainage because this mycobacterium can spread to humans. Most reported cases have occurred in aquarists, who contracted localized, open, papulopustular lesions on the hands and the arms after cleaning a contaminated tank; therapy is required for 12 to 24 months.[8] Sick or dead fish probably are best left in the garbage rather than flushed down the toilet—this disease occurs in freshwater and saltwater fish.

Vibrio infection, also called *red disease*, is most often caused by *Vibrio parahaemolyticus*. It occurs commonly in winter months in newly imported fish and new additions to tanks. Fish under stress during transport are more susceptible.[9]

Vibrio parahaemolyticus is closely related to the human pathogen *Vibrio cholerae*. *V. parahaemolyticus* is responsible for the human disease known as *seafood poisoning*, which is mostly limited to the Orient because of dietary preference. Like red disease in fish, seafood poisoning is a gastrointestinal disease in humans.[9] *V. parahaemolyticus* spreads from fish to fish in the same way that seafood poisoning is disseminated, through ingestion. The disease usually spreads during holding and transport in small amounts of water, which is also a high-stress period.

The bacteria replicate in the gastrointestinal tract and spread to other organs. Feces are often a pure culture of the bacteria, causing a bloody discharge and reddening of the cloaca. Distention and congestion of the liver, the spleen, and the intestine are common. Congestion and necrosis of the kidneys often complicate recovery even if bacterial replication can be halted.[9] The most noticeable lesions are bloody ulcerations on the skin, with loss of scales and muscular necrosis, surrounded by light-colored areas of freshly infected tissue. These lesions begin as small petechial hemorrhages and grow into lumps or boillike lesions (Figure 9). A tentative diagnosis can be made by examining the curved or S-shaped *Vibrio* organisms in fecal material or in a swab of a skin lesion (Figure 10).[9]

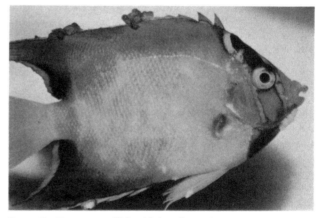

Figure 5—Queen angelfish with lymphocystis.

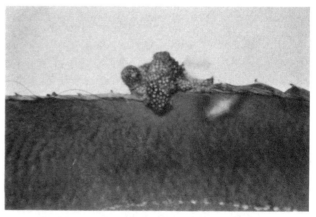

Figure 6—Close-up of Figure 5.

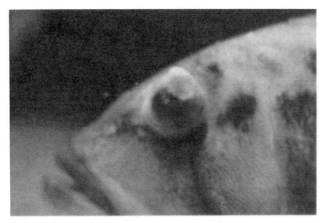

Figure 7—California rockfish with exophthalmos. The patient responded to tuberculosis therapy.

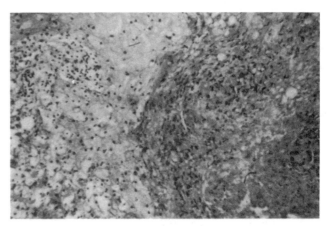

Figure 8—Piscine tuberculosis organisms.

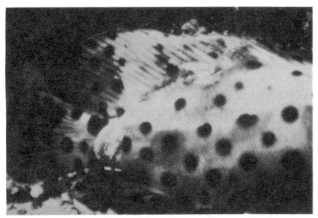

Figure 9—Panther grouper with *Vibrio parahaemolyticus* infection.

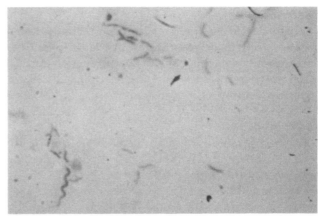

Figure 10—*Vibrio parahaemolyticus* organisms.

The condition is treated with antibiotics. Gentamicin or kanamycin used at a dose of 66 mg/L (250 mg/gal) probably is most effective. Nitrofurazone, at 25 mg/3.8L, or water also can be used.[9] Chloramphenicol has been recommended at a dosage of 13 mg/L (50 mg/gal) for seven days with a 50% water change each day.[4] Chloramphenicol is pH sensitive; it must be used at a pH of 8.0 or higher. Its effectiveness as a water bath treatment therefore is limited, but it might be helpful as an intraperitoneal injection.[9]

Vibrio anguillarum often is considered to be the cause of red disease.[6,10] This bacterium is a prevalent pathogen in marine food fish but rarely, if ever, occurs in marine hobbyist tanks.[6]

Fin rot is a disease the primary cause of which can be poor water quality, lack of oxygen, or poor circulation in extremities. Usually there are bacteria present that might play a primary role also. The bacterium involved is *Vibrio ichthyodermis* or *Pseudomonas ichthyodermis*—the classification is being debated.[11] An early sign is the fins and the tail turning white and cloudy. The affected areas eventually die and become torn and frayed. The skin mucus on the body is affected next, showing bloodshot epidermal patches.[6] These patches eventually ulcerate and lead to other serious secondary invasions.[11]

The frayed appearance of the tail and the fins must be differentiated from that caused by aggression or territorial fighting.

Acute fin rot rarely can be cured. Touching the affected area with copper sulfate can help in the early stages.[5] A streptomycin-penicillin combination given parenterally or oxytetracycline given in food also can be effective.[11] Tetracycline baths at a dose of 250 mg/3.8 L for one to two hours given for seven consecutive days also might effect a cure.[a] A nitrofurazone bath at a dose of 25 mg/3.8 L might be the preferred drug for this and all *Vibrio* spp. infections.[9]

Protozoal Disease

White spot disease, the marine counterpart to freshwater *Ichthyophthirius* (also called *Ich*), is caused by the ciliate protozoan *Cryptocaryon irritans* (Figure 11). The protozoan has a wide host range and a complex life cycle.[12]

Initial signs include loss of appetite, bizarre swimming behavior, and minor respiratory distress. The first lesions appear on the skin rather than the gills, as in oodinosis. The skin lesions are pinhead-sized, white to gray nodules caused by the trophonts burrowing into the epidermis (Figure 12). This burrowing causes severe irritation, excess mucus production, and hyperplasia of the epithelium. Large areas of the epithelium can fall off, exposing the fish to secondary bacterial invasion. If the eyes are affected, exophthalmos can be present; the eyes will turn cloudy, and blindness can result.[12] Death can occur with few or no gross disease signs.[a]

Diagnosis is made by scraping off a nodule and examining it for trophonts. This should be done early because the disease is highly contagious and fatal in three to five days.[12] The diseased fish should be removed to a sick tank immediately.

The encysted tomites are difficult to eliminate from an aquarium. An endless cycle will continue until all the fish die or develop acquired immunity. The water quality, the population density, and the stress level will determine which fish will prevail.[4]

Several treatments are available for white spot disease. Copper sulfate is used widely with moderate results. The treatment water should contain no invertebrates, which are highly susceptible to copper toxicity. A copper sulfate solution of 0.15 ppm (± 0.1 ppm) should be prepared in the treatment tank. The copper sulfate level, which never should rise above 0.3 ppm, can be tested with a colometric kit purchased from a pet store. The copper will kill the trophonts and the free-swimming tomites but not the encysted tomites, which emerge in two to eight days at 26.7°C (80° F). A copper sulfate bath lasting 14 days therefore will kill all infectious stages. Recurrence is not uncommon,[12] but new infections also can be introduced from unquarantined new arrivals.[a]

Coral fish disease, also called *marine oodinosis*, is a flagellate protozoal disease caused by *Oodinium ocellatum*. The early signs are rapid respiration, erratic swimming, and rubbing on gravel and coral. Initially the gills are parasitized heavily with small, dustlike, white nodules. A swab of the gills should reveal the organism (Figures 13 and 14). After respiratory signs are observed, the lesions can spread over the skin and are most visible on the fins and the tail.[13]

The disease has a rapid onset, and death occurs within two days after respiratory distress is noted. Death can be within 12 hours at higher water temperatures. Avoiding the pathogen by using ozone filters or ultraviolet light is recommended.[4] All incoming fish should be quarantined for two weeks. During this period, several freshwater baths, lasting a minimum of three minutes and as long as 15 minutes, should be given. Ten minutes is suitable for most species.[a] These baths cause the *Oodinium* organisms to rupture.[13] If the disease does occur, treatment with copper sulfate is effective. The regimen used for white spot disease can be followed.[4]

Brooklynella hostilis and *Uronema marinum* are look-alike ciliate protozoa that are gaining prevalence as severe, rapidly fatal diseases in marine aquariums.[a,b] *Uronema marinum* probably occurs more frequently than *Brooklynella hostilis*.[a] The majority of *Brooklynella hostilis* cases have been confirmed in the Philippine clownfish and in seahorses, but other fish are not immune.[14] Skin lesions on recent arrivals should be checked because they can be misdiagnosed as bacterial infections. The diseases are contagious, and fish can die within 12 hours from metabolic exotoxins produced by the organisms.

In both protozoa, infection initially is confined to the gills. Although the parasites do not burrow into the skin, they cause significant tissue irritation and damage. Infected fish demonstrate lethargy, lack of appetite, and excess mucus secretion that causes respiratory distress. Body lesions eventually appear as small, diffuse, discolored foci. The epithelium ultimately can slough, an important diagnostic sign[a,14] (Figure 15).

The parasites are confirmed by gill or skin smears; gill smears are necessary to confirm suspected fish not yet showing skin lesions. The living parasite is heart-shaped or kidney-shaped and has an oval macronucleus, several micronuclei, and numerous food vacuoles. The most recognizable structure of *Brooklynella hostilis* is a caudoventral adhesion organ used to attach to the host.[14] *Uronema marinum* is recognized by elongated caudomedial cilia.[a]

Copper sulfate solution used at 0.15 to 0.20 ppm has not been successful in eradicating the parasite,[14] but the

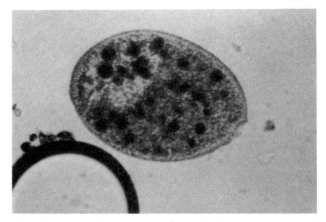

Figure 11—Ganbaldi skin scrape, demonstrating *Cryptocaryon irritans* ciliated tomite measuring 56 × 42 μ. (vital red stain, × 400)

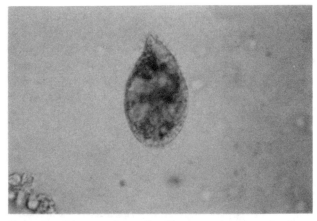

Figure 12—Skin smear from a Stoplite parrot, demonstrating *Cryptocaryon* trophont measuring 400 × 80 μ. (methylene blue stain)

solution has been effective at 0.25 ppm.[a] The infection can be controlled by using 50-minute baths of 1 ml of 37% formalin per 3.8 L. A single formalin treatment usually is required for *Brooklynella hostilis*[14]; *Uronema marinum* can necessitate more than one bath.[a] Freshwater dips lasting 10 minutes also are safe and effective. Malachite green baths at 0.13 to 0.15 ppm for 50 minutes can be useful. Patients with severe body lesions should be placed on antibiotic therapy to prevent secondary bacterial infections.[14]

Fungal Disease

Undetermined external fungi can grow filamentous projections from sites of external injury. Faulty environmental conditions, such as dissolved organic matter, low pH, or accumulation of organic substances, contribute to their occurrence. These fungi are rare and are much less common in marine aquariums than in freshwater tanks.[5]

Treatment is simple and effective: copper sulfate is touched to the site. In severe cases, a griseofulvin freshwater bath of 25 mg/L might be necessary.[5]

Ichthyophonus hoferi, a more common external fungus, also is rare. It infects vital organs, and the spores spread to other organs via the bloodstream (Figure 16). The fungus usually is not discovered until it has disseminated and the fish are dying. *Ichthyophonus hoferi* is found most often in the liver and the kidneys. Clinical signs can include exophthalmos, emaciation, abnormal swimming, abdominal swelling, fin decay, and blackish skin discoloration.[6] There is no known cure.

Some patients can survive by encapsulating the parasite. Raising the water temperature to 28° to 30°C (82° to 86°F), feeding vitamins A and B$_{12}$, and feeding food soaked in 1% solutions of phenoxyethanol or parachlorophenoxetol might overcome an acute crisis. The disease is likely to break out of encapsulation when the fish are stressed again. The fungus probably is introduced into a tank most often through feeder fish. It might be preventable by feeding frozen fish.[6] Because of its presenting signs, *Ichthyophonus hoferi* frequently is misdiagnosed as piscine tuberculosis.

Crustaceans and Worms

Most crustaceans that infest fish, such as copepods, are visible near the eyes or the gills. These crustaceans usually cannot reproduce in the aquarium and will eventually die off and disappear. A 15-minute bath of 1 ml of 37% formalin per L can be used if necessary.

The fish lice *Argulida*, which can reproduce in the tank, can cause serious problems. They can reach several millimeters in length and have a sucking disk. The mandibles sting the victim, and venom (which can kill a small fish) is released; the lice then live off of the wound's blood and mucus. The wound is a potential site for secondary bacterial infection.

The lice are hardy, and all treatments also are stressful and potentially fatal to the fish. The lice therefore should be pulled with tweezers.[4] Pet stores sell products that claim success in treating lice, but care must be exercised because such products probably will stress the fish.

Trematode worms of the genera *Gyrodactylus* and *Benedinia* can be observed near the eyes or the gills of fish. They are grayish white parasites up to 1.5 mm in

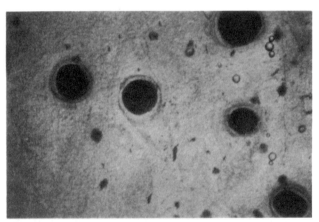

Figure 13—Swab from a Green sunfish gill, demonstrating *Oodinium limnetic* organisms. (× 1000)

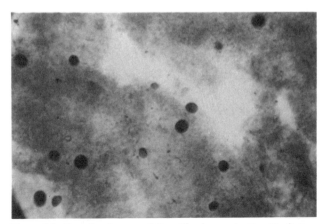

Figure 14—Sample of mucus from gills, demonstrating *Oodinium* organisms.

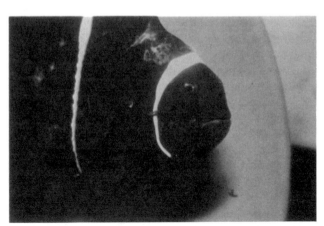

Figure 15—Maroon clownfish with *Brooklynella hostilis* infection.

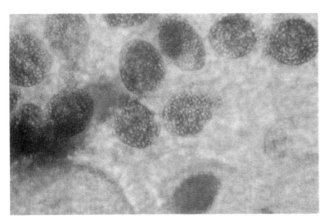

Figure 16—Liver squash smear from a Snook, demonstrating *Ichthyophonus hoferi* organisms. (unstained, × 100)

length. Infected fish demonstrate signs of heavy respiration and rubbing against rocks and gravel; their eyes might become inflamed, and they might hover in the water with fins clamped against the body. The condition is highly contagious and must be treated.[6]

Treatment is the same as that for crustaceans: a 15-minute bath of 1 ml of 37% formalin per L of salt water. A copper sulfate bath at 0.20 ppm also can be used until the parasite is no longer visible on the patient's gills.[6]

Summary

Management of a marine aquarium is not difficult but does require an understanding of the interaction of fish, waste, and water. Most general principles of medicine can be extended to aquarium fish. Veterinarians armed with medical knowledge, an awareness of aquarium management, and access to information on specific diseases can adequately diagnose and treat sick fish and unhealthy tank environments.

As with any medical problem, a proper history is essential. A data base consisting of water samples, microscopic examination (of skin or gill swabs, feces, or necropsy lesions), and keen observation is vital in treating specific diseases or avoiding potential problems.

Acknowledgments

The author thanks Dr. Roger Klocek at the John G. Shedd Aquarium in Chicago and Dr. Nelson Herwig, Curator of Fishes at the Houston Zoological Gardens, for supplying information and photographs and for making important corrections. Figures 5, 6, 8-10, 14, and 15 appear through the courtesy of Dr. Herwig; Figures 7, 11-13, and 16 appear through the courtesy of Dr. Klocek. Dr. Nathan Gabbert and Dr. James Coffman at Kansas State University also provided help and guidance in the writing of this article.

REFERENCES

1. Ford DM: Ornamental fish keeping and the veterinary profession. *Proc Kal Kan Symp Treatment Small Anim Dis*: 20, 1980.
2. Wickler W: *The Marine Aquarium*. Neptune City, NJ, Tropical Fish Hobbyist Publications, 1973, pp 23-24.
3. Axelrod HR, Burgess WE, Emmens CW: *Exotic Marine Fishes*, ed 4. Neptune City, NJ, Tropical Fish Hobbyist Publications, 1975, pp 26, 53-55.
4. Spotte S: *Marine Aquarium Keeping: The Science, Animals, and Art*. New York, John Wiley & Sons, 1973, pp 27, 28, 55-57.
5. Curry C: Management of salt water fish. *Iowa State Univ Vet* 38(2):76-79, 1976.
6. de Graff F, Spiekman J (trans): *Marine Aquarium Guide*. Harrison, NJ, Pet Library Ltd, 1973.
7. Dulin MP: An overview of the more prevalent marine and fresh water aquarium fish diseases. Unpublished paper, Kansas State University, Manhattan, KS, April 20, 1982.
8. Dulin MP: A review of tuberculosis (mycobacteriosis) in fish. *VM SAC* 74(5):731-735, 1979.
9. Herwig N: Disease prevention and control. *Fresh Water and Marine Aquarium* 2(3):38-39, 83-86, 1979.
10. Sinderman CJ: *Principal Diseases of Marine Fish and Shellfish*. New York, Academic Press, 1973, pp 18-19.
11. Curry C: Diseases of salt water fish. *Iowa State Univ Vet* 39(1):26-30, 1977.
12. Dulin MP: White spot disease (cryptocaryoniasis) of marine fish. Unpublished paper, Kansas State University, Manhattan, KS, April 20, 1982, pp 1-3.
13. Dulin MP: Marine oodinosis. Unpublished paper, Kansas State University, Manhattan, KS, April 20, 1982, pp 1-3.
14. Blasiola GC: Disease prevention and control. *Fresh Water and Marine Aquarium* 3(3):18-19, 82-83, 1980.

Medical Management of Disorders of Freshwater Tropical Fish

KEY FACTS

- Keeping freshwater tropical fish is an extensive hobby that is becoming increasingly popular.
- Proper husbandry, including good water quality and adequate nutrition, is the most important factor in keeping healthy freshwater tropical fish.
- Valuable diagnostic information can be quickly obtained with an accurate history in conjunction with simple biopsy or necropsy procedures.
- Many standard veterinary medications are useful in the treatment of sick freshwater tropical fish; however, routes of administration may be unusual.

North Carolina State University
Raleigh, North Carolina
Gregory A. Lewbart, MS, VMD

A CLINICIAN'S first responsibility in dealing with disorders of freshwater tropical fish is to obtain an accurate medical history. The first few cases of freshwater tropical fish disorders that clinicians encounter often send them frantically leafing through their reference books; an accurate history makes book work much easier. I have found several invaluable references that deal with diagnosis and treatment of freshwater tropical fish.[1-14]

There currently are hundreds (or perhaps even thousands) of species of freshwater tropical fish that are kept as pets throughout the world. When these figures are added to the many viral, bacterial, fungal, protozoal, helminthic, and dietary diseases of fish, the practicing clinician can soon be overwhelmed simply by trying to learn the new information that is associated with these diseases. In order to assist practitioners in sorting through the diseases, this article discusses diagnosis and treatment of disorders that most commonly affect freshwater tropical fish. The clinical appearance of some common disorders are shown in Figures 1 through 3.

OBTAINING THE HISTORY

When dealing with fish, the clinician must remember that, unlike most vertebrates, fish are constantly immersed in water. They feed in water, excrete wastes in water, reproduce in water, and (perhaps most important) breathe in water. Gills efficiently remove oxygen from water and introduce the oxygen to circulating erythrocytes. The fragile gill tissue is directly exposed to the aquatic environment and therefore is vulnerable to any noxious change in the water. The most common cause of disease among freshwater tropical fish is poor water quality; the clinician should target this area first when the history is taken. Stoskopf provides an excellent approach to obtaining the basic history.[9] Answers to the questions listed in Taking the History can provide clinicians with a solid foundation on which the differential diagnosis can be based.

It is important to know whether the client is an advanced hobbyist or a novice. Clients who have been keeping fish for a long time probably have already made or are at least aware of basic mistakes. These clients usually understand

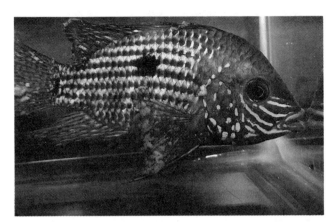

Figure 1—A green terror cichlid (*Aequidens rivulatus*) with a severe case of lymphocystis disease. The causative agent is an iridovirus called lymphocystis disease virus. The virus causes extreme hypertrophy of dermal connective tissue cells. Surgery is the only treatment known to be effective, but most cases are self-limiting.

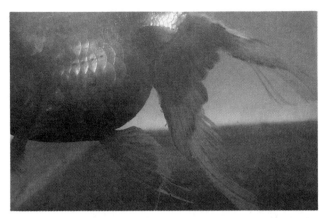

Figure 2—An oranda goldfish (*Carassius auratus*) with bacterial fin disease; the disorder usually is caused by motile gram-negative bacteria. Antibiotics and good water quality are sufficient to control the disease if it remains superficial.

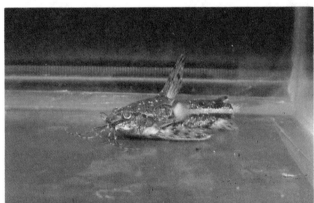

Figure 3A

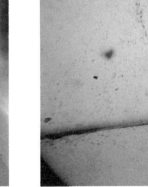

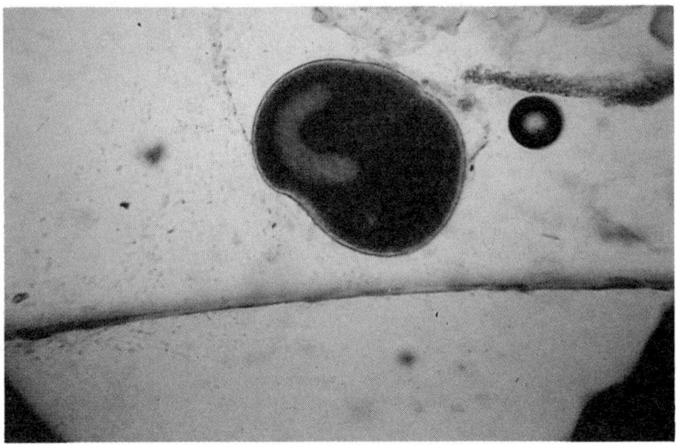

Figure 3B

Figure 3—(**A**) Talking catfish (*Acanthodoras spinosissimus*) infected with the protozoal ectoparasite *Ichthyophthirius multifilis* (small white spots) and the dermal fungus *Saprolegnia* species (tuft below dorsal fin). (**B**) Trophozoite or trophont stage of *I. multifilis*, which causes a disease commonly known as ich (pronounced *ick*). The protozoa can reach one millimeter in diameter. Each trophozoite may give rise to thousands of tomites; the tomite stage is the infective stage. The large, crescent-shaped macronucleus is characteristic of ich. (400×)

the importance of good water quality, and their problems may require immediate examination of the fish. Clinicians often need to devote more time to those clients who have recently obtained an aquarium.

The clinician's initial contact with the client is most likely to be over the telephone. If time permits, basic information can be immediately gathered; the clinician must also assess whether the client is serious about having the fish and a water sample from the tank or bowl examined. Although some basic problems may be solved over the telephone, if the clinician believes it to be necessary, the client should be asked to bring in the affected fish and approximately one quart of water from the tank. Either over the telephone or on arrival at the office, the client should

provide answers to the 10 questions listed in Taking the History. It also may be necessary for the client to bring the fish food container as well as possibly the boxes or (at least) written descriptions of the equipment of the aquarium, such as the heater, filter, and air pump. Most freshwater tropical fish can be safely transported for several hours in a sealed jar or plastic bag that contains half water and half air.

AFTER the client has arrived, the clinician can finish taking the history and can test the water. Educating clients, especially new ones, on the importance of clean water can

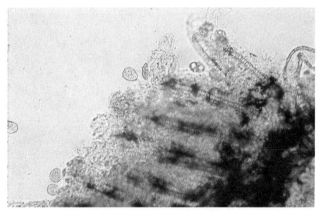

Figure 4A

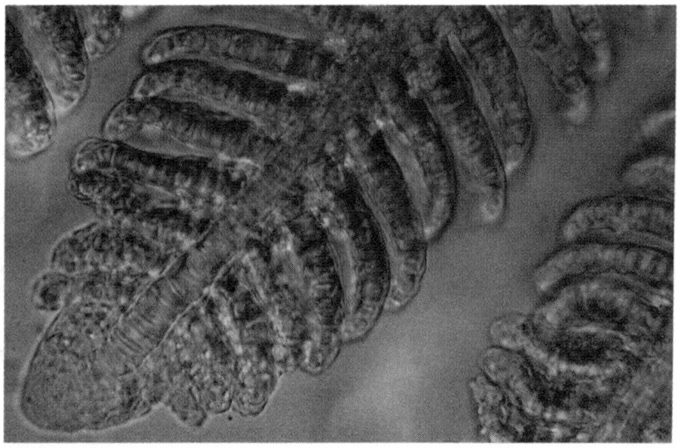

Figure 4B

Figure 4—(A) Necrotic, hyperplastic gill from an emperor tetra (*Nematobrycon palmeri*) infected with the protozoal ectoparasite *Chilodonella*. Secondary lamellae cannot be distinguished. (100×) **(B)** Normal gill of an algae eater (*Gyrinocheilos aymonieri*). Note the well-defined secondary lamellae that contain circulating erythrocytes. (400×)

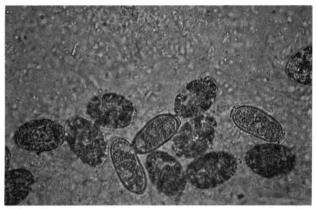

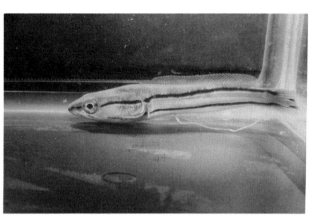

Figure 5A

Figure 5B

Figure 5—(A) Fecal smear of a red snakehead (*Channa micropeltes*). Cestode and nematode ova are evident. (400×) **(B)** The snakehead 30 minutes after tank treatment with 2.0 parts per million of praziquantel. Note the adult cestode protruding from the anus.

be done during preliminary proceedings. The clinician can also discuss any abnormal parameters of the water quality with the client after testing is completed.[10] The information contained in Water Quality Parameters presents normal values for components typically found in water.

An essential component of treating freshwater tropical fish on a regular basis is a basic kit that tests water quality. These kits, which are usually reasonably priced, can be purchased from a local pet store. The clinician needs to have equipment and kits that test levels of pH, ammonia, nitrite, chlorine, and dissolved oxygen. It also is helpful to have a test kit that provides values for water hardness, total alkalinity (i.e., the buffering capacity of the water), and dissolved carbon dioxide.

EXAMINATION

The fish is examined after the history has been taken and

the water has been evaluated. If the entire tank population is experiencing high morbidity and mortality, the client should be urged to sacrifice a debilitated fish for thorough necropsy. Because of rapid onset of autolysis, a fish that died before being presented to the clinician should be examined only as a last resort.

The first step in examination is a thorough visual inspection of the fish. Much valuable information can be obtained by taking the time to look carefully at the fish. Are the fins frayed? Are there areas of discoloration or depigmentation? Are there any visible ectoparasites? Is the fish swimming and breathing normally?

Handling the fish should be minimized. A routine skin, fin, and gill biopsy usually can be performed quickly and without anesthesia. Surgical procedures may require an anesthetic agent, such as tricaine methanesulfonate (MS-222). This agent is relatively safe and rapidly takes effect;

Recipe for Gelatinized Food[a]

The following recipe makes approximately 750 grams of food.

- Weigh 250 grams of a well-balanced flake food. Place in blender.
- Add 500 milliliters tap water. Mix well.
- To this slurry, add 25 milliliters cod liver oil and 25 milliliters vegetable oil (both optional).
- Add a can of sardines, tuna, or jar of spinach baby food (all optional).
- Blend well.
- Add any medication at this time, and mix.
- In a separate pan, heat 500 milliliters of tap water to boiling.
- Add 30 to 50 grams of powdered unflavored gelatin (8 to 10 normal-size packets) to the hot water, and stir well until gelatin is dissolved.
- Allow gelatin mixture to cool but not set.
- Add food mixture to gelatin mixture and stir well. Place mixture in separate bags and place in refrigerator. Food should be ready within an hour or may be frozen until needed. The food can be broken into bite-size pieces by using a cheese grater or potato peeler. Breaking up the food is important especially when the food is frozen.

[a]Courtesy of John Gratzek, DVM, University of Georgia

it also has the advantage of allowing a quick recovery. Many books on piscine diseases contain information on biopsy and necropsy procedures.[1-4]

Using a sterile scalpel, skin and fin tissues are firmly scraped. Resultant exudates are then suspended in a few drops of clean water and examined with a microscope. A small piece of gill tissue should be carefully obtained with a pair of scissors; gill tissue also can be examined using unstained wet-mount preparation. Biopsy samples are likely to demonstrate some type of pathology.

Protozoal and other ectoparasitic organisms are easily observed on any or all tissue (Figures 3 and 4A). Healthy gill tissue appears red, and the small secondary lamellae appear distinct and even (Figure 4B). Gill tissue that has been exposed to water of poor quality or an excessive number of bacteria appears blunt or fused because of hyperplasia; this condition is called bacterial or environmental gill disease. The existence of some bacteria on the tissue should be considered normal; however, a large number of motile bacteria on the skin and gills usually indicates that a problem exists. Such samples can be stained with Gram's stain or even cultured to obtain information regarding present bacteria and sensitivity. Combined disease processes in areas that were first compromised by parasites and then secondarily invaded by bacteria are common.

Much information can be obtained if a fresh specimen is available for necropsy. Most freshwater tropical fish can be quickly killed by severing the cervical spine with a scalpel or sharp scissors. Kidneys provide an excellent location from which to take a sterile bacterial culture if bacteremia or septicemia is suspected. The coelomic cavity and gastrointestinal tract can be examined for such abnormalities as internal parasites or neoplasia. An examination of the gills during necropsy allows for a more thorough examination than does a small biopsy from a live fish, and larger areas of the skin and fins can be scraped. Fresh feces can be easily obtained for fecal examination. The microscopic appearance of a fecal smear is shown in Figure 5. Although obtaining a fecal sample from a live fish is logistically difficult, this type of examination is a valuable diagnostic technique.

DIAGNOSIS

A differential diagnosis should be formed after information from the history, water tests, and biopsy or necropsy results have been evaluated. At this point, the clinician should begin therapy and/or encourage the client to modify current husbandry practices. In many cases, water quality deficiencies must be corrected before medical treatment is begun.

TREATMENT

Treating freshwater tropical fish can be much more challenging than treating mammals or birds. It is not always practical (or possible) to use injectable or oral routes of

TAKING THE HISTORY
Important Questions for the Client

- How long have you been keeping tropical fish?
- What are the problems with the fish?
- When did you first notice these problems?
- How long have you had the sick fish? Where was it obtained?
- Do you have other fish at home that appear healthy? Are these fish in the same tank as the sick fish or are they separated from it?
- What is the size of the tank? How is it heated, filtered, aerated, and lighted?
- What and how often do you feed your fish?
- Have the fish already been treated and, if so, with what and by whom?
- Do you have a water test kit and, if so, how often do you test the quality of the water? Do you know the current pH and ammonia readings for your tank?
- Who is responsible for the day-to-day care of the fish?

Water Quality Parameters

Temperature

Most freshwater tropical fish should ideally be kept between 24° and 27°C (76° and 80°F). Temperatures below this level can predispose freshwater tropical fish to numerous disease problems. Some common fish, such as guppies and goldfish, thrive at room temperature and do not require a heater in the tank.

pH

The actual pH value (i.e., logarithm of the reciprocal of the hydrogen ion concentration) is not nearly as important as the relationship of pH to other water chemistry parameters, such as the amount of ammonia present in the water. Ammonia is much less toxic to fish when the pH level is acidic (less than 7.0). Toxicity of a given level of ammonia is directly proportional to an increase in pH. The ideal pH level of freshwater aquariums generally is between 6.5 and 7.5. Many freshwater fish can withstand widely varying pH values as long as changes occur gradually. It is not uncommon for some species of South American fish to live in water with a pH of 3.0 to 4.0 in nature and still thrive in a home aquarium with a pH of 7.0. Abrupt changes, however, must be avoided.

Ammonia

Ammonia in water occurs in two forms: toxic un-ionized ammonia (NH_3) and the relatively nontoxic ionized form (NH_4^+). Both types of ammonia are measured to arrive at the total concentration of ammonia in water. The actual proportion of each compound depends on temperature, salinity, and most important, pH. A greater concentration of un-ionized ammonia is present when the pH value is increased. Nearly 10 times more un-ionized ammonia is present when the pH is 8.0 than when the pH is 7.0.[9] Most simple test kits measure the total ammonia level in the water. Under ideal conditions, no detectable ammonia should be present in an aquarium. Levels over 1.0 parts per million indicate a significant filtering deficiency. Certain species of fish tolerate ammonia better than do others, but high levels of ammonia can create problems and should be immediately corrected. A 30% to 50% water change should be performed as soon as possible if the level of ammonia in an aquarium is high. Clients should be educated on aspects of filtration and feeding to prevent accumulation of toxic levels of ammonia.

Nitrite

Nitrite is an intermediate compound in the nitrogen cycle and is converted to nontoxic nitrate by a healthy biological (one that utilizes nitrifying bacteria) filter. Nitrite levels that rise above 1.0 parts per million are likely to compromise the health of the fish. As in mammals, nitrite causes formation of methemoglobin in the blood and results in respiratory compromise. Affected fish display signs of oxygen starvation and may die of asphyxiation. Even very low levels of nitrite may have adverse effects on fish. Poor filtration is nearly always the cause of elevated nitrite levels.

Chlorine

Adding chlorine to municipal water supplies is a common means of sterilizing drinking water. Chlorine is harmless to humans; however, it can be deadly to freshwater tropical fish. The amount of chlorine in tap water can fluctuate but is usually between 0.5 and 1.0 parts per million. Chlorine can usually be bubbled out of the water by aerating it for several days. Any pet store that sells freshwater tropical fish probably also stocks a commercially prepared compound that contains sodium thiosulfate, which safely inactivates chlorine by a chemical reaction that results in formation of sodium chloride (three grams of pure sodium thiosulfate removes chlorine from 250 gallons of tap water containing 2.0 parts per million of chlorine).

Oxygen

Oxygen is the most important life-supporting element dissolved in the water. Most test kits measure total dissolved oxygen in water. Freshwater tropical fish generally require between 6 and 10 parts per million of dissolved oxygen. Most fish become stressed below six parts per million. Commercially available air pumps provide plenty of oxygen for fish. Being able to measure the level of oxygen in an aquarium is important in order to rule out aeration problems as a cause of disorders of the fish.

TABLE I
Common Disease Groups and Treatments

Agent	Dosage and Administration	Comments
Bacterial diseases		
Enrofloxacin	5 mg/kg given IM or IP q 48 h for 15 days; 5 mg/kg PO for 10–14 days or 0.1% in food and feed to fish for 10–14 days; 2.5 mg/L as a 5-hour bath, repeated q 24 h for 5–7 days, 50–75% water change between treatments.	Usually effective and safe. Good broad-spectrum activity and pharmacokinetics have been worked on in several fish species.
Erythromycin	Bath treatment of 200 mg/10 gallons of water; treat daily for 6 to 12 hours In feed, use 100 mg/kg per day for 14 to 21 days	No longer a first-choice antibiotic because of resistant strains; use water-soluble phosphate form
Nalidixic acid	Bath treatment of 500 mg/10 gallons of water for 1 to 4 hours; repeat as necessary	Can be toxic to some species; effective against many gram-negative bacteria
Nitrofurazone	Bath treatment of 400 mg/10 gallons of water for 6 to 12 hours; repeat as necessary	Commonly used and still considered to be fairly effective; absorbed well into bloodstream
Tetracycline	Bath treatment of 250 to 500 mg/10 gallons of water for 3 to 6 hours; some commercially prepared diets containing this antibiotic are available	Many resistant strains result from overuse; very brief half-life in water
Trimethoprim-sulfamethoxazole	Bath treatment of 960 mg/10 gallons of water for 6 to 12 hours; treat until signs of disease are gone Oral administration of 50 mg/kg for 10 days	Very effective and safe for most species
Fungal diseases[a]		
Formaldehyde (37%)	Bath treatment of 20 to 25 ppm for 12 to 24 hours, or 100 to 250 ppm for 30 minutes to 1 hour	Very effective for this purpose; more toxic in soft, acidic water; water must be well aerated and fish much be closely monitored; use care when handling
Malachite green	Bath treatment of 0.1 to 0.15 ppm for 12 to 24 hours; repeat as necessary	Use zinc-free preparations; may be toxic to some species of scaleless fish; works well when combined with formaldehyde at the listed dosage
Sodium chloride	30–35 ppt (g/L) as a 3- to 5-minute bath treatment. Artificial sea salt or food grade salt may be used.	Safe for the handler, inexpensive, and effective. Fish in salt solution need to be monitored closely for signs of stress. Smaller fish more sensitive. Salt bath is an alternative to quarantine when quarantine protocols cannot be followed. May be repeated as needed but not more often than every 24 hours. Concentrations of 1–3 ppt can be used as an indefinite bath in many species to help control ectoparsites and reduce stress.
Protozoal diseases		
Formaldehyde (37%)	Same dosage as for fungal diseases	Often advisable to combine this treatment with a broad-spectrum antibiotic to fight secondary bacterial invasion
Malachite green	Same dosage as for fungal diseases	Must be handled using gloves; can be combined with antibiotic treatment
Metronidazole	In feed, 10 to 15 mg/g of food for 5 to 10 days As a bath treatment, 10 mg/L for 6 to 12 hours repeated 1 to 2 times	Excellent for internal and external infestations of the flagellate *Hexamita*
Sodium chloride	Same dosage as for fungal diseases	
Monogenean trematode diseases		
Acetic acid (glacial)	Dip treatment of 8 ml/gallon for 30 to 45 seconds	Smaller fish are more sensitive to this treatment than are larger ones; treatment kills very debilitated fish

[a]The presence of a true fungal disease must be diagnosed by skin scraping because several other diseases grossly resemble dermal mycoses in fish. Most cases of fungal disease are secondary to some other disease that compromises protective epithelium. Supportive care (e.g., good water and nutrition) commonly enables the fish to slough fungal colonies without chemical treatment.

TABLE I (continued)

Agent	Dosage and Administration	Comments
Monogenean trematode diseases (*cont*).		
Formaldehyde (37%)	Same dosage as for protozoal diseases	Same considerations as for protozoal diseases
Praziquantel	5–10 mg/L as a 3- to 6-hour bath. Repeat in 7 days.	Remove fish to treatment tank if possible and aerate water well. Some marine species may be sensitive. Aquarium may still be infected; treated fish should be moved to new aquarium if possible. May not kill all species of monogeneans.
Sodium chloride	Same dosage as for fungal diseases	
Nematode diseases		
Fenbendazole	In feed, 250 mg/100 g of food fed daily for 3 consecutive days	Drug can be mixed into gelatinized food (see Recipe for Gelatinized Food)
Cestode diseases		
Praziquantel	Drug is dissolved in tank at a concentration of 2 to 3 ppm; fish remain immersed in bath for 3 hours	Safe and effective in eliminating gastrointestinal cestodes
Crustacean diseases		
Acetic acid (glacial)	Same dosage as for trematode diseases	Very effective against anchor worms (*Lernaea*); purges the host of fish lice (*Argulus*)
Trichlorfon	0.5 mg/liter, 3 treatments 10 days apart, 20–30% water change 24 to 48 hours following each treatment.	Use extreme caution when handling these organophosphate compounds. Liquid form commonly used to kill cattle grubs is easy to handle, measure, and dispense.
Sodium chloride	Same dosage as for fungal diseases	

drug administration. There are several informative references that provide detailed information on treating diseases of freshwater tropical fish.[1-3,7,8] Several basic but effective treatment protocols are included in Table I, which also contains information regarding some of the more commonly used and effective drugs.

When a single fish is ill, the fish usually can be placed in a hospital tank, either at the practice or in the owner's home. Isolating the sick fish reduces the risk of spreading disease to other fish and prevents healthy fish from being exposed to medication. In cases in which many or all fish are affected, especially with a contagious disorder (such as infestation with *Ichthyophthirius multifilis* [Figure 3]), the entire tank should be treated. During any type of tank treatment, carbon filtration should be discontinued because it nullifies the medication. If the tank contains a viable undergravel filter, the air lift tubes should be inactivated during treatment to protect nitrifying bacteria. An air stone can be used to aerate the water during treatment. After treatment, 30% to 50% of the water in the tank should be changed.

In some cases, examining and obtaining a biopsy from a fish is impossible. Making an accurate diagnosis and initiating effective therapy therefore becomes very difficult. In this type of situation, the shotgun approach to treatment can be used. An acceptable regimen per 10 gallons of water is 1.0 to 1.5 milliliters of 37% formaldehyde, 960 milligrams trimethoprim-sulfamethoxazole, and 250 milligrams metronidazole. After 8 to 12 hours of tank treatment, 30% to 50% of the water should be changed before the fish are treated again. If the agents are effective, three such treatments usually suffice.

CONCLUSION

Diagnosis and treatment of freshwater tropical fish can be very challenging; however, the greatest challenge facing the clinician is deciding to attempt to diagnose and treat the first patient. As soon as the decision has been made, successful treatment of freshwater tropical fish can be both clinically and financially rewarding.

About the Author

Dr. Lewbart is Assistant Professor of Aquatic Medicine with the College of Veterinary Medicine at North Carolina State University, Raleigh, North Carolina.

REFERENCES

1. Stoskopf M: Tropical fish medicine. *Vet Clin North Am [Small Anim Pract]* 18(2):474, 1988.
2. Post G: *Textbook of Fish Health.* Neptune, NJ, T.F.H. Publications, 1987, p 288.
3. Untergasser D: *Handbook of Fish Diseases.* Neptune, NJ, T.F.H. Publications, 1989, p 160.
4. Stoskopf MK: Anesthesia of pet fishes, in Kirk RW, Bonagura JD (eds): *Current Veterinary Therapy XII.* Philadelphia, WB Saunders Co, 1995, pp 1365–1369.
5. Herwig N: *Handbook of Drugs and Chemicals Used in the Treatment of Fish Diseases.* Springfield, IL, Charles C Thomas, 1979, p 272.

6. Roberts RJ: *Fish Pathology*, ed 2. London, Bailliere Tindall, 1989.
7. Gratzek JB: An overview of ornamental fish diseases and therapy. *J Small Anim Pract* 22:345–366, 1981.
8. Gratzek JB: Control and therapy of fish diseases. *Adv Vet Sci Comp Med* 27:297–324, 1983.
9. Stoskopf M: Taking the history. *Vet Clin North Am [Small Anim Pract]* 18(2):283–291, 1988.
10. Beleau M: Evaluating water problems. *Vet Clin North Am [Small Anim Pract]* 18(2):293–304, 1988.
11. Gratzek J: *Aquariology: The Science of Fish Health Management.* New Jersey, Tetra Press, 1992, p 330.
12. Lewbart GA: Emergency pet fish medicine, in Kirk RW, Bonagura JD (eds): *Current Veterinary Therapy XII*. Philadelphia, WB Saunders Co, 1995, pp 1369–1374.
13. Noga EJ: *Fish Disease: Diagnosis and Treatment.* Mosby-Yearbook, St. Louis, MO, 1996, p 367.
14. Stoskopf M: *Fish Medicine*. Philadelphia, WB Saunders Co, 1992, p 882.

An Introduction to Diseases of Nonhuman Primates

Theresa Y. Parrott, DVM
Pembroke Park Animal Clinic
Pembroke, Florida

During the past 12 years, laws restricting the importation of nonhuman primates into the United States have drastically reduced the numbers of primates appearing in the pet trade. Import bans have forced many private and public institutions to increase captive breeding efforts. An awareness of nutritional and medical problems in primate species can increase reproductive potentials and life expectancy.

Types of Nonhuman Primates Commonly Encountered

New World nonhuman primates are maintained in zoos and research facilities commonly. These animals also are the most frequent pet monkeys encountered in private veterinary practice. Distinguishing characteristics of New World primates include the presence of a prehensile tail and imperfectly opposable thumbs.[1,2] Sizes range from 150-g marmosets (*Callithrix*) (Figure 1) to 12-kg Woolly monkeys (*Lagothrix*). Other New World primates include the squirrel (*Saimiri*), spider (*Ateles*), and capuchin (*Cebus*) (Figure 2) monkeys.

Old World primates common in research and in private facilities include rhesus (Figure 3), pig tail, crab eating, and Japanese monkeys (*Macaca* spp.) as well as green monkeys (*Cercopithecus* spp.) and Patas monkeys (*Erythrocebus* spp.). These monkeys have ischial callosities and cheek pouches. On rare occasions, chimpanzees (*Pan*), baboons (*Papio*) and orangutans (*Pongo*) are seen outside zoologic institutions.

Examination Techniques

Examination procedures on smaller simian species can be conducted with minimal restraint. A pair of leather welder's gloves is excellent for marmosets and squirrel monkeys. The larger species can be handled with a pair of primate gloves.[a] Tranquilization will be necessary if the patient cannot be handled safely (i.e., if it exceeds 5 kg in weight) or if an adequate examination cannot be performed (Table I).

Respiratory rates and heart rates will be increased when the patient is restrained. If blood sampling is required, the femoral vein is easily accessible in an awake animal. Directing the needle slightly downward in the femoral triangle, the clinician can obtain enough blood to run a complete blood count and panel. Clipping the patient's nails to obtain blood smears is painful and

[a]Primate Imports Inc., PO Box 416, Port Washington, NY 11050.

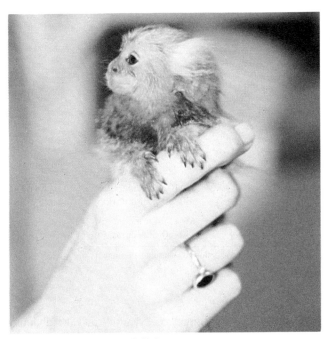

Figure 1—A marmoset (*Callithrix*).

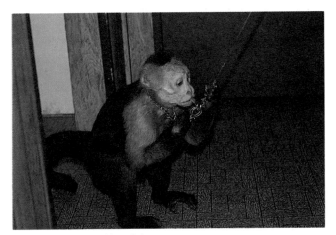

Figure 2—A capuchin (*Cebus*).

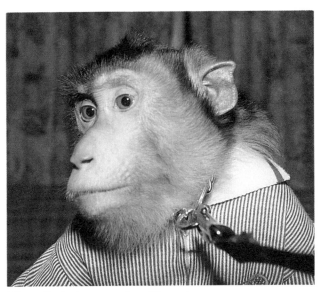

Figure 3—A rhesus monkey (*Macaca*).

should be avoided. The cephalic veins might be difficult to expose for venipuncture because of the heavy forearm musculature and the relatively small vessels in nonhuman primates. In certain instances, lateral cephalic and saphenous veins are used to take small to moderate amounts of blood from tranquilized patients, especially in smaller primates. Normal physical and hematologic values are listed in Table II.

Common Ailments
Vitamin C Deficiency

Patients with vitamin C deficiency present with poor haircoats, bleeding mucous membranes, and general debilitation. A history of a diet lacking in vitamin C is common. Oral vitamin C given at 15 to 25 mg/kg of body weight daily will correct the deficient state. Ascorbic acid can be given by injection at an initial rate of 7 to 10 mg/kg.[3,4]

Calcium/Vitamin D₃ Deficiency

Deficiency of calcium and/or vitamin D_3 will cause rickets and osteomalacia in young nonhuman primates.[4,5] Acute lameness is the most common complaint made by owners. Radiographs show skeletal demineralization, and scoliosis/kyphosis often is evident. Folding fractures also are common. A chronically deficient state will induce fibrous osteodystrophy of the mandible, with loss of dentition. Correction of the diet and oral calcium and vitamin D_3 are indicated. Because New World monkeys do not synthesize vitamin D_3, it must be given daily as a dietary additive.[3,4] Calcium carbonate is preferable to bone meal because of the unwanted phosphorus in the latter.

Inadequate Caloric Intake

Inadequate caloric intake can cause chronic catabolism and hypoglycemia.[5] When a depressed or comatose primate is presented, this should be one of the primary working diagnoses. An intravenous catheter should be inserted; the author prefers sites in the following order: lateral saphenous, metatarsal/metacarpal, and cephalic veins. The size of the smaller primates can restrict the clinician's access to the larger vessels. Intravenous dextrose should be given in addition to lactated Ringer's solution for treatment of shock. Intravenous prednisolone should be given at a dose of 3 to 5 mg/kg. Blood should be drawn, and the blood glucose level should be determined (normal is 60 to 110 mg/dl).[5] Rectal temperature should be taken; if it is below normal, treatment for hypothermia is initiated. If the intravenous set must be maintained for more than a few hours, the patient's hands should be wrapped and a restraining collar applied around its neck. This will prevent removal of the set by the patient.

Gastrointestinal Disorders
Internal Parasites

Among the most common internal parasites encountered

TABLE I
Common Immobilizing Agents for Primates[a]

Agent	Route	Dose	Induction and Duration
Ketamine hydrochloride	Intramuscular	10–30 mg/kg	3–10 min induction, 30–50 min duration
Diazepam	Intramuscular	1–3.5 mg/kg	15–30 min induction, 60–90 min duration
Promazine hydrochloride	Intramuscular	5 mg/kg	3–8 min induction, 40–80 min duration
Meperidine hydrochloride	Intramuscular	12 mg/3.5–10 kg	3–10 min induction, 30–90 min duration
Fentanyl citrate and droperidol (Innovar)	Intramuscular	1 ml/18 kg	3–15 min induction, 30–60 min duration

[a]Other agents are available, but most require intravenous use. Halothane and methoxyflurane are inhalation agents.

in captive nonhuman primates are *Strongyloides* spp.[4,6,7] An animal with chronic diarrhea, dull haircoat, and weight loss should be suspected of being parasitized with this genus. Other parasites encountered include ascarids, acanthocephalans, and *Dipetalonema* spp.[4,6,7] Table III lists worming agents and dosages.

Dietary Indiscretion

The usual clinical presentation of dietary indiscretion is acute onset of diarrhea with a history of recent ingestion of substances normally not included in the patient's diet. Foods incriminated most commonly include cooked or processed meats, milk, and abundant greens. Treatment should include fluid replacement therapy in dehydrated patients, parenteral antibiotics, and withholding of food for a period of 24 hours.

Bloat

Ingesting moderate to large amounts of fluids after eating monkey biscuits or other water absorbent substances can lead to gastric dilatation. The patient will present depressed or comatose, with shallow, rapid respirations. The

mucous membranes might be cyanotic, and the abdomen usually is distended. (Woolly monkeys commonly have a potbellied appearance; care should be taken not to confuse this with gastric dilatation.) Treatment consists of passage of a gastric tube to relieve vascular and respiratory compromise. Gastric lavage using warmed lactated Ringer's solution often is rewarding. Treatment for shock should include intravenous prednisolone, replacement fluids, and dextrose. Solid food should not be offered for at least 48 hours. Fruit juices and oral electrolyte mixtures can be given.

Infectious Diseases
Influenza

Signs of influenza in primates include depression, emesis, diarrhea, and fever.[4,5,7] A careful history might show that the handler or the owner also has been ill recently. Treatment should be symptomatic, and care should be taken to maintain the patient's hydration.

Herpes Simplex

Herpes simplex usually is transmitted from the handler

TABLE II
Physical and Hematologic Values of Primates[4,5,6]

	Weight	Rectal Temperature (°C)	Respiratory Rate (breaths/min)	Heart Rate (beats/min)	Packed Cell Volume (%)	White Blood Cell Count (10 × 3/mm³)	Red Blood Cell Count (10 × 6/mm³)
Marmoset	235–250 g	35.4–39.7	20–50	240–350	36.1–60.7	7.1–14.7	4.04–7.70
Squirrel monkey	750–1000 g	33.5–38.8	20–50	225–350	42.0–57.0	5.0–16.0	7.4–11.3
Capuchin	1.7–4.0 kg	37.0–38.5	30–50	165–225	40.0–63.0	6.3–34.3	4.15–6.68
Woolly monkey	6–8 kg	36.0–39.0	15–30	80–180	35.0–40.0	11.0–14.0	—
Spider monkey	6–8 kg	36.0–39.0	18–35	210	34.0–47.0	8.9–31.2	3.50–4.92
Rhesus monkey	10–25 kg	36.0–40.0	10–25	150–333	37.0–42.0	8.64–15.50	5.0–6.0

TABLE III
Worming Agents Used in Primates in Clinical Practice[4,5,6]

Agent	Spectrum	Dosage
Thiabendazole (Mintezol®— Merck Sharp & Dohme)	Intestinal nematodes	50–100 mg/kg
Mebendazole	Intestinal nematodes	3 mg/kg for 10 days or 15 mg/kg for 2 days
DDVP (Task®—Solvay Veterinary)	Intestinal nematodes and *Trichuris* spp.	16–20 mg (active ingredient)/kg—two doses 24 hours apart
Diethylcarbamazine citrate	Filarids (*Dipetalonema* spp.)	6–20 mg/kg for 6–15 days

to the nonhuman primate. Acute depression and death are the usual clinical signs.[5,7] Treatment is symptomatic. Strict hygiene methods are essential.

Measles and Pox

Natural outbreaks of measles and pox have been reported in primates.[4–6] The clinical signs and course resemble that of humans. A vaccine for measles is available (Attenuated live measles—Merck Sharp & Dohme). Measles virus is important because it has an immunosuppressive effect and can cause a false-negative tuberculin reaction. Pox virus can be transmitted to the handler.

Infectious Hepatitis

Infectious hepatitis has been reported in chimpanzees and can be transmitted to man.[4,5] Gloves always should be worn by people working with soiled materials from these animals. Precautions also should be taken with sharp objects (e.g., needles and scalpel blades) contaminated with blood or other body fluids.

Tuberculosis

All newly acquired primates should be tested with 0.1 ml of Old Tuberculin (the Tine test®—American Cyanamid, or the Mantoux test®—Coopers Animal Health); human purified protein derivatives can show only an obscure reaction compared with mammalian tuberculin. Intradermal test sites include the ventral forearm, the chest, and the eyelid. The test should be read at 48 and 72 hours[5,6]; reactions should be investigated. Clinical signs include chronic debilitation and cough. Old World primates are more susceptible to tuberculosis than New World primates are.

Salmonella

Various *Salmonella* spp. cause violent diarrhea and vomiting, with leukocytosis usually present. The feces should be cultured; the patient can be started on antibiotics (sulfonamides or cephalosporins) while the culture is pending. With diarrhea caused by *Salmonella*, as well as other infectious diarrheas, fluid therapy is as important as antibiotic therapy.

Surgery
Lacerations

Nonhuman primates housed in groups commonly fight among themselves. Most of the superficial wounds will heal by second intention without complications. Deep cuts or punctures need to be thoroughly cleaned and debrided. As with other animals, closure of the wound should follow normal tissue tension planes. Buried sutures are managed more easily in primate patients. The hardest part of wound management is patient cooperation. To ensure wound healing, the primate probably will need to be kept away from the surgical site for at least three to five days after closure. Collars, bandages, and tranquilization have been used successfully.

Dental Procedures

Removing or blunting the canine teeth in nonhuman primates often is requested for safety. In blunting, the canines are cut off to be even with the incisors. The pulp is removed, and the pulp cavity is filled with amalgam. Maintenance can be a problem with this procedure. The filling often will fall out, and the patient will need to be tranquilized again for repair work. This can be a major problem in large colonies of captive primates. Tooth extraction is permanent. The teeth must be elevated adequately before removal is attempted. Care must be taken when extracting canine teeth. Dental flap techniques are recommended and resemble those used in dogs. The roots on the canine teeth of primates are long, and fracture of the tooth or the alveolar bone is common if elevation and removal is not done carefully. Removing canine teeth from the great apes can be difficult and disfiguring. When properly performed, canine cutting followed by partial pulpectomy gives good results.

Rectal Prolapse

Primates with acute diarrhea, colitis, and obstipation commonly prolapse their rectums. Reduction of the prolapsed portion can be accomplished with corn starch, sugar, or sulfa-urea granules. After replacement, a purse-string suture using a nonabsorbable suture material is placed in the mucocutaneous junction. The suture ends should not protrude because of the risk of picking by the patient. The purse-string suture should be slack enough to allow feces to pass. It should be removed after 7 to 14 days.

Sterilization

Sterilization is not performed routinely in nonhuman primates. Neoplasia, metritis, or intractable hormone problems usually are the reasons for castration or ovariohysterectomy. The anatomy of the female nonhuman primate is similar to that of a woman; surgery should not be attempted without first studying the specific anatomy of the primate. Castration of the male can be performed as it is in canids. Care must be taken to inhibit self-mutilation after surgery.

REFERENCES

1. Chiarelli AB: *Taxonomic Atlas of Living Primates.* New York, Academic Press, 1972, pp 10–30.
2. Napier JR, Napier PH: *Handbook of Living Primates.* New York, Academic Press, 1967, pp 3–7.
3. *Nutrient Requirements of Nonhuman Primates,* ed 14. Washington, DC, National Research Council, National Academy of Sciences, 1978.
4. Johnson D, Russell RJ, Stunkard JA: *A Guide to Diagnosis, Treatment and Husbandry of Nonhuman Primates.* Edwardsville, KS, Veterinary Medicine Publishing Co, 1981, pp 6–20.
5. Wallach JD, Boever WJ: *Diseases of Exotic Animals.* Philadelphia, WB Saunders Co, 1983, pp 3–123.
6. *UFAW Handbook on the Care and Management of Laboratory Animals,* ed 4. Baltimore, The Williams & Wilkins Co, 1972, pp 374–423.
7. Griner LA: *Pathology of Zoo Animals.* San Diego, Zoological Society of San Diego, 1983, pp 332–337.

UPDATE

IMMOBILIZING AGENTS

Tiletamine hydrochloride/zolazepam hydrochloride—Dosage is dependent on degree of tranquilization.

Intramuscular: Small primates (marmosets) 5-8 mg/kg
Medium primates (capuchins) 4-6 mg/kg
Large primates (baboons) 3-4 mg/kg

In certain instances when the clinician cannot grasp or catch the animal, an oral dose of this medication will give a degree of relaxation. The absorption from the gastrointestinal tract is variable depending on stomach contents. An initial dose of 10 mg/kg is recommended.

Isoflurane inhalation can be done in a small cage within a plastic bag or induction chamber. Flow rates of 4% to 5% are needed for induction. When relaxed, the animal can be changed to a face mask or intubated and the flow rate decreased to 1% to 2%. Smaller primates may need recovery in an incubator. Pediatric uncuffed endotracheal tubes are commonly used.

PARASITIC DISEASES

Parasitic infections may be present in the primate at the time it is bought or imported. Human parasites also may be transmitted to the animal by feeding them food that is contaminated with human feces.

Entamoeba histolytica can cause severe diarrhea and dehydration. Some animals are asymptomatic carriers. Treatment with metronidazole is recommended (17.5 to 25.0 mg/kg bid for 10 days). If this drug cannot be administered due to the bitter taste, paromomycin at 10 mg/kg tid orally for 10 days can be administered.

Giardia is frequently suspected in clinical and research settings in both new and old world primates. The parasite is not easy to find in feces when the primate is admitted with diarrhea. Treatment with metronidazole at 17.5 to 25.0 mg/kg bid for 10 days usually will clear the infection. Toxoplasma gondii has been seen with increasing frequency in marmosets (*Callithricidae*). Diarrhea with neurological signs and death has been seen. Treatment of choice is with

sulfadiazine at 100 mg/kg/day in combination with pyrimethamine 2 mg/kg/day for the first three days then 1 mg/kg/day. Supplementation with folinic acid is advised, which should be continued for 30 days.

Nematodes
Levamisole, 10 mg/kg
Ivermectin, 200 µg/kg

Oxyuris, Other Pinworms
Pyrantel pamoate, 11 mg/kg once

HERPES B VIRUS *(Herpesvirus simiae)*

Herpesvirus simiae is an infectious disease in macaques and is transmissible to humans. Recently, there have been many outbreaks of the virus in research facilities, which have been transmitted to workers and veterinarians alike.[1] The animals do not have to be clinically ill to spread this virus to humans. Oral and fecal transmission is common. All macaques should be considered infected. Proper protective clothing and face shields should be worn when handling macaques. The signs in humans are frequently flu-like. A fever and lethargy are common. Neurological signs, which can lead to encephalitis and death, manifest as the disease progresses. Treatment with antiherpes drugs, such as acyclovir, is effective.

TUBERCULOSIS

Tuberculosis is more common in old world primates, such as the great apes, baboons, and macaques. All primates should be tested on a routine basis. Most animals are tested at least yearly in practice. The intradermal injection of mammalian tuberculin in the eyelid, chest, or ventral forearm should be read at 48 and 72 hours. If there is a reaction, the patient should again be assessed at 96 and 120 hours consecutively. Animals with a questionable test reaction should be retested after a minimum of two weeks has elapsed. The second test should be done at a different one or two sites on the body. An animal that gives a second positive result should be isolated and considered infected. There have been reports of marmosets (*Callithrix jacchus*) being infected with *Mycobacterium avium.*[2]

VITAMIN C DEFICIENCY

The formation of collagen, osteoid, and dentin are all roles of L-ascorbic acid (vitamin C). Primates (human and nonhuman) depend on exogenous sources. In new world monkeys such as the squirrel monkey (*saimiri*), rough hair coats, bleeding gums, and subdural hematomas are common with vitamin C deficiency. Nonhuman primates often will present with a classic normocytic and normochromic anemia. This may be due to multiple hemorrhages at different sites with resulting blood loss. Young animals will have bone deformities as a result of the defective production of the osteoid matrix. Treatment as stated earlier can initially be parenteral doses of ascorbic acid followed by the oral route.

VITAMIN D₃ (Activated 7-dehydrocholesterol; cholecalciferol) DEFICIENCY

This deficiency is very prevalent in new world primates such as marmosets (*Callithrix*) and tamarins (*Sanguinus*) fed a diet other than commercial marmoset food or gel. It is seen commonly in practice with pet capuchins (*Cebus*) and spider monkeys (*Ateles*). The animals are often presented paralyzed, with radiographic changes consisting of decreased mineralization (cortical thinning) and widened epiphyses with large irregular processes of cartilage extending toward the shaft of the bone. In areas of membranous bone, mineralization of the new osteoid tissue fails to occur and is accompanied by increased vascularization and fibrosis. The degree of deformity depends on the severity of the deficiency and the growth rate of the monkey. In young primates, an excess of osteoid tissue produces "frontal bossing" with a very square appearance to the head. The chest also becomes deformed with the sternum and anterior portion of the rib cage tending to protrude. The paralysis may come from folding fractures of the legs or spine deformities. The treatment for the deficiency is initial supplementation at 1.25 IU per gram of diet followed by proper commercially mixed diets suggested for that species.[3]

Vitamin D₃ toxicity also has been seen in these animals when an excess has been given. Hypercalcemia with hypercalciuria is encountered. Many of these animals die from subsequent renal disease and wasting. The mobilization of skeletal calcium may also lead to osteoporosis, which becomes worse with the age of the animal.

REFERENCES

1. Centers for Disease Control, B virus infections in humans. Pensacola, Florida. *MMWR* 36:289–90, 96–106, 1987.
2. Hatt JM, Guscetti FL: A case of mycobacteriosis in a common marmoset (*Callithrix jacchus*). *Proceedings of the Assoc. of Zoo Veterinarians,* 1994, pp 241–243.
3. Wallach JD, Boever WJ: *Diseases of Exotic Animals.* Philadelphia, WB Saunders, 1983, pp 26–27.

Practical Medicine of Primate Pets

KEY FACTS

- Primate species are in general not suitable as companion animals.
- Proper husbandry is important in prevention of common health problems.
- Semiannual physical examination and tuberculin testing are recommended.
- Primate owners and handlers (including veterinarians and veterinary staff) must be made aware of the many potential zoonoses carried by primates.

The Philadelphia Zoo
Department of Animal Health
Philadelphia, Pennsylvania
Donna M. Ialeggio, DVM

NONHUMAN PRIMATES cannot be imported into the United States for use as pets,[1,2] although captive-bred nonhuman primates of species that are not classified as endangered may be kept as pets. Whether legally or illegally kept, however, primate species are not suitable as companion animals. Although this article presents a practical approach to the care of these species, it is not intended to encourage the practice of keeping primate pets.

Because they are smaller and have lower maintenance costs, new world primates are kept more often as pets than are old world species.[3] The most commonly kept species include squirrel monkeys (*Saimiri sciureus*); capuchin or "organ-grinder" monkeys (*Cebus* species); spider monkeys (*Ateles geoffroyi*); marmosets (*Sanguinus* species and *Callithrix* species); dourocoulis (*Aotus trivirgatus*), which are also known as owl or night monkeys; and titi monkeys (*Callicebus* species). The bush baby or galago (*Galago senegalensis*), an old world prosimian, has also been a popular pet.[3,4]

MANAGEMENT OF PRIMATE PETS

With proper management, many health problems can be avoided; those that occur may be recognized relatively early in their course. Nonhuman primates should be maintained at ambient temperatures between 18.3 °C (65 °F) and 26.7 °C (80 °F)—optimally, 21.1° to 25.6 °C (70° to 78 °F).[3-5] Although most primate species can be gradually adapted to colder ambient temperatures, rapid temperature changes are stressful and predispose the animal to respiratory problems, to which new world species are particularly susceptible.

For most primate species, the relative humidity should be between 55% and 70%. Marmosets require slightly higher (70% to 80%) atmospheric moisture.[3-5] Relative humidity below this range may result in skin and haircoat problems; excessively high humidity encourages bacterial and fungal growth.

Myriad laws, guidelines, and regulations govern minimum dimensions of cages for research animals. If primate pets are to be caged, these guidelines should be considered. Cage height should be at least 2.5 times that of the animal; cage width should be at least five times the animal's arm span. Suitable adjustments are necessary when several primates are housed together. Cage bars should be spaced so that the animal can neither escape nor become trapped between them.

Each cage should have at least one perch per animal plus one additional perch (e.g., for two animals, there should be three or more perches). Conspecific groups housed together should be offered several food pans to decrease the likelihood that dominant animals will prevent subordinates from feeding.

PRIMATES OF different species should not be housed together because diseases that are benign in one species can be lethal to others. For example, herpesvirus T, which produces latent to mild infection in squirrel and spider monkeys, is often fatal to marmosets and dourocoulis.[3-6]

Climbing ropes, tree limbs, or similar occupational devices encourage exercise and constructive activity and help prevent the development of stereotypical or destructive behaviors. Hiding places or sight barriers help decrease stress associated with continuous exposure. Marmosets do not thrive without nest boxes.[3] Special lighting is required if nocturnal species, such as dourocoulis, are to be active during daylight instead of nighttime hours. A false floor or grill facilitates the removal of feces, urine, and other cage waste and helps prevent coprophagy, which can lead to reinfection with such gastrointestinal parasites as *Entamoeba histolytica* and is aesthetically unappealing.

Primates tend to mouth, taste, or ingest various other items. Paints should therefore be free of heavy metals,[7] and substances that might cause intoxication or gastrointestinal obstruction should be kept out of reach. Cages and waste pans should be cleaned twice daily with detergent and bactericidal solutions of phenolic compounds or organic iodides.[4] Weekly cleaning of pans in acid solution to remove nitrogenous buildup and monthly high-pressure cleaning of the entire cage are also recommended.

Nutrition

Nutritional disorders (e.g., nutritional secondary hyperparathyroidism,[4,8-10] scurvy,[10-12] or protein-deficiency disease[5,10]) can easily be prevented.[13] Primates daily consume approximately 4% of their body weight (as fed rather than on a dry-weight basis).[3-5] Because they waste food, however, a greater quantity should be offered. Dividing the total ration into several feedings decreases the amount of food wasted and may prevent acute gastric dilatation.[4,14-16]

Several commercial feeds as well as canned marmoset diets are available. Commercial feeds for old world species tend to contain approximately 15% protein. Those for new world species contain at least 25% protein because new world monkeys appear to have a higher requirement for protein.[3,17]

NEW WORLD MONKEYS require cholecalciferol (vitamin D_3), whereas ergocalciferol (vitamin D_2) or cholecalciferol can sustain old world species.[17] New world feeds provide vitamin D as cholecalciferol; many, but not all, old world feeds contain cholecalciferol.

With the possible exception of some of the prosimians, primates cannot synthesize vitamin C. If monkey biscuits are soaked in fruit juice, milk, or water to encourage their consumption, the use of excessive liquid—more than just enough to make the biscuits spongy—will result in leaching of vitamin C from the biscuits.

Improper or excessively long storage results in decreased vitamin potency. A diet based on commercially available feeds (e.g., the canned diet for marmosets) supplemented with small amounts of fruit and vegetables is suggested. Supplementary mealworms, crickets, and neonatal mice should be considered for squirrel and spider monkeys, marmosets, and galagos.[3] Canned or moistened dog food may also be used to supplement squirrel and spider monkey diets. Fresh, clean water should be available at all times.

Restraint and Handling

Primate pets should be examined by a veterinarian at least twice each year. This schedule allows for semiannual tuberculin testing in accordance with current guidelines of the Infectious Disease Committee of the American Association of Zoo Veterinarians.[18] For the safety of other clients and hospital personnel, the examination room should be equipped with securely closing doors. For primates weighing more than 5 kg, a squeeze-back cage is ideal but is infrequently available.[3,5,19] At least two people—a handler and the veterinarian—are required to complete the physical examination.

The primate should be grasped firmly from behind, just proximal to the elbows. The arms are then gently rotated laterally and dorsally and the elbows brought nearly into contact behind the animal's back (Figure 1). The use of excessive force may result in humeral fractures; for malnourished animals, even minimal force may be excessive. Once the primate's arms have been positioned as described, the restraint can be maintained with one hand. The free hand is then used to extend the hindlimbs much as one would restrain a cat.

Nonhuman primates larger than 12 kg require at least two handlers.[3,20,21] Heavy leather gloves may be worn, but such gloves do not protect against bite wounds. A strong net or a rabies pole may be sufficient to restrain the animal to allow the practitioner to carry out minor procedures or may provide sufficient physical restraint to allow the administration of chemical restraints.

Practitioners should be aware that anything directed at a nonhuman primate can be grabbed and redirected back at the handler; for this reason, the use of pole syringes on larger, unrestrained primates should be avoided. Hospitalized primates must be kept in escape-proof cages with double-locking doors.[19] The type of cage used in most small animal practices will not contain an alert primate.

Chemical Restraint and Anesthesia

Intramuscular injection is the only practical administration route for restraint drugs in nonhuman primates. Ketamine hydrochloride is, at present, the drug of choice.[3,4,20,22] At a dose of 8 to 10 mg/kg intramuscularly, ketamine hydrochloride provides adequate restraint for such minor procedures as venipuncture and tuberculin test-

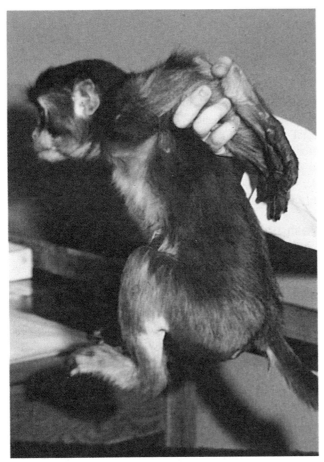

Figure 1—Manual restraint of a small primate. Examination gloves should be worn when handling any ill nonhuman primate. (Courtesy of Lloyd Dillingham, DVM, Cornell University)

ing; a dose of 15 to 20 mg/kg produces surgical anesthesia.[3,23,24] Smaller or younger primates require a larger perkilogram dose than do larger or older animals.[25]

If the volume of ketamine hydrochloride required is too large to administer rapidly as a single intramuscular dose, the calculated dose may be divided into two or more smaller doses. When the patient has become more tractable after the initial administration, it should be physically restrained and the remaining ketamine hydrochloride given. Atropine sulfate (0.02 to 0.04 mg/kg intramuscularly)[25] may be given to decrease hypersalivation and prevent bradycardia. If seizure activity or excessive muscle rigidity is present, intravenous or intramuscular diazepam (0.25 to 0.5 mg/kg) may be used. Fixed combinations of fentanyl and droperidol (Innovar-Vet®—Pitman-Moore; 1 ml per 18 kg intramuscularly) and of tiletamine and zolazepam (Telazol®—A. H. Robins; 2 to 6 mg/kg intramuscularly) are also used.[3,20,25] Telazol® is licensed for use in nonhuman primates and may have advantages over ketamine hydrochloride in restraint of nonhuman primates.[23]

Inhalation anesthesia is preferred over injectables for prolonged procedures. Anesthesia is induced with either intramuscular ketamine hydrochloride or a fixed combination of tiletamine and zolazepam. The pharynx and larynx are sprayed with local anesthetic (e.g., Cetacaine®—Cetylite),[5] and the animal is intubated. Halothane gas is introduced at a concentration of 2% to 4%. Once the desired plane of anesthesia is attained, the animal is maintained at 0.5% to 1.5% halothane[3,26] with a 50:50 mixture of nitrous oxide and oxygen at a fresh gas flow rate of 2 L/min (in larger primates, 4 L/min[26]).[3,5,25] A pediatric circle semiclosed system is recommended.[5]

PREVENTIVE MEDICINE

The primate pet should be examined by a veterinarian at least twice each year. The basic semiannual veterinary visit should include a physical examination, complete blood count, fecal examination, and tuberculin testing.[5]

Physical Examination

Rectal temperatures of 37.2° to 40.2°C (99.0° to 104.4°F), an average of 38.8°C (101.8°F),[3] may be expected. Small primates have pulse and respiratory rates of 165 to 240 beats/min and 20 to 50 breaths/min, respectively; larger animals will have pulse rates of 95 to 112 beats/min and respiratory rates of 12 to 20 breaths/min.[3] Careful abdominal palpation and palpation of the femoral lymph nodes are extremely important. Splenomegaly, intraabdominal lymphadenopathy, and femoral lymphadenopathy with or without suppuration may indicate tuberculosis, even if the tuberculin test is negative.[5,27,28] The differential diagnosis of tuberculosis includes avian tuberculosis, meliodiosis, and systemic mycosis.

Complete Blood Count

The most common sites of venipuncture are the cephalic, saphenous, and femoral veins.[20] The jugular vein is also used; however, jugular venipuncture usually requires sedation. The packed cell volume should be approximately 40% to 45%.[3-5] Serum from samples drawn during the initial examination should be frozen so that a baseline sample is available should serologic testing become necessary in the future.[5] Douroucoulis, because of a naturally high concentration of antithrombin III in their blood, have longer clotting times than other primate species have.[3]

Fecal Examination

The most commonly found gastrointestinal parasites are nematodes of the genera *Strongyloides* and *Oesophagostomum*[5,10,29,30] (Figure 2). Thiabendazole (two oral doses of 100 mg/kg two weeks apart) is effective against these parasites,[5,31] and semiannual prophylactic deworming is recommended. Ivermectin 1% at a dose of 200 μg/kg subcutaneously is also effective. Other commonly found gastrointestinal parasites include such protozoans as *Entamoeba* and *Balantidium*, against which iodoquinol (650 mg orally daily for 10 to 20 days) is effective[5]; *Trichuris* species, which respond to two-day treatment with dichlorvos or mebendazole[31]; and pinworms (*Enterobius* species), which are treated with 100 mg/kg of piperazine.[30,31]

No available treatment is effective against *Prosthenorchis elegans* infection. This acanthocephalan burrows

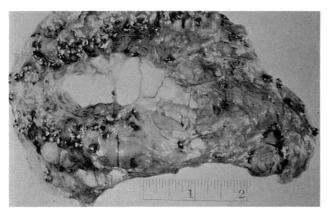

Figure 2—Intestinal lesions of *Oesophagostomum* infection. (Courtesy of Lloyd Dillingham, DVM, Cornell University)

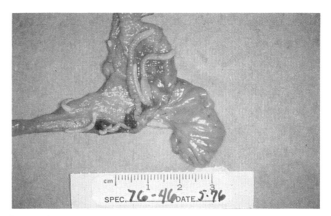

Figure 3—Intestinal lesions of *Prosthenorchis elegans* in a squirrel monkey. (Courtesy of Lloyd Dillingham, DVM, Cornell University)

into the gut wall and occasionally penetrates into the peritoneal cavity, thus causing acute peritonitis (Figure 3). The best preventive measure is cockroach control because the cockroach is the intermediate host of this parasite.[5]

Tuberculin Testing

The tuberculin test[18,27] is arguably the most important part of the examination of a nonhuman primate. State accreditation is required in order to perform the test, which consists of an intradermal injection of 0.1 ml of mammalian old tuberculin. Although the upper eyelid (Figure 4) is frequently used as the test site, intradermal injection in the skin of the abdomen or forearm seems to be more acceptable to the pet owner. The test site is examined at 24, 48, and 72 hours after injection. An animal with an inconclusive response should be retested in 14 days.

ALTHOUGH ONLY a positive culture is pathognomonic of tuberculosis, a single positive reaction or two inconclusive responses in a nonhuman primate are sufficient for presumptive diagnosis of tuberculosis and a recommendation for euthanasia.[4,28] Thoracic radiographs are minimally rewarding diagnostically because calcium is rarely deposited in pulmonary tubercular lesions in nonhuman primates.[4] Treatment of tuberculosis in pet primates is not indicated because treatment will result in diminished response to the tuberculin test despite failure to eliminate the animal's ability to transmit the disease.[28]

The intradermal test may produce a negative response for nonhuman primates truly free of the disease, anergic animals (i.e., those in advanced stages of the disease), primates with measles infection or any debilitating illness, animals that are receiving corticosteroid medication, or those that have recently been immunized. An anergic animal may show a so-called flash reaction (transient positive response) to the intradermal injection. Animals with an inconclusive response to the initial test should be observed for a transient positive response at two and eight hours after injection in the retest.[5,18,28]

Other Routine Procedures

Vaccination of nonhuman primates is controversial. Annual tetanus prophylaxis is recommended; however, fatal cases of tetanus in vaccinated nonhuman primates have been reported.[32] Apes should be vaccinated against poliomyelitis. In 15 zoos that responded to a survey, apes receive annual doses of modified live virus poliomyelitis vaccine.[a] Vaccination against measles (modified live virus vaccine) may be considered if the danger of exposure to the disease exists[a,6]; human hyperimmune serum globulin has also been used prophylactically and as a supplement to treatment. Although the American Veterinary Medical Association does not sanction rabies prophylaxis in nondomestic species, several zoos in rabies-endemic areas vaccinate resident nonhuman primates against the disease.[a,33]

COMMON REASONS FOR PRESENTATION

Ailing nonhuman primates are typically presented with gastrointestinal or respiratory signs. Gastroenteritis is among the most common of gastrointestinal disorders. Although the causes of gastroenteritis in nonhuman primates vary, the most common bacterial agents are *Shigella* and *Salmonella*.[4,10,34] A presumptive diagnosis of *Shigella* or *Salmonella* enteritis can be based on the finding of bloody diarrhea; and fluid and antibiotic therapy can be instituted. Examination of fecal smears may be supportive; in one study involving human patients, the presence of fecal leukocytes was found to be more reliable than culture in the diagnosis of enteric shigellosis.[34]

It has been suggested[35] that antimicrobial therapy should be reserved for more severe cases of *Shigella* or *Salmonella* gastroenteritis because antibiotic use in less severe cases may facilitate the development of carrier states. Unconfirmed cases of *Shigella* or *Salmonella* enteritis often respond well to subcutaneous trimethoprim-sulfadiazine (24%, 1 ml/10 kg daily) or intramuscular gentamicin (2 mg/kg three times daily) for 7 to 10 days. In addition to gastroenteritides, nonhuman primates may show gastrointestinal signs related to intestinal parasitism, dental dis-

[a]Heuschele W: Personal communication, Zoological Society of San Diego, San Diego, California, 1988.

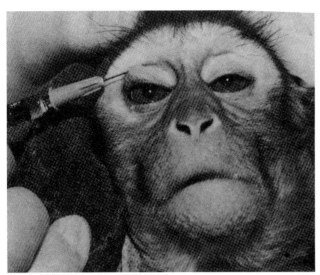

Figure 4—Intradermal injection of tuberculin (0.1 cc of mammalian old tuberculin) into the upper eyelid of a nonhuman primate. In a pet primate, intradermal injection into the skin of the forearm or abdomen is preferred. (From Whitney RA Jr, Johnson DJ, Cole WC: *Laboratory Primate Handbook*. New York, Academic Press, 1973. Reproduced with permission.)

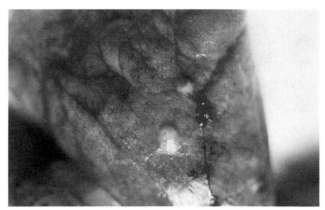

Figure 5—Lesions of pulmonary *Pneumonyssus* infection in a rhesus monkey. (Courtesy of Lloyd Dillingham, DVM, Cornell University)

ease, and acute gastric dilatation (bloat). Bloat is common in research colonies and is most often associated with overeating following a period of food deprivation.[5,14,15,36] Treatment consists of decompression and subsequent supportive care. Several small feedings instead of a single daily feeding may be preventive.

Respiratory signs are most frequently attributable to pneumonia.[37] Pneumonia may be primary or secondary to measles or such metazoal parasites as the lung mite *Pneumonyssus*. Abnormal findings on auscultation of the lungs in conjunction with an elevated white blood cell count are the most reliable aids to diagnosis of pneumonia. Because anorexia may accompany respiratory signs and because small new world species are particularly susceptible to hypoglycemia, nutritional supplementation should be strongly considered.

DEMONSTRATION OF *Streptococcus pneumoniae* in sputum confirms the diagnosis of pneumococcal pneumonia,[3] which is a lobar pneumonia often accompanied by empyema.[10] The disease may be acute (leading to death in 6 to 10 days if untreated) or chronic and usually responds well to treatment with parenteral penicillin, chloramphenicol, or trimethoprim-sulfadiazine.[3]

Panophthalmitis or bacterial meningoencephalitis may occur with or as sequelae of pneumococcal pneumonia. Signs may include ptosis, palpebral edema, nystagmus, torticollis, ataxia, and paraplegia. Treatment of pneumococcal meningoencephalitis consists of chloramphenicol administered at a dose of 110 mg/kg four times daily for 5 to 10 days intramuscularly (intrathecal administration of

aqueous penicillin has also been successful) and can be instituted based on clinical signs or demonstration of the organism in cerebrospinal fluid.[3]

Presumptive diagnosis of pulmonary *Pneumonyssus* infection (Figure 5) may be based on radiographic evidence (i.e., diffuse interstitial densities or discrete opaque densities away from the region of the hilus of the lungs).[38] A single dose of ivermectin (200 μg/kg subcutaneously) appears to be effective in treatment of this infection.[38]

PREVENTION OF ZOONOSES

The primate owner should be advised of zoonoses[39] that can be transmitted from a primate pet. These include tuberculosis[28]; shigellosis, salmonellosis, and amoebiasis[4]; measles[9]; infectious hepatitis[40,41]; parasitic infections; and rabies and other viral diseases.[6] Two extremely important viral zoonoses are herpesvirus B and Marburg virus. Both viruses occur naturally in primates of old world species—herpesvirus B in Asian macaques and Marburg virus in African monkeys. Both are associated with high mortality in humans. In humans, herpesvirus B produces a fatal encephalitis whereas Marburg virus produces fatal hemorrhagic disease.

Any macaque with ulcers of the lips or oral cavity may be presumed to have and be capable of transmitting herpesvirus B and should therefore be euthanatized.[6] More than 80% of wild-caught adult macaques have significant antibody titers to herpesvirus B. In African species, a herpesvirus (SA8) that cross-reacts with herpesvirus B may be found; but SA8 has not been documented as a public health problem.

For the primate owners or handlers (including veterinarians and veterinary staff), the following preventive measures are strongly recommended[42]:

• Preexposure serum sample for freezing
• Preexposure thoracic radiographs
• Tuberculin testing every four to six months
• Annual radiographs for individuals vaccinated with BCG vaccine

- Testing of all exposed personnel after identification of a positive tuberculin seroconversion in a nonhuman primate
- Tetanus boosters every 10 years or after exposure if the previous booster was received more than five years before.

Vaccination against smallpox, polio, rubella, and rabies should be considered. For personnel working with chimpanzees, a semiannual prophylactic administration of hyperimmine serum globulin to protect against infectious hepatitis is recommended.

ACKNOWLEDGMENTS

The author gratefully acknowledges the contributions of Lloyd Dillingham, DVM, of the New York State College of Veterinary Medicine, Cornell University, Ithaca, New York; Jeffrey Wimsatt, DVM, who is affiliated with the Regional Primate Research Center at Davis, California; Keith Hinshaw, DVM, MPH, of the Philadelphia Zoological Society; Werner Heuschele, DVM, from the San Diego Zoological Society; and the reviewers of this article and offers special thanks to Robin Gleed, MVSc, of the New York State College of Veterinary Medicine, Cornell University.

About the Author

Dr. Ialeggio is Associate Veterinarian at the Department of Animal Health for the Philadelphia Zoo, Philadelphia, Pennsylvania.

REFERENCES

1. Meyers NM: Government regulation of nonhuman primate facilities. *J Med Primatol* 12:169–183, 1983.
2. Johnson DK, Morin ML: U.S. laws, regulations and policies important to managers of nonhuman primate colonies. *J Med Primatol* 12:223–238, 1983.
3. Wallach JD, Boever WJ: *Diseases of Exotic Animals: Medical and Surgical Management.* Philadelphia, WB Saunders Co, 1983, pp 3–133.
4. Johnson DK, Russell RJ, Stunkard JA: *A Guide to Diagnosis, Treatment and Husbandry of Nonhuman Primates.* Edwardsville, KS, Veterinary Medicine Publishing, 1981.
5. Whitney RA Jr, Johnson DJ, Cole WC: *Laboratory Primate Handbook.* New York, Academic Press, 1973.
6. Ott-Joslin JE: Viral diseases in nonhuman primates, in Fowler ME (ed): *Zoo and Wild Animal Medicine,* ed 2. Philadelphia, WB Saunders Co, 1986, pp 674–697.
7. Zook BC, Sauer RM, Garner FM: Lead poisoning in captive wild animals. *J Wildl Dis* 8:264–272, 1972.
8. Miller RM: Nutritional secondary hyperparathyroidism in monkeys, in Kirk RW (ed): *Current Veterinary Therapy IV.* Philadelphia, WB Saunders Co, 1971, pp 407–408.
9. Resnick S: Bone disease in pet monkeys. *JAVMA* 159(3):557–559, 1971.
10. Ruch TC: *Diseases of Laboratory Primates.* Philadelphia, WB Saunders Co, 1959.
11. Kupper JL, Britz WE: The squirrel monkey, in *Selected Topics in Laboratory Animal Medicine,* vol XVIII. Brooks Air Force Base, TX, United States Air Force School of Aerospace Medicine, 1972, pp 4–5.
12. Lehner NDM, Bullock BC, Clarkson TB: Ascorbic acid deficiency in the squirrel monkey. *Proc Soc Exp Biol Med* 128:512–514, 1968.
13. Harris RS (ed): *Feeding and Nutrition of Nonhuman Primates.* New York, Academic Press, 1970.
14. Pond CL, Newcomer CE, Anver MR: Acute gastric dilation in primates: A review and case studies. *Vet Pathol* 9(Suppl 7):126–133, 1982.
15. Vickers JH: Gastrointestinal diseases of primates, in Kirk RW (ed): *Current Veterinary Therapy IV.* Philadelphia, WB Saunders Co, 1971, pp 408–411.
16. Smith AW, Casey HW, LaCroix JT, et al: Acute bloat syndrome (gastric dilatation) in *Macaca mulatta. JAVMA* 155(7):1241–1244, 1969.
17. Martin DP: Feeding and nutrition, in Fowler ME (ed): *Zoo and Wild Animal Medicine,* ed 2. Philadelphia, WB Saunders Co, 1986, pp 661–663.
18. Ott-Joslin JE: Tuberculin testing recommendations for primates, in *Minutes, Infectious Disease Committee.* Philadelphia, PA, American Association of Zoo Veterinarians, 1983.
19. Harris JE: Restraint and physical examination of monkeys and apes, in Kirk RW (ed): *Current Veterinary Therapy IV.* Philadelphia, WB Saunders Co, 1977, pp 721–722.
20. Martin DP: Restraint and handling, in Fowler ME (ed): *Zoo and Wild Animal Medicine,* ed 2. Philadelphia, WB Saunders Co, 1986, pp 663–667.
21. Altman R: Handling monkeys, in Kirk RW (ed): *Current Veterinary Therapy IV.* Philadelphia, WB Saunders Co, 1971, p 404.
22. Drake KJ: Initial experiences with ketamine anesthesia in nonhuman primates. *Lab Primate News* 11(2):18–27, 1972.
23. Cohen BJ, Bree MM: Chemical and physical restraint of nonhuman primates. *J Med Primatol* 7:193–210, 1978.
24. Veracruysse J Jr: The chemical restraint of apes and monkeys by means of phencyclidine or ketamine. *Acta Zool Pathol Antwerp* 70:211–220, 1978.
25. Cramlet SH, Jones EF: Anesthesiology, in *Selected Topics in Laboratory Animal Medicine,* vol V. Brooks Air Force Base, TX, United States Air Force School of Aerospace Medicine, 1976, pp 78–83.
26. Krahwinkel DJ Jr: Primate anesthesiology. *J Zoo Anim Med* 1(1):4–9, 1970.
27. Ott JE: Tuberculin testing in primates. *Proc Am Assoc Zoo Vet*:75–81, 1979.
28. Martin DP: Infectious diseases, in Fowler ME (ed): *Zoo and Wild Animal Medicine,* ed 2. Philadelphia, WB Saunders Co, 1986, pp 669–673.
29. Toff JD II: The pathophysiology of the alimentary tract and pancreas of nonhuman primates: A review. *Vet Pathol* 19(Suppl 7):44–92, 1982.
30. Sedgewick C: A clinical view of exotic animal practice. *J Zoo Anim Med* 2(4):5–16, 1971.
31. Martin DP: Parasitic diseases, in Fowler ME (ed): *Zoo and Wild Animal Medicine,* ed 2. Philadelphia, WB Saunders Co, 1986, pp 700–701.
32. Kessler MJ, Martinez HS: Treatment of tetanus in the rhesus monkey (*Macaca mulatta*). *J Zoo Anim Med* 10:119–122, 1979.
33. Kessler MJ, Summer JW, Baer GM: Evaluation of a killed rabies vaccine for rhesus monkeys (*Macaca mulatta*). *J Zoo Anim Med* 13:74–77, 1982.
34. Nelson JD, Haltalin KC: Accuracy of diagnosis of bacterial disease by clinical features. *J Pediatr* 78:519–522, 1971.
35. Kollias GV Jr: Diagnosis and management of salmonellosis and shigellosis in nonhuman primates, in Kirk RW (ed): *Current Veterinary Therapy VIII.* Philadelphia, WB Saunders Co, 1984, pp 666–669.
36. Newton WM, Beamer PD, Rhoades HE: Acute bloat syndrome in stumptailed macaques (*Macaca arctoides*): A report of four cases. *Lab Anim Sci* 21(2):193–196, 1971.
37. Vickers JE: Respiratory diseases of primates, in Kirk RW (ed): *Current Veterinary Therapy IV.* Philadelphia, WB Saunders Co, 1971, pp 412–414.
38. Joseph BE, Wilson DW, Henrickson RV, et al: Treatment of pulmonary ascariasis in rhesus macaques with ivermectin. *Lab Anim Sci* 34(4):360–364, 1984.
39. Fiennes R: *Zoonoses of Primates: The Epidemiology and Ecology of Simian Diseases in Relation to Man,* ed 2. Ithaca, NY, Cornell University Press, 1972.
40. Friedman CTH, Dinnes MR, Bernstein JF, et al: Chimpanzee-associated infectious hepatitis among personnel at an animal hospital. *JAVMA* 159:541–545, 1971.
41. Davenport FM, Hennessey AV, Christopher N, et al: A common source multi-household outbreak of chimpanzee-associated hepatitis in humans. *Am J Epidemiol* 83:146–151, 1966.
42. Martin DP: Preventive medicine, in Fowler ME (ed): *Zoo and Wild Animal Medicine,* ed 2. Philadelphia, WB Saunders Co, 1986, pp 667–669.

UPDATE

The demographic profile of nonhuman primate (NHP) species commonly held as pets appears to have changed from that stated at the beginning of the preceding article. I am unaware of current statistics relating to numbers and types of privately owned primates; my impression is that preferences are shifting away from smaller (< 1 kg) new world species and toward larger (< 15 kg) new and old world monkeys.

In reference to the use of nest boxes, these should be provided for many of the smaller primate species. Most primate species will benefit from the addition of hiding spots to their holding areas.

While research into the nutritional requirements of various NHPs continues, the question of whether new world species have a higher dietary requirement for protein remains unanswered at this time. According to recent information, the feeding of neonatal mice to callitrichids (marmosets and tamarins) may place them at increased risk of exposure to lymphocytic choriomeningitis virus (a.k.a. callitrichid hepatitis virus), which could result in fatal hepatitis in these species.[1,2]

Immobilization of NHPs may be achieved using tiletamine/zolazepam, fentanyl/droperidol, combinations of ketamine hydrochloride with acepromazine, diazepam, midazolam, or xylazine (all administered intramuscularly), or propofol (administered intravenously).[3-5] In the author's own anecdotal experience, droperidol (injectable) delivered *orally* in juice to chimpanzees, orangutans, and gorillas 20 to 60 minutes prior to the intramuscular administration of ketamine hydrochloride resulted in sufficient restraint to allow hand-injection of a reduced dose of ketamine.

Reference ranges are available for hematologic and serum chemical values of some NHPs.[4-7] An extensive list of resources available to the primate practitioner may be found in reference 5.

In addition to those parasiticides considered in the preceding paper, the following therapeutics have been used in the treatment of parasitisms in NHPs:[5,8] fenbendazole, mebendazole, levamisole, pyrantel pamoate (nematodes); praziquantel (cestodes, trematodes); and metronidazole and sulfa-containing drugs (protozoans). In one study in free-ranging rhesus macaques (*Macaca mulatta*), ivermectin administered *topically* (injectable solution applied to the skin of the perineum) at a dosage of 500 μg/kg was as effective in the elimination of fecal shedding of *Strongyloides, Trichuris,* and *Ascaris* as was the standard subcutaneous dosage of 200 μg/kg.[9]

The potential for zoonotic transmission of disease from NHPs is very real. It has been suggested that NHPs are inappropriate companions for children under five years of age, geriatric persons, and individuals who are immunocompromised by disease and/or chemotherapeutics. In addition to those listed in the preceding articles, disease organisms that may be carried by NHPs (sometimes asymptomatically) and are of particular importance to immunocompromised humans include *Campylobacter* species, *Cryptococcus neoformans, Pneumocystis carinii, Mycoplasma pneumoniae, Giardia* species, *Toxoplasma gondii,* and cytomegalovirus.[4-7,10]

REFERENCES

1. Montali RJ, Scanga CA, Pernikoff D, et al: A common-source outbreak of callitrichid hepatitis in captive tamarins and marmosets. *J Infect Dis* 167:946–950, 1993.
2. Scanga CA, Holmes RJ, Montali RJ: Serologic evidence of infection with lymphocytic choriomeningitis virus, the agent of callitrichid hepatitis, in primates in zoos, primate research centers, and a natural reserve. *J Zoo Wildl Med* 24(4):469–474, 1993.
3. Sainsbury AW, Eaton BD, Cooper JE: Restraint and anaesthesia of primates. *Vet Rec* 125:640–643, 1989.
4. Satterfield WC, Voss WR: Nonhuman primates and the practitioner, in JE Harkness (ed): *Vet Clinics of North America, Exotic Pet Medicine*. Philadelphia, WB Saunders, 1989, 17(5):1185–1202.
5. Johnson-Delaney C: Primates, in Quesenberry KE, Hillyer EV (eds): *Vet Clinics of North America, Exotic Pet Medicine II. Philadelphia, WB Saunders,* 1994, 24(1):121–156.
6. Wallach JD, Boever WJ: *Diseases of Exotic Animals: Medical and Surgical Management.* Philadelphia, WB Saunders, 1983, pp 3–133.
7. Fowler ME: *Zoo and Wild Animal Medicine, ed. 2.* Philadelphia, WB Saunders, 1986, pp 523–552.
8. Wolff PE: Parasites of new world primates, in Fowler ME (ed): *Zoo and Wild Animal Medicine, Current Therapy 3.* Philadelphia, WB Saunders, 1993, pp 378–389.
9. Bercovitch FB, Rodriquez JF, Nieves P, et al: A non-invasive technique for the control of intestinal parasites in rhesus macaques (*Macaca mulatta*). *J Med Primatol* 21(7–8): 363–365, 1992.
10. Fowler ME: *Zoo and Wild Animal Medicine, Current Therapy 3.* Philadelphia, WB Saunders, 1993, pp 340–373.

INDEX

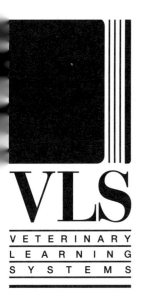

PRACTICAL RESOURCES FOR YOUR CLINIC FROM VLS

SMALL ANIMAL/EXOTICS

- ☐ Atlas of Feline Ophthalmology (Ketring, Glaze)
- ☐ Emergency Medicine in Small Animal Practice
- ☐ Exotic Animals: A Veterinary Handbook
- ☐ Gastroenterology in Practice
- ☐ Head and Neck Medicine & Surgery
- ☐ Managing the Veterinary Cancer Patient (Ogilvie, Moore)
- ☐ Ophthalmology in Small Animal Practice
- ☐ Pet Skin and Haircoat Problems for Veterinary Technicians (Ackerman)
- ☐ Practical Avian Medicine
- ☐ Practical Exotic Animal Medicine
- ☐ Radiology in Practice
- ☐ Readings in Companion Animal Behavior (Voith, Borchelt)
- ☐ Renal Disease in Small Animal Practice
- ☐ The Exotic Animal Drug Compendium: An International Formulary (Marx, Roston)
- ☐ The Pocket Guide to Antimicrobial Therapy (Ford)
- ☐ Veterinary Laboratory Medicine in Practice

EQUINE

- ☐ Abdominal Disease in Equine Practice
- ☐ A Guide to Equine Hoof Wall Repair (Moyer, Sigafoos)
- ☐ A Guide to Equine Joint Injection (Moyer)
- ☐ A Guide to Equine Acute Laminitis (Moyer)
- ☐ A Guide to Equine Field Radiography (Watrous)
- ☐ Lameness in Equine Practice

FOOD ANIMAL

- ☐ Food Animal Surgery (Noordsy)
- ☐ Infectious Disease in Food Animal Practice

CROSS SPECIES

- ☐ Pulmonary Function in Healthy, Exercising and Diseased Animals (Lekeux)

For more information call, FAX or write:
Veterinary Learning Systems • 425 Phillips Blvd. #100 • Trenton, NJ 08618
609-882-5600, 800-426-9119, Fax: 609-882-6357, email: books.vls@medimedia.com